THE TREATMENT
OF WAR WOUNDS IN GRAECO-
ROMAN ANTIQUITY

STUDIES IN
ANCIENT MEDICINE

EDITED BY

JOHN SCARBOROUGH

VOLUME 21

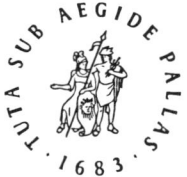

THE TREATMENT OF WAR WOUNDS IN GRAECO-ROMAN ANTIQUITY

by

CHRISTINE F. SALAZAR

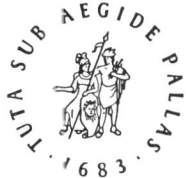

BRILL
LEIDEN · BOSTON · KÖLN
2000

This book is printed on acid-free paper.

Library of Congress Cataloging-in-Publication Data
The Library of Congress Cataloging-in-Publication Data is also available.

Die Deutsche Bibliothek - CIP-Einheitsaufnahme
Salazar, Christine F.:
The treatment of war wounds in Graeco-Roman antiquity / by Christine F. Salazar. – Leiden ; Boston ; Köln : Brill
 (Studies in ancient medicine ; Vol. 21)
 ISBN 90–04–11479–3

ISSN 0925–1421
ISBN 90 04 11479 3

© *Copyright 2000 by Koninklijke Brill NV, Leiden, The Netherlands*

All rights reserved. No part of this publication may be reproduced, translated, stored in a retrieval system, or transmitted in any form or by any means, electronic, mechanical, photocopying, recording or otherwise, without prior written permission from the publisher.

Authorization to photocopy items for internal or personal use is granted by Brill provided that the appropriate fees are paid directly to The Copyright Clearance Center, 222 Rosewood Drive, Suite 910 Danvers MA 01923, USA. Fees are subject to change.

PRINTED IN THE NETHERLANDS

Matri dilectissimae

CONTENTS

Acknowledgements	ix
Abbreviations	xi
List of Illustrations	xiii
Illustrations	xv
Introduction	xxiii

PART ONE

WOUNDS AND THEIR TREATMENT

Chapter One: Sources	1
Chapter Two: Surgical Aspects of Wound Treatment	9
Chapter Three: Pharmaka	54
Chapter Four: Medical Services in Armies	68
Chapter Five: Expert and Layman	84

PART TWO

WOUNDING AS A CODE

Chapter Six: The *Iliad*	126
Chapter Seven: Beautiful Death; the Adjustment of an Ideal	159
Chapter Eight: Alexander the Great	184
Chapter Nine: Epilogue	209

PART THREE

NON-TEXTUAL MATERIAL

Chapter Ten: The Archaeological Evidence	230
Conclusion	248
Bibliography	250
Index locorum	277
General Index	297

ACKNOWLEDGEMENTS

Since this book is the revised version of my PhD thesis, I take the opportunity to thank my supervisor, Professor Sir Geoffrey E. R. Lloyd, for his valuable advice while I was a research student. I also wish to thank Dr Andrew R. Cunningham, my MPhil supervisor, who helped me change the way I looked at the past.

For help and advice with the first version I am indebted to Professor Antony M. Snodgrass, Drs Angie Hobbs, Richard Hunter, Ralph Jackson, Ernst Künzl, John N. W. R. Prag, Jonathan Walters and Gareth Williams as well as Bill G. Zajac, who took the photographs for Figs. 6 and 7. I also thank Professor Philip J. van der Eijk for his advice on editorial matters. Research would not be possible without certain institutions, and I should like to thank the staff of the Cambridge University Library, the Classics Faculty Library (Cambridge), the Library of the Institut für klassische Philologie (University of Vienna), the British Museum and the Kunsthistorische Museum, Vienna. I am greatly obliged to Dr Bruce Fraser without whose editing and formatting skills this book would not have achieved its final shape, as well as to Ms Gera van Bedaf at Brill, who has been immensely helpful and patient. I am also very grateful to my friend Dr Sachiko Kusukawa for her help and advice (and, occasionally, criticism) over many years. Any remaining shortcomings are, of course, my own responsibility.

Last but certainly not least, I wish to express my gratitude towards my mother, Mag. phil. Christiana Fiedler, whose support – both moral and material – enabled me to do my PhD. This book is dedicated to her.

ABBREVIATIONS

ANRW	*Aufstieg und Niedergang der römischen Welt /Rise and Decline of the Roman World* (various eds.), Berlin/New York 1972-
CIG	*Corpus Inscriptionum Graecarum* (various eds.), Berlin 1923-
CIL	*Corpus Inscriptionum Latinarum* (various eds.), Berlin 1828-
CMG	*Corpus Medicorum Graecorum* (various eds.), Leipzig/Berlin 1927-
CML	*Corpus Medicorum Latinorum* (various eds.), Leipzig/Berlin 1915-
D--K	H. Diels and W. Kranz, eds. *Die Fragmente der Vorsokratiker*. 6th edition. Berlin, 1951-2.
K	C. G. Kühn, ed. *Claudii Galeni Opera Omnia*. 22 vols (first edn.: 1821). 2nd edition. Hildesheim. 1964-86.
L	E. Littré, ed. *Oeuvres complètes d'Hippocrate*. 10 vols. Paris 1839-61.
RE	G. Wissowa, *et al.*, eds. *Paulys Realencyclopädie der classischen Altertumswissenschaft,* Stuttgart 1913-
SEG	*Supplementum Epigraphicum Graecum* (various eds.), Leiden 1923-
Z	S. G. Zerbos, ed. ΑΕΤΙΟΥ ΛΟΓΟΣ ΠΕΝΤΕΚΑΙΔΕΚΑΤΟΣ (Book XV. of Aetius), *Athena* XXI, 1909.

ILLUSTRATIONS

Fig. 1: Achilles tending the wounded Patroklos. Attic wine cup by the Sosias painter, c. 500 BC. Antikenmuseum, Berlin (Inv. F 2278). From: Deutsches Archäologisches Institut, ed., *Antike Denkmäler*, vol. I, Berlin 1887, pl. 9.

Fig. 2: Treatment of casualties. Trajan's Column, second century AD. From: C. Cichorius, *Die Reliefs der Trajanssäule*. Berlin 1896-1900, pls. XXX & XXXI.

Fig. 3: Warrior protecting a wounded comrade with his shield. So-called Fugger Sarcophagus, depicting a battle between Greeks and Amazons. Greek, late fourth century BC. Kunsthistorisches Museum, Vienna (Inv. 1 169); photograph taken by the author.

Fig. 4: Iapex attempts to extract an arrow from Aeneas' thigh (*Aen*. XII.391-404). Wall-painting from the Casa di Sirico, Pompeii, first century AD, now at the Museo Nazionale Archeologico, Naples. From: F. Noack, 'Amazonenstudien', *JDI* 30 (1915), p. 159, fig. 9.

Fig. 5: Roman surgical instruments from Vindonissa (Windisch, Switzerland). By courtesy of the Schweizerische Landesmusem, Zurich.

Fig. 6: Treatment of a leg wound. Plaster cast of a Graeco-Roman gem. From: A. Furtwängler, *Die antiken Gemmen: Geschichte der Steinschneidekunst im klassischen Altertum*, Leipzig/Berlin 1900, pl. XXIII.18.

Fig. 7: a) Treatment of a wounded warrior. Plaster cast of a Graeco-Roman gem. From: Ib., pl. XIII.19. b) Childbirth scene. Roman (?) ivory carving from Pompeii. From: E. Holländer, *Plastik und Medizin*. Stuttgart 1912, p. 270, fig. 163.

Fig. 8: Two warriors assisting a wounded comrade. Graeco-Roman gem. Courtesy British Museum, London.

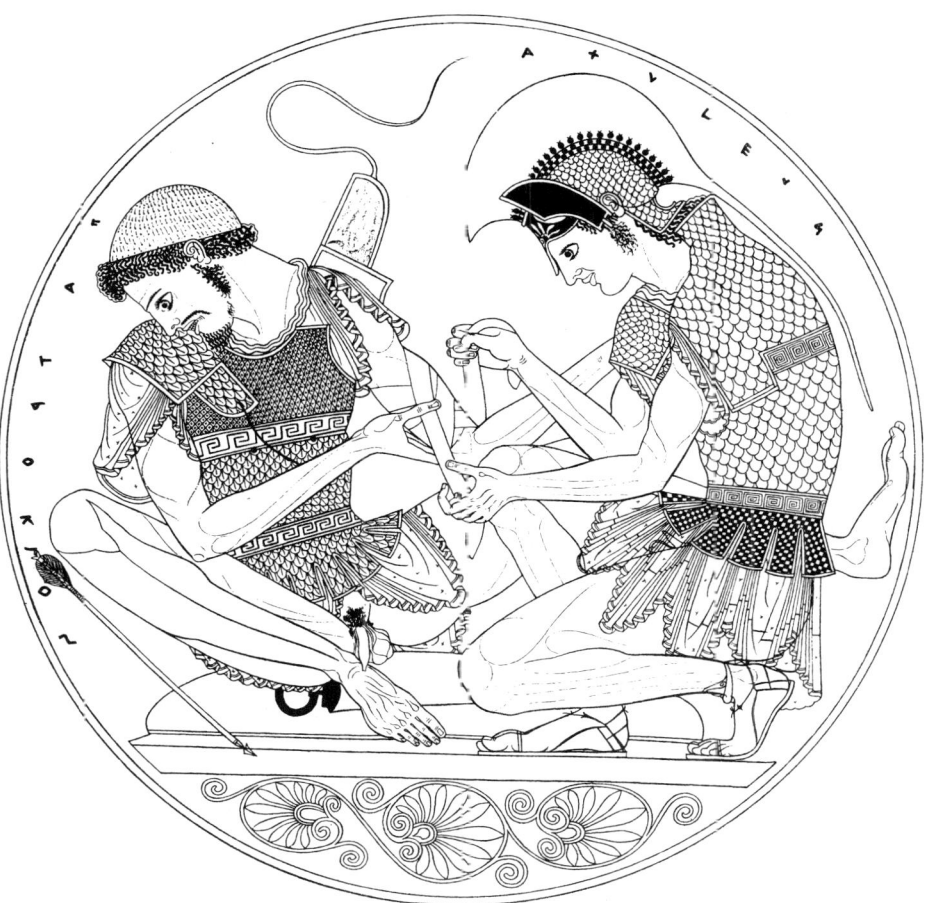

Fig. 1: Achilles tending the wounded Patroklos. Attic wine cup by the Sosias painter, *c.* 500 BC.

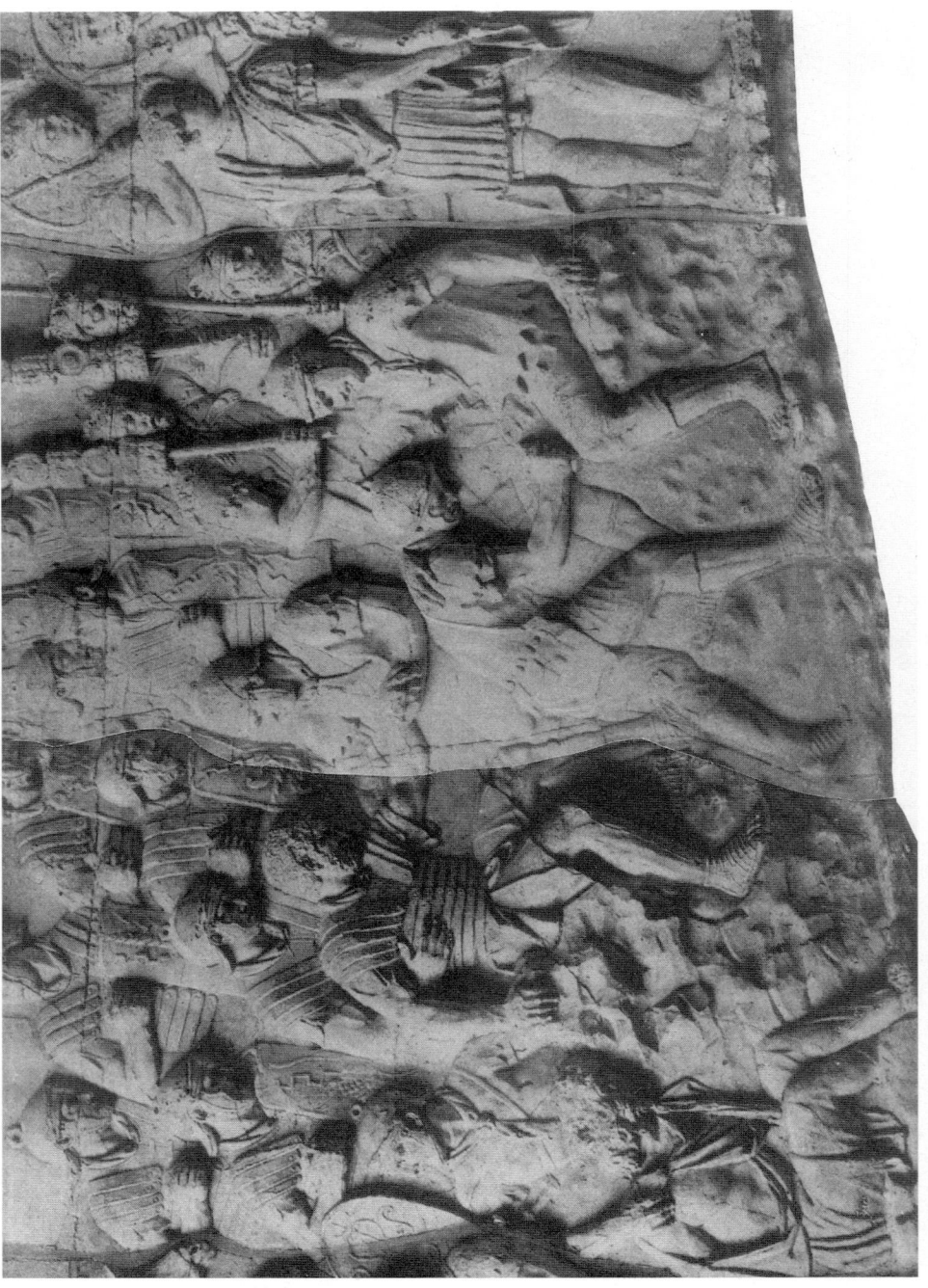

Fig. 9. Treatment of casualties. Trajan's Column, second century AD.

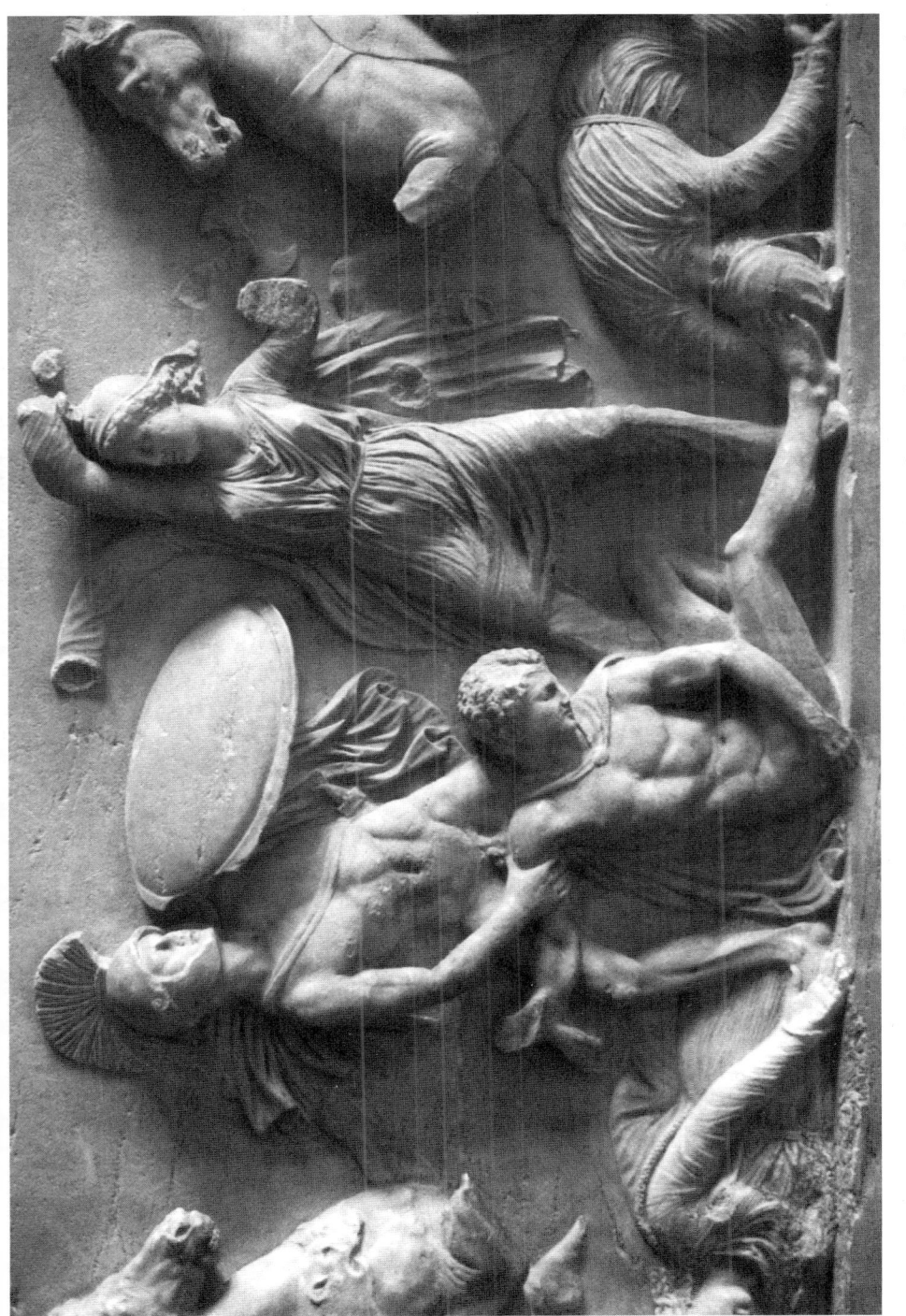

Fig. 3: Warrior protecting a wounded comrade with his shield. So-called Fugger Sarcophagus, depicting a battle between Greeks and Amazons. Greek, late fourth century BC.

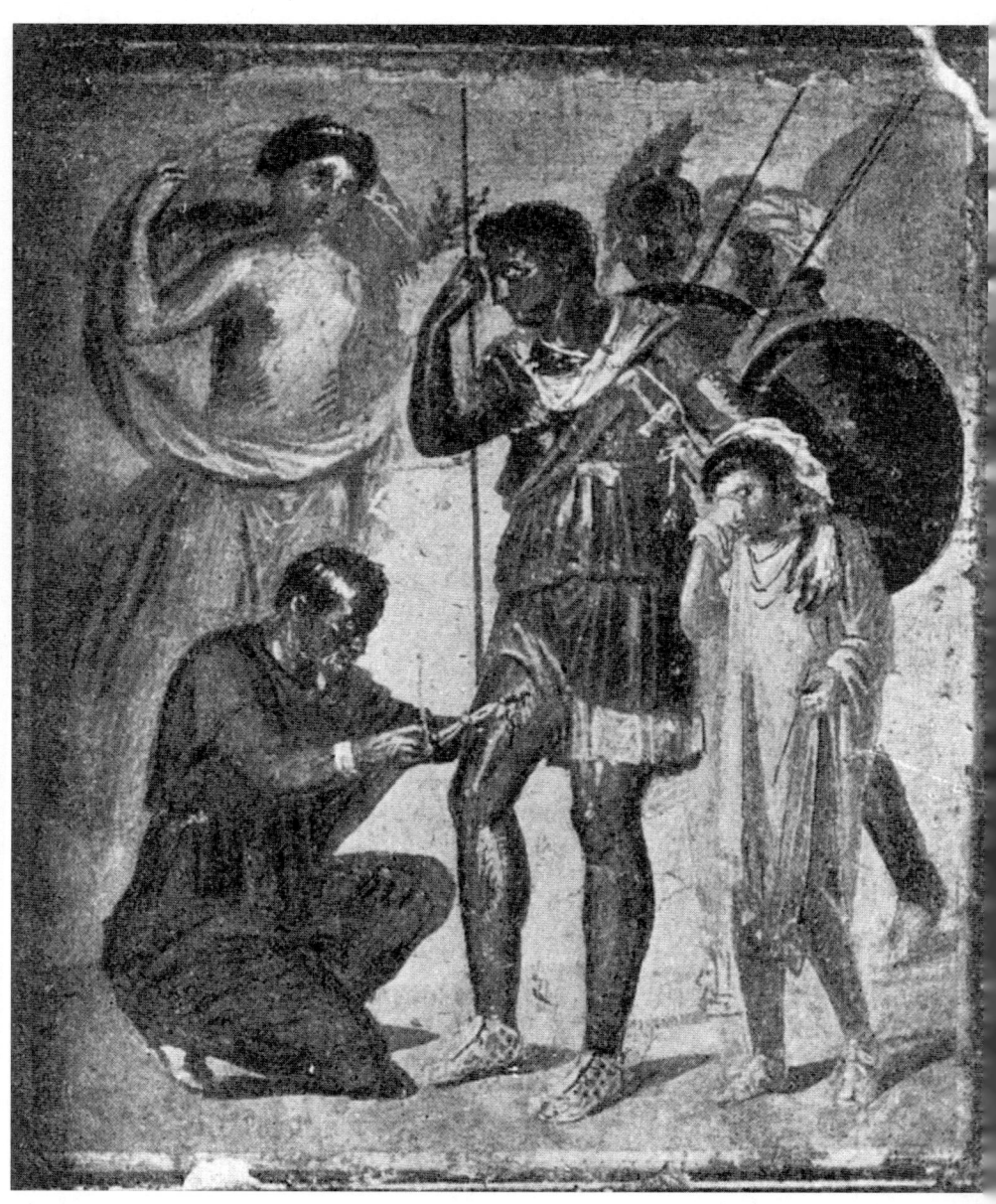

Fig. 4: Iapex attempts to extract an arrow from Aeneas' thigh (*Aen.* XII.391-404). Wall-painting from the Casa di Sirico, Pompeii, first century AD.

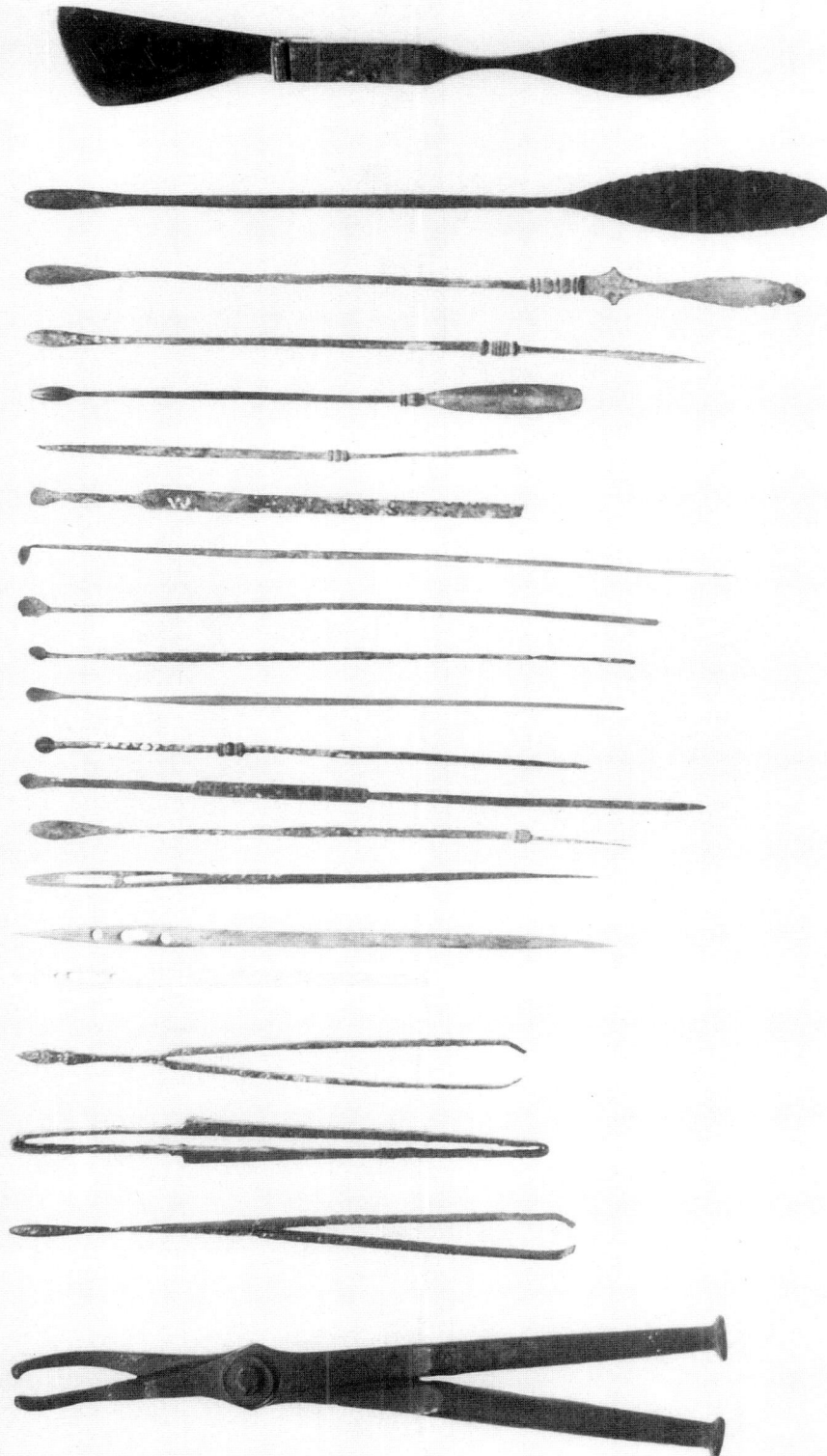

Fig. 5: Roman surgical instruments from Vindonissa (Windisch, Switzerland).

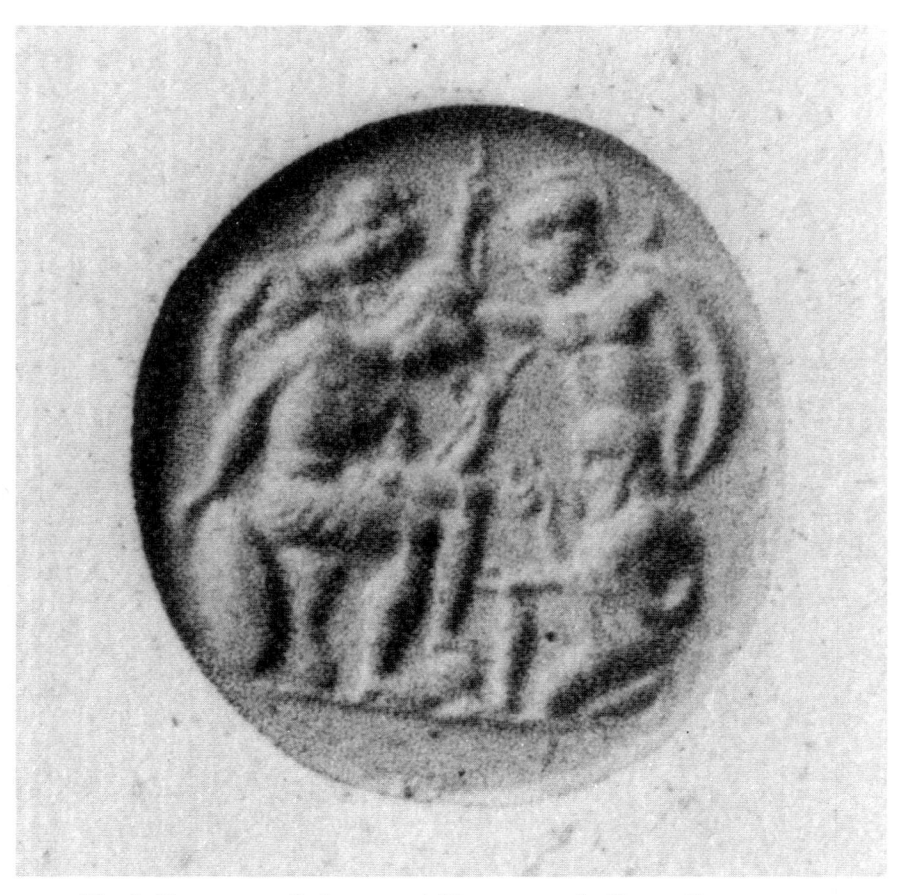

Fig. 6: Treatment of a leg wound. Plaster cast of a Graeco-Roman gem.

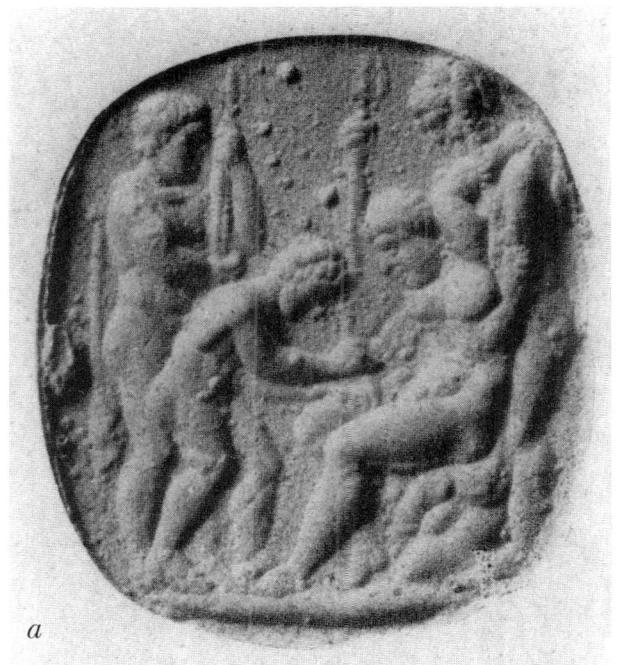

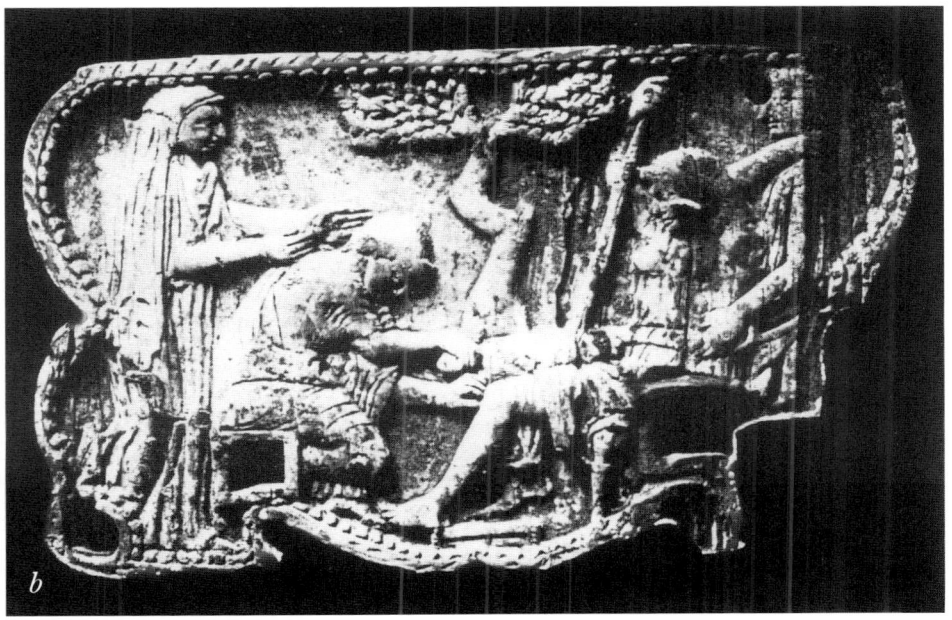

Fig. 7: a) Treatment of a wounded warrior. Plaster cast of a Graeco-Roman gem.
b) Childbirth scene. Roman (?) ivory carving from Pompeii.

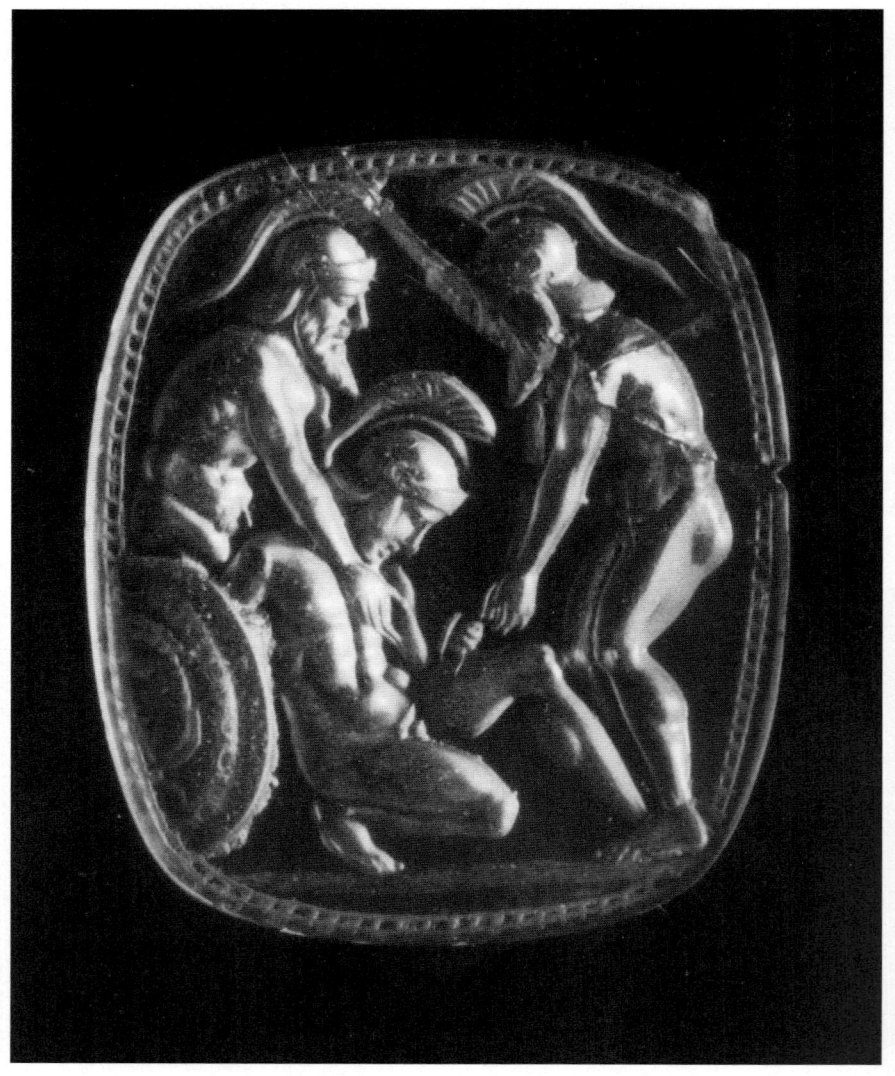

Fig. 8: Two warriors assisting a wounded comrade. Graeco-Roman gem.

INTRODUCTION

"War is continuous for all men throughout their lives."[1] These words, uttered by the Cretan Kleinias in Plato's *Laws*, will have rung true for most Greeks and Romans. Indeed, classical literature leaves the reader with the overriding impression of continuous armed conflict: there appears to have been practically no period in antiquity during which there was not some fighting going on involving Greek or Roman armies.

Given this situation, the risk of being wounded at some point in their lives must have been fairly high for most men, whether fighting for their city or country or as mercenaries. Consequently, doctors were very likely to find themselves in the position of having to deal with battle wounds and therefore needed to be acquainted with their treatment. In fact, the treatment of war wounds is the only kind of medical activity mentioned in the *Iliad*, the earliest Greek source available. It stands for what a healer does - most explicitly so in the much-quoted praise of the physician at XI.514f., stating that he is "a man worth many others, for cutting out arrows and applying soothing remedies".[2]

However, despite its undeniable high profile during antiquity, the importance of 'army surgery' - to use an anachronistic term for the sake of convenience - appears not to have been recognised by scholars studying ancient medicine[3] and the field has not been given the credit which it deserves. One of the reasons for this indifference may be a certain reluctance of scholars in the second half of this century (in the Anglo-Saxon world in particular) to deal with practical aspects of ancient medicine, *Realien* rather than medical theories, the latter being considered a more rewarding object of scholarly endeavour. Another reason may well be the absence of surviving medical treatises dealing exclusively with war wounds.

Within the extant medical writings only head injuries are treated in detail in a separate treatise in the Hippocratic Corpus, namely *On Wounds in the Head*[4] (*VC*). Needless to say, not all, or not even the

---

[1] πόλεμος ἀεὶ πᾶσιν διὰ βίου συνεχής ἐστι ...: Pl., *Leg.* 625e.
[2] ἰητρὸς γὰρ ἀνὴρ πολλῶν ἀντάξιος ἄλλων, / ἰοὺς τ' ἐκτάμνειν ἐπι τ' ἤπια φάρμακα πάσσειν.
[3] An exception is G. Majno, whose *The Healing Hand* (1970) deals exclusively with the treatment of trauma, albeit mainly with injuries other than battle wounds.
[4] *De capitis vulneribus*.

majority of the injuries discussed in it are battle wounds. However, not only is there valuable information scattered throughout the works of most medical writers, but it has generally been overlooked that much insight is to be gained from non-medical sources.[5] It appears legitimate therefore to include passages from non-medical authors in the discussion of the medical aspects of our topic.

A further point, which has been disregarded by practically all scholars, is the fact that scenes of wounding in non-medical literature are not merely an inevitable accessory of realistic description - something that was described because it was there. It would appear on the contrary that such scenes are used by the authors with a certain purpose in mind: in some cases this was done in order to bring an air of sensationalism into an account, but more often as a key element of the hero-image. The more an author is concerned with representing a hero, the more often he is likely to use scenes of wounding - even of fatal wounds - or wound treatment as a device to emphasise the hero's excellence.

My aim in this monograph is to examine all the various aspects of the treatment of war wounds as reflected in Greek and Roman literature - medical or other - as well as in non-textual material. This approach is novel and different from other scholars' in its combination of very heterogeneous evidence, whereas so far only individual facets, if any, of the topic have been examined. As this study should make apparent, an approach which focuses only on one or two aspects of so complex a subject is bound to gain only limited insight, and it is therefore necessary to examine the topic in its totality. Given the vast amount of material, this has still meant being selective and choosing particularly relevant examples, as not every single occurrence of wounding in Graeco-Roman literature can be quoted.

The questions to be addressed and, as far as possible answered here, are the following:

i) What wounds would result from battles fought with Greek or Roman equipment, and how were they treated (both surgically and pharmacologically)?

ii) Was medical treatment for casualties provided in Greek and Roman armies and, if so, of what kind was it?

iii) What difference, if any, was there between a medical expert and a layman in antiquity? (Given the extensive use made of non-medical literature, the question is of great relevance for this topic.)

---

[5] Only the *Iliad* has been looked at from a medico-historical point of view: see in particular Daremberg (1865), Frölich (1879) and Körner (1929).

iv) Was there something which we would call medical terminology in antiquity, and were any attempts made to create such terminology?
v) Why do scenes of wounding appear in non-medical literature, and is it possible to reconstruct the intentions the authors pursued in including those scenes?
vi) Is there some information - or confirmation of results obtained from the literary material - to be gained from archaeological evidence?

The goals are therefore:
i) to describe the modes of treatment for different types of war injuries;
ii) to examine the affinity and/or difference between medical and non-medical writing and the different degrees of inter-penetration; and to investigate such steps as were taken towards the creation of something that one might call technical terminology;
iii) to explore the ideological and socio-cultural framework behind the literary and artistic reflection of battle wounds and their treatment.

The contents and structure of this book are as follows: opening with a brief discussion of the sources (Ch. 1), Part I is concerned with the practical side of 'army surgery', describing the various kinds of wounds and the way they were treated by surgery (Ch. 2) or pharmacological applications (Ch. 3) as well as ways in which care for casualties was organised in Greek and Roman armies (Ch. 4). Chapter 5, investigating the degree to which medical knowledge was available to laymen and the use of a specific terminology in medical writings, serves as a bridge between Part I and Part II. The latter considers the use of wounding as a metaphor for heroism in non-medical literature - in particular in the *Iliad* and the literature about Alexander the Great - and is followed, in Part III, by a survey of the archaeological evidence.

It should become clear that the treatment of war wounds is marked off from other sections of ancient medicine, concerned with either disease or injury in everyday life or illness in war, by the particular mythology attached to wounds and death in battle. It therefore seems to me not merely justified but necessary that it should be treated separately, and that this study should be focused on this one branch of medicine.[6]

---

[6] This is not meant to suggest that in antiquity the treatment of wounds was considered a separate 'branch' of medicine, or indeed that there was such a concept as medical specialisation, since even the division between the practice of surgery and that of internal medicine did not appear until Hellenistic times.

While this specific field has not attracted the attention of any other scholars since the first half of this century, much research has been done recently in the general area of ancient medicine. Two aspects in particular have been a focus of scholarly interest: the socio-cultural background of medicine in the widest sense, and linguistic aspects of medical writings. Numerous contributions in these fields are at least marginally relevant for my topic and will be referred to in the text. For a general idea, examples of the former field can be found, e.g., in Ph. J. van der Eijk, H. F. J. Horstmannshoff, P. H. Schrijvers (eds.), *Ancient Medicine in its Socio-Cultural Context*, Amsterdam/Atlanta 1995 (2 vols.). Questions concerning the language of medical writings and the influence of literacy are discussed, for example, in contributions to G. Baader, R. Winau (eds.), *Die hippokratischen Epidemien. Theorie - Praxis -Tradition*, Berlin 1989; W. Kullmann, M. Reichel (eds.), *Der Übergang von der Mündlichkeit zur Literatur bei den Griechen*, Tübingen 1990; or W. Kullmann, J. Althoff, M. Asper (eds.), *Gattungen wissenschaftlicher Literatur in der Antike*, Tübingen 1998; as well as in articles or monographs by U. Capitani (1975), P. Easterling (1985), J. B. Hofmann (1926), D. Langslow (1991), I. Mazzini (1978), C. de Meo (1986), P. Mudry (1991), J. Pigeaud (1988), P. Rodriguez Fernandez (1973) and A. Setaioli (1983), to name only some. R. Wittern, P. Pellegrin (eds.), *Hippokratische Medizin und antike Philosophie*, Hildesheim/Zurich/New York 1996, covers aspects of both approaches.

In order to make the quoted writings accessible for non-classicists as well, Greek and Latin passages are quoted in translation and the original texts are relegated to footnotes. When Greek words are used in transcription, long vowels are indicated by circumflexes, and subscript iotas are rendered as *is* (e.g. *anthrôpôi* for ἀνθρώπῳ). Greek proper names have been transcribed without indication of vowel length. Where possible, I have preferred not to use Latinized spelling for Greek names (e.g. Patroklos, not Patroclus), but some are so well established in their Latinized form (e.g. Socrates or Hippocrates) that, despite the resulting inconsistency, it has seemed inevitable to use the latter. Secondary literature in languages other than English is also quoted in translation; unless specifically mentioned, all translations are the author's.

For Greek and Roman sources the abbreviations are those used in Liddell and Scott's *Greek-English Dictionary* and Lewis and Short's *Latin Dictionary* respectively; for the titles of periodicals the abbreviations are those of *Année Philologique* where available. At their first occurrence, the titles of works from the Hippocratic collection and of those by Galen will appear in their full form followed by the standard Latin abbreviation in square brackets; for any further occurrences only the abbreviation will be used. The references for both authors are to the Littré and Kühn edition respectively, these being the only complete editions to date. These volume and page numbers can be found also in the margins of those works that have appeared in the *CMG* so far.

References to Aretaeus, Celsus, Oribasius, Paul of Aegina and Soranus are followed by *CML / CMG* page and line numbers, preceded by the volume number where there are several volumes. In order to keep these references within a manageable length, the abbreviations *CML* and *CMG* are not repeated after each of them, nor is the volume number within the respective *Corpus* cited. Thus, for example, 'Paul II.180' refers to page 180 in the second volume, i.e. in *CMG* IX.2.

Terms such as 'doctor', 'physician', 'practitioner' and 'surgeon' are unsatisfactory renderings of the Greek *iatros* and the Latin *medicus*, but since there is little alternative, they will be used interchangeably throughout. It should also be stated here that those performing the treatment of war wounds will be referred to as 'he' throughout; given that none of our sources ever mention female practitioners in this context, inclusive language would be not merely pointless but misleading.

PART ONE

WOUNDS AND THEIR TREATMENT

CHAPTER ONE

SOURCES

The written sources can be divided roughly into three groups - this is, of course, by making a subdivision according to modern genre boundaries. The first consists of the works of authors considered as 'medical writers'; we will accept them as such here, for the sake of argument, although many of them would not fit this category in the modern sense. The other two groups are, on the one hand, the purely literary texts, such as historical writings or poetry, and, on the other, texts of the kind that would now be called scientific or technical. It is likely that the Greeks or Romans themselves distinguished between different categories of texts according to their purpose; thus Galen writes in his work on anatomy, *On Anatomical Procedures*[1] [*De Anat. Admin.*],[2] that one should not read it "for pleasure"[3] like the *Histories* of Herodotus. The distinction between the two latter groups is not clearly drawn: they may be distinguished in some cases, but most of the time there is some overlap between them.

It cannot be stressed enough that what writings we have at our disposal are merely the survivors against the ravages of time and the vicissitudes of textual transmission, a fraction of the quantity of texts that existed in antiquity. Quotes from lost works in our extant authors are a constant and painful reminder of this fact.

1. *Medical authors*

The oldest collection of Greek medical writings, and no doubt the most famous in European history, is the Hippocratic Corpus. We know practically nothing about the 'great' Hippocrates of Cos, the son of Heracleidas, who lived in the fifth century BC, a slightly younger contemporary of Socrates, and is considered the founder of what is now referred to as 'Hippocratic medicine' in the widest sense. Several *Lives* of Hippocrates have come down to us as well as some fictitious letters, but these were all written considerable time after his death and are hagiographical rather than

---

[1] *De anatomicis administrationibus.*
[2] III. 9/II. 393 K.
[3] ἕνεκα τέρψεως.

biographical.[4] The way in which Plato mentions "Hippocrates of the Asclepiad family"[5] without further explanations suggests that he was already a famous figure by that time. This explains why, when a motley collection of medical writings - purportedly from the island of Cos - was assembled into a corpus in Hellenistic Alexandria, the name of Hippocrates was attached to it.

The disparate writings contained in the collection have all been transmitted with their respective titles, which they may have had from before the compilation, but without any reference to authorship. It is beyond doubt that they are by a variety of authors and some may even be the work of more than one. It would seem that even by the third or second century BC it was no longer possible to attribute any of the works to a particular author, and the debate about the 'genuine' works of Hippocrates continued unabated from antiquity until the earlier part of this century. It now has to be admitted that with the material available to us it is impossible to arrive at a definitive answer concerning Hippocratic authorship. Nevertheless, claims are still being made concerning Hippocrates' son-in-law Polybus.[6]

Information on the treatment of wounds can be found in several Hippocratic works, especially the following: *Epidemics* [*Epid.*][7] V and VII, *Diseases* [*Morb.*],[8] *Affections* [*Aff.*],[9] *Prorrhetics* [*Prorrh.*][10] (II in particular), *Aphorisms* [*Aph.*],[11] *On Wounds* [*Ulc.*],[12] *In the Surgery* [*Off.*],[13] *Fractures* [*Fract.*][14] and *The Physician* [*Medic.*].[15] As mentioned above, *VC* is devoted entirely to the topic of trauma.

With the exception of some cases in *Epid.* V and VII,[16] exact dating of the approximately seventy extant works in the Corpus is impossible, but most of them are assumed to have been written in the (late) fifth and fourth centuries BC. Some of them, such as

---

[4] For an overview, see R. Pinault, *Hippocratic Lives and Legends*, Leiden/New York/Cologne 1992.
[5] *Phaedr.* 270c; *Prot.* 311b.
[6] See Grensemann (1968).
[7] Ἐπιδημίαι/ De *morbis popularibus*. Some identical passages appear in both V and VII.
[8] *De morbis*.
[9] *De affectionibus*.
[10] *De praedictionibus*.
[11] *Aphorismi*.
[12] Περὶ ἑλκῶν/*De ulceribus*; this can also be translated as *On Ulcers*. The word *helkos* originally meant 'wound' and gradually acquired the meaning 'ulcer': see below, Ch. 4. 2.
[13] *De officina medici*.
[14] *De fracturis*.
[15] *De medico*.
[16] See below, Ch. 4, n.15.

Medic., may belong to the third century. Furthermore, the collection cannot be treated as a homogeneous entity, not only because of the multiplicity of authors, but also because of the variety in purposes and audiences. Thus, e.g., *Epid.* could have been a doctor's personal notes, *Aff.* appears to have been written mainly for a lay public, *Medic.* could have been meant for students at an early stage of their training and *Prorrh.* II for students at a more advanced stage or even practitioners.

Two of the extant ancient sources[17] also mention a treatise belonging to the Hippocratic Corpus dealing exclusively with wounds - or possibly two works which were also at times transmitted together. The sources do not quite agree on the title(s), but one variety for the combined title is Περὶ τραυμάτων καὶ βελῶν (*On Wounds and Arrows*), so it would seem that arrow wounds were a particular concern of the treatise(s). Tantalizingly, all that has come down to us are the title variants and some isolated words in a later glossary.[18] One can only hope that these writings have survived in an Arabic translation in some as yet unedited MS.

Chronologically the next major source is Dioscorides' *De Materia Medica*, the oldest surviving work devoted entirely to pharmacology. (There are some references to medicinal properties in the *Historia Plantarum* of Theophrastus, written in the late fourth or early third century BC, but pharmacology is not the main interest of the work.) Dioscorides, born in Cilicia in Asia Minor in the first century AD, acquired his knowledge of plants and minerals on his extensive travels - possibly as an army physician[19] - and his work contains numerous remedies for wounds.

The earliest (or at least earliest extant) Roman treatise on medicine is Aulus Cornelius Celsus' *De Medicina*, written during the reign of Tiberius, in the first half of the first century AD. Celsus, who may or may not have had first-hand medical experience, although he certainly did not practice medicine professionally, wrote the *De Medicina* as part of an extensive body

---

[17] Galen in three passages, two in his commentary on the Hippocratic *Aph.*, *In Hippocratis aphorismos commentarius* [*In Hipp. Aph.*], XVIII.A.28 and 30 K, and one in his glossary of Hippocratic works, *Linguarum seu dictionum exoletarum Hippocratis explicatio* [*Ling. Expl.*]/ XIX.116 K, and Erotian's glossary of Hippocratic terms (Ilberg ed., Leipzig 1893, p. 136). On the glossary, see Lara Nava (1988) and López Férez (1991).

[18] Galen, *Ling. Expl.*, XIX.62-157 K. For a more detailed treatment of the evidence, see Salazar (1997).

[19] Cf. *Mat. Med.*, praef. 4, where he refers to his 'military life': ἡμῖν στρατιωτικὸν τὸν βίον.

of writings, including works on agriculture and rhetoric, but all the other works in the collection have perished. Book VII, which discusses surgery, contains the oldest detailed passage on arrow wounds that we have, obviously drawing upon older material.[20]

Galen, born in Pergamon in (approximately) 129 AD, has left the most extensive collection of Greek medical literature written by one single author,[21] part of it consisting in commentaries on Hippocratic treatises. His is the most unmistakeably individual voice among the extant medical writers, by its combination of passion for 'the art' and for Hippocrates with biographical anecdotes and tetchy swipes at colleagues and predecessors (displaying far more animus than the criticisms expressed in the Hippocratic Corpus). Although in *De Anat. Admin.* he mentions the importance of anatomical knowledge for surgery,[22] none of his extant treatises is devoted entirely to surgical operations. He did not lack the necessary experience, however,[23] at least as far as the treatment of trauma is concerned, having worked as a doctor to the gladiators in Pergamon for five seasons from the age of twenty-nine,[24] and relevant details can be found in many of his numerous works.

Some information about wounds and their treatment can be found in the *Quaestiones Medicinales*,[25] written by Rufus of Ephesus[26] in the second century, as well as his *On Names*.[27] It is likely that there was more of it in his lost works *On Wound Remedies* and *On Wounds of the Joints*.[28]

---

[20] VII.5.1A-3B/308.6-310.28. It is impossible to tell to what extent Celsus modified the, presumably Greek, material available to him, and he does not name his sources. It has been argued (Wellmann [1913]) that Celsus merely translated a Greek original, but there is no compelling evidence for such a claim.

[21] Some of his works were lost, but what survives fills twenty-two volumes in the bilingual (Greek with a Latin translation) Kühn edition or, as Nutton (unpubl. lecture, Cambridge) puts it, claiming 'more space on the library-shelf than in the affection of classical scholars'.

[22] II/II.283f. K.

[23] At *De Anat. Admin.* III/II.345 K, in a discussion of lack of sensation after an injury, he emphasises the extent of his experience: "The day would be too short if I were to tell you how many such [cases] I have seen in the feet or hands, on soldiers wounded in wars as well as on those whom they call gladiators, ...". (ἐπιλείποι δ' ἄν με ἡ ἡμέρα διηγούμενον, ὅσα τοιαῦτα τεθέαμαι κατὰ τοὺς πόδας καὶ τὰς χεῖρας, ἐπί τε στρατιωτῶν ἐν πολέμοις τετρωμένων, καὶ τουτωνὶ τῶν καλουμένων μονομάχων, ...).

[24] Galen emphasises with obvious pride the young age at which he was entrusted with this responsibility: *De compositione medicamentorum per genera* [*Comp. Med. Gen.*], III/XIII.599 K. Cf. Scarborough (1971).

[25] Ἰατρικὰ ἠρωτήματα.

[26] On Rufus, see Ilberg (1930).

[27] Περὶ ὀνομασίας [*Onom.*], which can also be translated as *On Language*.

[28] Περὶ τραυματικῶν φαρμάκων. and Περὶ τραυματισμοῦ ἄρθρων.

The writings of Oribasius (fourth century AD), the friend, and eventually the court physician, of the emperor Julian, are a voluminous compendium culled from earlier sources (he cites some texts verbatim, including quotes from works that are now lost), on every aspect of medicine, including wounds. While the *Collectiones Medicae* are a lengthy and detailed work and the *Eclogae Medicamentorum* a collection of remedies compiled for Julian, the *Synopsis ad Eustathium* and *Libri ad Eunapium* are shorter introductions.[29]

The most recent author to be used for this study is Paul of Aegina. Although he wrote his untitled work[30] as late as the seventh century, he often refers to earlier material and has left us the only complete chapter on arrow wounds written in Greek - which may well have been derived in part from the lost Hippocratic treatise on this topic.[31]

The authors mentioned here are those whose works are directly relevant for our topic. However, information on wound treatment can also be found in less obvious authors, such as the second-century (AD) author Soranus (*Gynaecia / De fasciis / De signis fracturarum*), Scribonius Largus (first century AD), the author of *Compositiones Medicamentorum*, Aretaeus of Cappadocia (equally of the second century AD),[32] and Caelius Aurelianus (fifth century AD), whose *Acutae Passiones* and *Tardae Passiones* appear to be translations of two lost works by Soranus.

2. Literary sources

Homer's *Iliad*, by far the oldest and one of the most important non-medical sources, will be treated separately (Ch. 6), together with the later scholia to the *Iliad*. Some use can also be made of later epic poets who often model themselves on Homer, such as Virgil, Silius Italicus, Statius, Quintus Smyrnaeus and Nonnos.

Another main group of sources consists in the historians writing about Alexander the Great, namely Plutarch in his *Life* of Alexander (his other works are also very useful source material,

---

[29] For more detail on Oribasius, see Bouffartigue (1992), especially pp. 24, 51, 319, 483-6, 606.
[30] In the prooemium (*CMG* IX.I, p. 3) he refers to it as his *pragmateia* and as a *synagôgê*, so either may have been intended as a title.
[31] See Salazar (1998b) for a detailed discussion of Paul and a translation of his chapter on arrow wounds.
[32] On Aretaeus, see Kudlien (1964).

particularly for Part II), Arrian, Quintus Curtius and - to some extent - Diodorus Siculus, Justin, and even Pseudo-Callisthenes.

Apart from more obvious sources like the historians Herodotus, Xenophon, Polybius, Dionysius of Halicarnassus, Florus, Livy, Tacitus, Dio Cassius, Ammianus Marcellinus and Procopius, occasional references to wounds (and sometimes their treatment) are to be found in a wide range of authors. There is practically no literary genre that does not mention wounds or wound treatment either as an element of the narrative or in a metaphorical sense. Thus - to name just a few examples - the topic appears in philosophical writings (e.g. Plato, Aristotle, Seneca, Cicero), poetry (Pindar, Ovid, Lucan, etc.), tragedy (Sophocles) and even comedy (Aristophanes, Menander, Plautus).

Two further types of textual evidence may constitute only a quantitatively small part of the sources, but occasionally they provide important insights, namely epigraphical material and papyri. The former includes the descriptions of healing miracles from the temple of Asclepius at Epidaurus[33] and inscriptions thanking doctors for their services.[34] As for papyri, a not insignificant number contain some form of medical writings, recipes, doctors' bills, etc., so that they, too, can provide some important information.[35]

3. *Non-medical 'scientific' texts*

A number of writers who deal with technical or scientific material - this is a distinction by content, not by style - form a separate, but far from clearly distinguished, category. (The relationship between technical and non-technical literature will be treated in Chapter 5.)

It seems natural that one should find information on medical treatment in Theophrastus' *Historia Plantarum*, mentioned above, or Pliny's *Historia Naturalis*, compiled in the first century AD, but other authors are less obvious sources. Thus it may seem surprising that some passages of the pseudo-Aristotelian

---

[33] Published in, e.g., Herzog (1931) and the more recent, but less scholarly, edition of LiDonnici (1995).
[34] See Ch. 4.1 and, e.g., Sokoloff (1904).
[35] For some examples, see Marganne (1981), especially pp. 52, 54, 76, 141, 204, 278, 280, 285, 303, 343 for references to wounds (albeit none of them explicitly battle wounds); Roberts (1950); Boswinkel (1956); Fischer (1982).

Problemata deal with surgery[36] and that the problem of casualties is mentioned by the authors writing about tactics: Aeneas Tacticus (fourth century BC), Philo (third century BC), Asclepiodotus (first century BC), Heron (first century AD) and Aelianus Tacticus (late first and early second century AD). Vegetius also refers to the topic in his *Epitoma rei militaris*, written in the fourth century AD.

4. *Non-textual evidence*

The last class of our sources is constituted by all material other than writings, hence by archaeological finds and artefacts. These include:

i) weapons and also protective armour (as the latter would determine the probability of certain body areas being wounded);

ii) skeletal finds - to a very limited degree for this topic, since they can only give evidence of injuries to the bones;

iii) surgical instruments;

iv) buildings and inscriptions;

v) artistic representation of wounding - on paintings and gems, in sculpture, etc.

This group of material is also of considerable relevance, but since archaeology is not the main concern of this monograph, it will have to take second place to the textual evidence.

---

[36] I.32-6/863a-b. On similarities between the Hippocratic *Epid.* and the *Problemata*, see Bertier (1989).

CHAPTER TWO

SURGICAL ASPECTS OF WOUND TREATMENT

The question of how a Greek or Roman doctor would have treated battle injuries needs to be preceded by another: What type of wounds was he likely to encounter during or after a battle? The vast majority of wounds would have been made by the most common weapons, namely swords, spears, javelins and arrows, but also by other missiles used by slingers, such as stones or lead bullets. The treatment varied considerably according to the type of injury, so we first have to examine the different categories, although the boundaries between them fluctuate and varying criteria are used for categorising. The distinctions that I am making here or similar ones can be found in the writings of several authors.

1. *Types of trauma*

1.1. *Flesh wounds*

"What is in the flesh is the least dangerous of all."[1] This is Celsus' opinion (V.26.3B/216.15f.) on wounds in the flesh taken in a very narrow sense, excluding not only wounds to the bones and cartilages, but also those to the membranes, muscles, 'nerves' and 'arteries'.

Although the problem of medical terminology will be discussed at a later point,[2] the difficulties accompanying the translation of anatomical and medical terms call for a brief discussion here. In attempting to render Celsus' categories we have to admit that the only unequivocal distinction is the one between bones and soft tissues. *Nervus* and *arteria*, as well as the Greek νεῦρον (*neuron*) and ἀρτηρία (*artêria*), are prime examples of words which defy translation or which, at least, cannot be equated with any *one* English word, and - as with other terms - we can also see switches in significance between different authors and periods. Moreover, terms may lose connotations or effect a shift in reference in the process of translation from Greek into Latin. In some cases, such

---

[1] *Tutissimum omnium, quod in carne est.*
[2] Ch. 5.2.

as *artêria*, τένων (*tenôn*) or ἀορτή (*aortê*),[3] the etymology of the word may give us some clues as to the properties which a thing called by it is expected to have and thus to its meaning, but this method is not always applicable.

The word *neuron* is a particularly striking example of a wide range of references attached to one single word. Looking at medical contexts only, we find it used of sinews or tendons (*Art.* 11/IV.110 L, etc.), nerves (*Coan Prognostics*[4] [*Coac.*] IV.XXIX.494, ib.498, etc./V.696f. L) and even veins (*On the Use of Liquids*[5] [*Liqu.*] 2/VI.124 L; Rufus, *Onom.* 208). Galen, following Erasistratus, distinguishes between nerves, as organs of sensory perception, and tendons, but in *On the Bones for Beginners* (*De ossibus ad tirones* [*Oss.*]), II.739 K, he lists the tendons as one of the three types of *neura*:

> They said that there were three types of *neura*... Some they call intentional, namely the ones which grow from the brain and the spinal marrow; some [they call] connective; their origin is from the bones. The third variety is called *tenôn*, and it grows from the muscle.[6]

Even in post-Galenic writers it is difficult to be confident about the reference. Thus when Paul of Aegina speaks of a *neuron* in his discussion of the extraction of arrows (VI.88.3/II.131.3), this could be either a nerve or a tendon. If one takes into consideration the non-anatomical uses of the word[7] - cord, bow-string, string of a lyre, plant fibres - there seems to be one common element of "stringy-ness" and a certain elasticity that makes it possible to use it for those different objects. If one then accepts Irigoin's etymology[8] for *artêria* - i.e. as related to ἄρθρον (*arthron*) and ἀρτύς (*artys*) - it is slightly less surprising that a list given by Rufus of Ephesus (*Onom.* 208) of words used by others for what he calls *artêria* includes *neuron*, as the terms may have some associated ideas[9] in common. It is, however, impossible to give a consistent translation, as there are no single English terms covering all the possible meanings held by *neuron* and *artêria*.

---

[3] Cf. Irigoin (1980), pp. 254f.
[4] *Coacae Praenotiones.*
[5] *De liquidorum usu.*
[6] τρία τοίνυν εἶναι τῶν νεύρων ἔφασαν γένη. ... καλοῦσι δὲ τὰ μέν τινα προαιρετικά, τὰ ἐξ ἐγκεφάλου καὶ νωτιαίου πεφυκότα· τὰ δέ τινα συνδετικά· τούτων δὲ ἡ γένεσις ἐκ τῶν ὀστῶν· ἡ τρίτη δὲ αὐτῶν διαφορὰ καλεῖται μὲν τένων, ἐκφύεται δὲ ἐκ μυός. Caelius Aurelianus follows a similar line at *Acut.* II. 80/I.180.12, where he speaks of "the nerves which are called tendons" (... *nervis, quos tenontas appellant*).
[7] Cf. Lloyd (1979), p. 352.
[8] (1980), pp. 254f.
[9] In the sense of *Vorstellungen*: cf. Frege (1892), p. 25.

These two words are also examples of how in some cases discoveries made through dissection found repercussions in the use of already existing terms for a new reference. Even when the signification of a word changes, there remains a permanent core, consisting of certain elements or characteristics based on the original reference, the latter being thus crucial for the later sense.

In the aforementioned passage in Celsus we can see that *caro* has a very strictly defined reference - secured by exclusion - apparently referring only to what we would call subcutaneous adipose tissue and connective tissue. He makes the same distinction at V.26.30B/225.31: "... if nerves or muscles are wounded, or also if the flesh [is wounded] in depth",[10] while in other passages[11] *caro* is only contrasted with *membrana*, *ossa* or *cartilago* and he also uses it (*passim*) as a generic term for the soft tissues or the flesh of the body in general. Thus we can see that fluctuations in meaning are possible even within the works of one single author.

The distinction that one most commonly finds made by classical authors is that between wounds to the soft tissues and wounds to the bones (e.g. Paul, VI.88.3 and ibid. 5/II.130.25-131.5: "if it [i.e. the arrow] is fixed in the flesh ... if the missile has struck a bone, ...",[12] and within the flesh wounds (as it thus seems legitimate to call them) those involving large muscles, tendons or nerves are considered more dangerous and, as we shall see later, potentially disabling. Galen, too, appears to distinguish between mere flesh wounds and wounds to the *neura*, the latter being more serious and requiring specific treatment and medication. He devotes the entire book III of *On the Composition of Remedies according by Kinds* (*De compositione medicamentorum per genera* [*Comp. Med. Gen.*]) to the treatment of those wounded in the *neura* (νευροτρώτοι). For example, at XIII.599 K he describes a successful dressing which he developed for such wounds. (The passage is quoted by Oribasius, *Ecl. Med.* 87.10./IV.265.21-31) Celsus (V.26.3.B5/216.12-15) and Paul (IV.54/I.376-80) also have comments specifically about wounds to the 'nerves'.

A flesh wound was frequently made by a sword, especially when it was used with a cutting rather than a thrusting movement - according to Polybius the former was the Gaulish way of fighting. The Romans were well aware of the greater efficacy of a sword-thrust and trained their soldiers accordingly: cf. Vegetius, *Mil.*,

---

[10] *si nervi musculive vulnerati sunt; etiam si alte caro.*
[11] E.g. V. 28.12B/243.7f. or VII.15.1/332.17ff.
[12] εἰ μὲν ἐν σαρκὶ πέπηγεν ... εἰ δὲ τὸ βέλος ἐν ὀστῷ παγείη, ...

I.12: "For a cut, with whatever violence it may come, does not often kill ... but, on the other hand, a stab, thrust in two inches deep, is fatal."[13] A flesh wound could also be made by a spear when the point was slightly deflected and this type of lesion was very common, in particular in the areas not protected by armour or shield, such as the legs and the right arm.[14]

The passages quoted above highlight the necessity of investigating the problems concerning the use of literary texts as evidence. We are faced with very diverse material, and its value of evidence is both varied and problematic, but it is impossible to draw a clear line with pure fantasy on one side and an objective rendering of reality on the other. To take the extreme ends of the spectrum: neither are the largely fantastical accounts from the Epidaurus inscriptions invented from nothing, given that they show knowledge of ordinary medical procedures, nor are even the most down-to-earth accounts in the Hippocratic Corpus to be taken at face value, since fashions and current medical theories influence even the description of surgery, although to a far lesser degree than that of other branches of medicine.

Scenes in the *Iliad* - such as those of swords and spears cutting through or piercing bones at great ease - show identifiable modes of exaggeration, which are mirrored (and in some cases magnified) in later authors, but alongside with those we find anatomically realistic descriptions of wounds. In the same way, later literature displays varying degrees of relation to reality and it would be rash to discard all except medical writings in a narrow sense as worthless and unfit for evidence. One *can* use them, but with caution, keeping in mind that different literary criteria will lead to a varying choice of topics. So, for example, the description of certain types of wounds may be preferred in different periods, and one can thus be misled into drawing inferences about actual frequency of wounds - e.g. decapitation and traumatic amputation in Homeric times. Even knowing that all our evidence is biased, it is still difficult to establish, for example, how far heroisation would influence what was told and how (this concern is particularly relevant in treating the material concerning Alexander the

---

[13] *Caesa enim, quovis impetu veniat, non frequenter interficit, ... , at contra puncta duas uncias adacta mortalis est.*

[14] Plutarch (*Aem. P.*, XIX.5) relates a case in which the spear only causes a bruise: "It did not touch with its point, but ran transversely across the left side, and by the force of its passing the tunic was cut through and the flesh turned purple by a dark weal." (τῇ μὲν ἀκμῇ μὴ θιγεῖν, ἀλλὰ πλάγιον παρὰ τὴν ἀριστερὰν πλευρὰν παραδραμεῖν, ῥυμῇ δὲ τῆς παρόδου τόν τε χιτῶνα διακόψαι καὶ τὴν σάρκα φοινίξαι τυφλῷ μώλωπι). Literally, a 'blind weal', which presumably means that the skin was not broken.

Great[15]). There still remains the question whether medical literature, with its different agenda, was any more factual.

1.2. *Bone injuries*

With a slashing stroke the weight of the sword may occasionally have fractured a bone - particularly in places where the overlying muscle tissue was not very thick, but it will have been rare for an ancient sword to cut through to the bone. It did happen,[16] however, and so did traumatic amputations,[17] although they must have been infrequent, the blades not having the razor-like sharpness of later weapons such as Damascene or Japanese swords. Battle-axes, such as those used by the Dacians (or the Amazons on Greek vase paintings) will have been more effective in this respect, as demonstrated by the fact that the Romans adopted an arm-guard for the sword-arm in the Dacian campaigns.

It was far more likely for a spear or missile than for a sword to injure a bone, given the greater impact and speed of the weapon. This is reflected in Celsus' and Paul's chapters on arrow wounds and is also described in non-medical literature on various occasions, for example Procopius, *Goth.* VI.1.26f., where the arrow hitting a man in the shin is believed to have grazed the bone.[18]

1.3. *Head injuries*

Even when wearing a helmet, a soldier's head was not fully protected and one reads of swords cutting through helmets, or rather cracking them by the force of the blow, e.g. Alexander's at the battle at the Granicus (Plu., *Alex.* XVI.9f.; Arr., *An.*, I.15.7; D.S., XVII.20.6). Often lighter-armed troops wore only leather caps or no head protection at all, and from the description (Thuc., IV.XXXIV.3) of the Spartans on Sphacteria it would seem that

---

[15] See Ch. 8.
[16] Skeleton no. 21 from the Romano-British Cirencester cemetery (McWhirr [1982], p. 171) shows the marks of a blade on the inside of the humerus, a likely place for a right-handed fighter to be wounded from below when lifting his sword. If the cut reached the bone in this place, it would cause fatal haemorrhage from the brachial artery.
[17] E.g. Livy, IV.XXVIII.7 f.: "... the consul who had his arm cut off ..." (... *brachium abscisum consulem* ...). Decapitation is mentioned, e.g., in Virgil, *Aen.* XII.380ff.
[18] τούτῳ ἐνομίσθη εἶναι ἄκρου ὀστέου τὸ βέλος ἀψάμενον.

they were only wearing felt caps,[19] which were easily pierced by the Athenians' arrows.

Cuts, thrusts or shots to the head would often lead to eye injuries, since even on a fully armed hoplite the face was one of the unprotected areas, the percentage that was exposed depending on the type of helmet he wore. Although eye wounds were dangerous, they were not necessarily fatal: *Epid.* V.49/V.236 L describes the case of a man hit in the eye, apparently through the eye-lid (κατὰ τοῦ βλεφάρου); the arrow is removed and the casualty recovers quickly, without losing the eye (ὁ γὰρ ὀφθαλμὸς διέμεινε). There are many testimonies in non-medical literature, too, for men losing an eye in battle but surviving the wound (e.g. Herodotus, III.78.2).[20] The most famous example is Philip of Macedon, who was hit in the eye with an arrow (or catapult bolt) at the siege of Methone in 353 BC.[21] Of course, one possible consequence of injuries in and around the eye was blindness: cf. *Coac.* IV.XXIX.500/V.698 L: "The sight is obscured in wounds to the eye-brow and [those] slightly above it."[22]

Even a bronze helmet could not be relied upon to protect its wearer against stones shot either by slingers or by artillery engines, and because of their speed of impact these would cause the kind of injuries, in particular cranial fractures, described in the Hippocratic *VC. VC* 4-8 (III.194-210 L) distinguishes between five kinds of injuries to the skull: that is, contusions, fractures, *hedrai* or combinations of those. There is no English equivalent for the term *hedra* (ἕδρα), as there no longer is such a concept: it designates the mark left on the skull by a weapon but without depression of the bone. In his introduction, E. T. Withington, the translator of vol. III of the Loeb *Hippocrates*,[23] argues that the term covers what is now called a 'scratch fracture'. Each of the five types is subdivided into several 'forms' (ἰδέαι) of fractures, such as 'narrow', 'wider', 'straight' or 'curved'. In his chapter on skull fractures and their complications (VI.90/II.136.4-143.6), based partly on Galen, Paul, too, lists five types of head injuries as well as a sixth one that "some add". It is called τριχισμός (*trichismos*), a

---

[19] We are presumably meant to imagine them wearing the caps usually worn under the helmet because they had been taken by surprise by the Athenian attack. A cap of this kind can be seen on Fig. 1.

[20] Cf. Esser (1934).

[21] See D.S. XVI.34; Justin 7.6; and for an overview of the sources, Riginos (1994).

[22] τὴν δὲ ὄψιν ἀμαυροῦνται ἐν τοῖσι τρώμασι τοῖσιν ἐς τὴν ὀφρὺν καὶ μικρὸν ἐπάνω.

[23] (1968), p. 4.

hairline fracture, which, he writes, is often fatal because it is not noticed. This is reminiscent of *Epid.* V.27 (V.226 L), where the author admits his own failure to recognise a fracture because "it escaped my notice that the lesion of the missile [a stone] was in the very sutures".[24]

Wounds of this category were potentially fatal,[25] as were those of the following category.

1.4. *Penetrating chest and abdominal wounds*

Together with the aforementioned, these were the most dangerous wounds, caused either by a sword-thrust or - more often - by a spear, javelin or arrow. Even high-quality body armour was no perfect protection, as its weight had to be kept within limits so as not to make movement overly cumbersome. Shock, haemorrhage and infection would often make chest and abdominal wounds fatal,[26] but this was not necessarily so and there are examples of successful treatment. However, in most of the cases described in ancient authors it is extremely difficult, if not impossible, to determine whether these wounds involved lesions to the internal organs or were merely superficial injuries.

Perhaps the most written-about case (written about in antiquity, that is) is Alexander's most serious wound, sustained in India in 326 BC (Arr., *An.* VI.10.1-11.2; Curt., IX.V.9-30; Plu., *Alex.* LXIII.5-13; Plu., *Fort. Al.* 341C, ib. 344F), but, e.g., Plutarch also writes[27] of Epaminondas being wounded in the chest with a spear in a battle in his youth and surviving (the fatal wound he sustained at Mantineia was also a spear wound to the chest). The fact that, when Cato commits suicide by stabbing himself - "below the breast"[28] according to Plutarch - his doctor makes some attempt to save him (by stitching the wound) may suggest that recovery in such cases was not unknown.

However, the strongest evidence for survival after penetrating chest wounds comes from the Hippocratic Corpus. In *Morb.* I.21 (VI.180 L) the author speaks of those who suffer from *empyêma*

---

[24] ἔκλεψαν δέ μευ τὴν γνώμην αἱ ῥαφαὶ ἔχουσαι ἐν σφίσιν ἑωυτῆσι τοῦ βέλεος τὸ σίνος.

[25] E.g., *Epid.* V.60/V.240 L (=VII.32/V 400f. L), a stone-throw to the head.

[26] For example some of the casualties in *Epid.* V and VII: V.21/V.220 L (a lance thrust from the back to the abdomen); V.95/V.254 L = VII.121/V.466 L (a wound of the diaphragm); V.61/V.240 L = VII.33/V.402 L (a javelin wound to the side); V. 98/V.256 L = VII.29/V.400 L and V.99/V.256 L= VII.30/V.400 L (both arrow wounds to the abdomen).

[27] *Pel.*, IV.5 .

[28] ὑπὸ τὸ στῆθος (*Cat. Min.* LXX.5f.).

(that is, a collection of pus in the chest) as the long-term effect of a chest wound made by a spear, a dagger, or an arrow, the wound having healed on the surface but not on the inside. In this passage the author has no case to make for his treatment of chest wounds, but is merely speaking of the long-term consequences. It is therefore unlikely that he should attempt to make the survival rate better than it was, and we can assume that in reality many survived such wounds, although they may often not have recovered completely. Supporting evidence comes from one of the Epidaurian inscriptions: XXX[29] tells the story of Gorgias, "shot in the lung with an arrow in some battle",[30] still carrying the arrowhead in his chest a year and a half later. The wound has not healed and is chronically purulent - the same word *empyêma* is used as in the passage from *Morb.*, and this is the kind of case the author of the latter had in mind. (Gorgias is lucky, however, and Asclepius removes the arrow and cures him.)

Abdominal wounds are described also in Galen's *On the Method of Healing* (*De methodo medendi* [*MM*]), where he writes about some of the wounds he treated when in charge of the gladiators at Pergamon.[31] At X.410-23 K he discusses abdominal wounds and the specific difficulties in repositioning intestines when they prolapsed through the wound, and ibid. 345 he writes of wounds to the diaphragm. (In the fatal case at *Epid.* V.95/V.254 L=VII.121/V.466 L it is also the diaphragm that is wounded - or at least that is what the author believes.)

1.5. *Wounds complicated by foreign bodies*

This is not so much a category of its own as rather a subdivision running through all the aforementioned categories, representing an aggravating factor in all of them. These were the wounds that required the highest degree of surgical skill as well as a number of instruments and clearly went beyond the limit of what help soldiers could give one another. If the missile had pierced the body-armour, the surgeon was faced with an additional problem, for if the arrow had barbs and could thus not be pulled out through the armour, it would hinder the removal of the armour, effectively nailing it to the body. Plutarch (*Alex.* LXIII.11, *Fort.*

---

[29] Herzog (1931), p. 20.
[30] ἐμ μάχαι τινὶ τρωθεὶς εἰς τομ πλεύμονα.
[31] Walsh (1937), p. 37, suggests that Galen may also have been involved in treating gladiators in Rome, during the reigns of Commodus (AD 181-93) and Septimius Severus (from 193 onwards). While this possibility cannot be excluded, it is not supported by any evidence in Galen's extant writings.

Al. 344F-45A) and Curtius (IX.V.22f.) describe how the surgeons had to saw off the shaft of an arrow that had wounded Alexander in order to enable them to remove his breastplate.

Most of the time foreign bodies were - as one would expect - arrows or parts thereof (i.e. mainly the metal point), javelins and spears, but it is not so well known that at times they were also lead bullets, pebbles or shells used by slingers.[32] These were not lethal as often as other missiles, but their extraction presumably caused more problems and necessitated the intervention of an experienced surgeon. Surprisingly there are no written records (whether strictly medical or not) of pieces of clothing or armour having to be removed from a wound. This leads one to suppose that - although it must have happened at times - it was not as frequent an occurrence as it would become with gun-shot wounds. Given their cutting edge, spears and arrows would presumably cut through fabric rather than carrying it into the wound with them. Slingers' missiles, on the other hand, were more likely to have the effect of long-range gun-shot wounds.

Before proceeding to a discussion of the modes of treatment, it seems appropriate to shed some light on the dangers and problems accompanying the treatment of war wounds.

2. *Problems and complications*

Here one has to distinguish between two sets of 'problems': 1) those directly related to the wound and its more or less immediate consequences - in other words those directly concerning the casualty, and 2) the problems the doctor was faced with, i.e. in particular the difficulty of correct diagnosis and prognosis and difficulties arising from having to treat wounds in the conditions of an army at war.

2.1. *Consequences of the wound*

2.1.1. *Haemorrhage*

Bleeding was no doubt the greatest immediate danger with any major wound, given the relative inefficacy of the methods available for dealing with it. The dangers were well known to everyone and loss of blood is mentioned again and again in all types of literature, where to become ἔξαιμος (*exaimos*) or

---

[32] See Paul VI.88.9/II.134.24f. and Celsus VII.5.4.A/310.4f.

exsanguis is mostly related to fainting and danger of death, e.g. in Celsus, V.26.3.A/216.9f.: "Wounds are also dangerous wherever the blood-vessels are large, because they can exhaust the person by an effusion of blood."[33] This concern was obviously based on experience and sound evidence, but it should not be forgotten that blood also carried a heavy load of ideological associations, since it was seen as a life force and loss of it would therefore be all the more alarming for those without medical knowledge.

Such a belief is described by the author of *On the Nature of Man* (*De natura hominis* [*Nat. Hom.*]), when he writes (VI.44 L) that some people claim that blood is the sole essence of man, because "seeing men being cut down and seeing the blood flowing from the body, they believe that this is the soul for man."[34]

2.1.2. *Difficulties in the extraction of the missile*

At an early stage of the treatment, difficulties in locating the foreign body, and later problems in removing it, must have been fairly common. It seems that quite often the attachment of the shaft was deliberately made just about strong enough to keep the arrow together until it hit its target. This would have been done for varying reasons. It may have been done (Paul, VI.88.2/ II.130.13ff.) with the intention of complicating the extraction - as it was common knowledge that this would be more difficult without the shaft - or, according to Ammianus Marcellinus (XXXI.15.11), to prevent the enemy from reusing one's own arrows. This could easily be done if both sides had bows of similar strength. In Xenophon, *An.* IV.II.28, we even hear of the Greeks using the Carduchians' large arrows as javelins. The two passages in Paul and Ammianus Marcellinus are a salutary reminder of how an author's intellectual backgound and the contents and aims of his work can influence his view of things. Two sources discussing the same event can interpret it in entirely different ways.

According to Paul (loc. cit.), some would go even further in their attempt to make their arrows more troublesome: he describes two types of arrowheads, one having barbs moveable by hinges that would unfold at the attempt to pull out the arrow, and the other type having small pieces of metal set into grooves at the side of the point, which would remain inside the wound when the point

---

[33] *Periculosa etiam vulnera sunt, ubicumque venae maiores sunt, quoniam exhaurire hominem profusione sanguinis possunt.*
[34] ὀρέοντες ἀποσφαζομένους τοὺς ἀνθρώπους καὶ τὸ αἷμα ῥέον ἐκ τοῦ σώματος, τοῦτο νομίζουσιν εἶναι τὴν ψυχὴν τῷ ἀνθρώπῳ.

was removed. Dio Cassius (XXXVI.5)[35] also mentions the latter type, but so far no arrowheads corresponding to this description have been found. The only possibility, a rather remote one, is to see them in a certain type of pyramidal point found at several locations in Greece and Asia Minor. These arrowheads, of which there are some in the collections of the British Museum, have a small hole which need not necessarily have served for attaching it to the shaft, but may have held an extra piece of metal. (Paul's description does not make it clear what shape these "pieces of metal" would have been.)

The disintegrating arrowhead could well be the result of poor manufacturing, but on the other hand it would be an effective device and far less labour-intensive than the first type. It is also very unlikely that Paul should copy this particular detail from Dio Cassius, given that the former's chapter about arrow wounds contains much information about different types of arrowheads - either culled from Paul's own experience or from another source. Even if the two independent passages regarding composite arrowheads do not give us sufficient proof that the latter were manufactured with the intention of complicating the wound, they certainly show that this was widely believed about them. Needless to say, these accounts leave open the question whether Paul and Dio are reporting commonly accepted facts or whether these are their personal ideas on how and why these arrowheads were used.

When, for whatever reasons, an arrow no longer had a shaft attached to it, the only way the surgeon could detect it was by using his tactile sense, either by direct palpation or, more often, by using a probe. Given the frequency of the recourse to probing - the probe is probably the instrument most frequently mentioned by medical authors and the most common in finds of surgical instruments - and the fact that it was the only diagnostic means available for wounds, this technique was developed to a degree

---

[35] "And the wounds were severe and difficult to heal, for they used double arrowheads and furthermore poisoned them, so that the arrows, whether they remained in the bodies or even when they were extracted, most swiftly destroyed them; for the other iron [point] was left inside, not having any means for withdrawing it ." (καὶ ἦν τὰ τραύματα χαλεπὰ καὶ δυσίατα· ταῖς τε γὰρ ἀκίσι διπλαῖς ἐχρῶντο, καὶ προσέτι ἐφάρμοττον αὐτάς, ὥστε τὰ βέλη, εἴτε ἐμμένοι πῇ τοῖς σώμασιν εἴτε καὶ ἐξέλκοιτο, τάχιστα αὐτὰ διολλύναι· τὸ γὰρ ἕτερον σιδήριον ἔνδον, ἅτε μηδεμίαν ἀνθολκὴν ἔχον, ἐγκατελείπετο.)

difficult to imagine nowadays,[36] when it has been replaced by other methods.

2.1.3. *Injuries to vital organs*

These would often occur together with the first two points and were one of the dangers of head, chest and abdominal wounds in particular. Lists of fatal and dangerous places to be wounded can be found in several authors (*Prorrh.* II.12/IX.32 L; *Aph.* VI.18/ IV.566f. L; *Coac.* IV.XXIX.499/V.698 L; *Morb.* I.3/VI.142f. L; Galen's *In Hipp. Aph.* VI.18/XVIIIA.27-31 K; Celsus V.26.2f./ 215.28-216.3; Paul VI.88.5/II.132.23-133.9). Given that this knowledge was based on experience, it is not surprising that they largely agree, in particular on the brain, heart, liver, large blood vessels and the bladder. The passage in Galen is a discussion of *Aph.* VI.18 rather than an independent list, questioning whether these wounds are necessarily fatal: "That wounding of the heart necessarily brings about death is one of the things that are agreed upon, but concerning the others there is no consent that every wound brings inescapable death, but only [those that are] large and deep [reading βάθους for Kühn's πάθους], [which is] what appears to be meant by the expression 'cut through' ." (loc. cit., 28).[37] These lists were a response to certain demands put on doctors which will be discussed in section 2.2. The above are merely the passages containing complete lists, but many remarks on how to recognise dangerous injuries are scattered throughout medical texts, e.g. *VC* 19/III.250-4 L, on the signs for impending death from a head wound.

2.1.4. *Fainting*

There is something ambiguous about the concept of fainting, even within medical literature, almost as though there were two co-existing concepts - both of the loss of consciousness as a concomitant factor and of fainting as something aggressive and dangerous. The latter is initially surprising: fainting cannot have been a rare occurrence, given the considerable blood-loss

---

[36] See, for example, the wide spectrum of tactile sensations transmitted by the probe in the examination of fistulae described by Celsus V.28.12.C-E/ 243.18-27. On the use of palpation and probing, cf. also Michler (1970).

[37] ὅτι μὲν οὖν ἡ τῆς καρδίας τρῶσις ἐπιφέρει θάνατον ἐξ ἀνάγκης ἕν τι τῶν ὁμολογουμένων ἐστίν, οὐ μὴν ἐπί γε τῶν ἄλλων ὡμολόγηται πᾶσα τρῶσις ἄφυκτον ἔχειν τὸν θάνατον, ἀλλ ἡ μεγάλη καὶ μέχρι βάθους, ὅπερ εἰκός ἐστι σημαίνεσθαι πρὸς τῆς διακοπέντι φωνῆς, ...

accompanying most major wounds as well as the absence of anaesthetics for surgical operations. And indeed, for Aetius, for example, it is something to be expected, when he writes about an operation that one has to make the patient lie down, because "the seated position is most quickly conducive to fainting" (XV, p.19 Z).[38] This expresses the more obvious theory of seeing fainting as one of many symptoms - if a striking one - of certain conditions such as loss of blood, severe pain, head injuries, etc. However, even Aetius' injunction appears to contain the idea that fainting is something to be avoided whenever possible. Losing consciousness during an operation may after all not have been such a bad thing for the patient, and it appears that, e.g., in the late eighteenth and early nineteenth centuries arm amputations were deliberately performed with the patient in a seated position with the intention of causing a faint.[39]

It would go beyond the scope of this section to discuss in depth the question of the etymology of the words used to express the loss of consciousness, but it is worth noting how clearly the life-threatening aspect of fainting appears in them. The Greek λ(ε)ιποψυχία (l[e]ipopsychia) and λ(ε)ιποθυμία (l[e]ipothymia), as well as the Latin *animae defectio*, all eloquently express the loss of life-force, i.e. of ψυχή (*psychê*), θυμός (*thymos*) or *anima*, which would normally be lost only at the moment of death. Thus the words themselves show how strongly the concept of fainting was equalled with danger in Greek or Roman thought.

We can find fainting as a symptom mentioned by many authors, medical as well as non-medical. The author of *VC*, for example, lists being stunned and falling down[40] as one of the symptoms which should make the doctor suspect a fracture or contusion (III.238 L). According to Paul (V.13/II.16.9), fainting is also one of the symptoms of viper bite.

Fainting associated with wounds appears in many passages in non-medical literature, where it is mentioned in a matter-of-fact way. To quote but a few of the numerous examples: in Diodorus Siculus the Spartan Brasidas faints from loss of blood after having sustained numerous wounds (XII.61.4),[41] we hear of Alexander losing consciousness when wounded (e.g., Curt. IV.VI.20), and Plato's *Laws* (944a) contain the speculation on what would have happened in the *Iliad* if Patroklos had only been unconscious and

---

[38] τὸ γὰρ καθέδριον σχῆμα εἰς λιποθυμίαν τάχιστα προτρέπει.
[39] Mann (1988), p. 20.
[40] ἐκαρώθη καὶ κατέπεσεν.
[41] διὰ τῶν τραυμάτων αἵματος ἐκχυθέντος πολλοῦ, καὶ διὰ τοῦτο λιποψυχήσαντος αὐτοῦ ...

had recovered after having been brought back to his tent, "as it has happened to ten thousands".⁴²

In his commentary on *Off.*, *Hippocratis de medici officina liber at Galeni in eum commentarius* [*In Hipp. Off.*], Galen (XVIII.B.686 K) speaks of fear as a cause of fainting: "There are some", he writes, "who are so fearful in respect to surgical treatment, that they faint before they are cut, from the anticipation of the pain."⁴³

In speaking of anodynes in *On the Method of Healing for Glaucon* (*Ad Glauconem de medendi methodo* [*Glauc.*]), Galen (XI.114 K) asserts that to do some small harm to a patient's health by administering a strong analgesic is preferable to allowing him to faint from the pain.⁴⁴ In this statement one can see the loss of consciousness as a symptom and consequence of severe pain, but at the same time also the second notion, of fainting almost as a hostile, harmful power.

This is expressed more clearly by the author of *Art*. In the context of traumatic amputation he says (LXVIII/IV.282 L): "What is cut off completely at the joints of the fingers/toes, is without danger, unless the patient has taken harm [by] fainting at the moment of injury".⁴⁵ The passage regarding amputation in cases of gangrene (ib. LXIX/IV.284 L) is even more explicit on the effects of fainting. The author warns against amputation in the live part of the limb, because, if the patient suffers pain during the operation, "there is great danger that he may faint from the pain, and swoons of this kind have already killed many suddenly".⁴⁶ In the case of the first passage one could object that the grammar is ambiguous, but the second makes the active, aggressive, character of *leipothymia* unmistakable.

Galen expresses the same concern with the consequences of fainting in his *In Hipp. Aph.* (XVII.B.802 K), when he says: "... for haemorrhage is followed by fainting, and fainting by death".⁴⁷ Celsus seems to be following suit when he states on the same topic

---

⁴² οἷον δὴ μυρίοις συνέπεσεν.

⁴³ εἰσὶ γάρ τινες οὕτω δειλοὶ πρὸς τὰς χειρουργίας, ὡς λειποψυχεῖν πρὶν τμηθῆναι διὰ τὴν τῆς ὀδύνης προσδοκίαν.

⁴⁴ ... ἀλλὰ πρὸς τὸ κατεπεῖγον ἐνιστάμενος αἱρήσῃ μετὰ μικρᾶς βλάβης σῶσαι τὸν ἄνθρωπον ὑπὸ τῆς ὀδύνης μεγέθους συγκοπτόμενον.

⁴⁵ ὅσα δὲ κατὰ τὰ ἄρθρα τὰ κατὰ τοὺς δακτύλους ἀποκόπτεται τελείως, ταῦτα ἀσινέα τὰ πλεῖστά ἐστιν, εἰ μή τις ἐν αὐτῇ τῇ τρώσει λειποθυμήσας βλαβείη.

⁴⁶ κάρτα κίνδυνος ὑπὸ τῆς ὀδύνης λειποθυμῆσαι· αἱ δὲ τοιαῦται λειποθυμίαι πολλοὺς παραχρῆμα ἤδη ἀπώλεσαν.

⁴⁷ Or possibly "haemorrhage is followed by fainting and by death through fainting": ἕπονται δὲ ταῖς αἱμορραγίαις λειποθυμίαι καὶ ταύταις ὁ θάνατος.

as the Hippocratic author (VII.33.1/361.8f): "for often they die during the operation itself, either from the bleeding or from the fainting",[48] and even goes so far as to say, in a discussion of wounds and abscesses (VII.3.2/305.2f.), that "to lose consciousness, either during the treatment or after it, is the worst of all",[49] a statement that seems both excessive and unrealistic.

We can see a similar idea reflected in non-medical literature as well, e.g. in two passages in Plutarch. In *Ages.* (XXVII.2) he speaks of "a deep [or repeated?] faint and acute danger from it"[50] and in *Alex.* (LXIII.12) he relates how Alexander is "brought close to death by his [repeated] fainting".[51]

It has to be admitted that in some of the quoted texts the grammar and syntax may make the meaning ambiguous, especially the use of the dative in Greek and of the ablative in Latin, but in some there is no question as to the idea the author wanted to express, and the sheer number of examples justifies the assumption that the same underlying idea is expressed in all of them.

The key to understanding the diverging statements about fainting may lie in the perception of differing stages of its intensity. Thus Galen in *On Venesection against the Erasistrateans Residing in Rome* (*De venae sectione adversus Erasistrateos Romae degentes* [*Ven. Sect.*]), XI.289 K, uses the expression "such a faint that [the patient] could not be resuscitated",[52] thus suggesting an idea of (measurable?) degree. This appears to be valid for several consequences of wounds - haemorrhage, inflammation, suppuration and fever. While they are not an evil in themselves, they become so when they go beyond a certain just measure and thus become incontrollable.

While fainting appears in the texts fairly frequently, one cannot fail to notice the absence of other symptoms which we would associate with shock, such as pallor, weakening of the pulse, cold and clammy skin and shallow breathing. If one were to treat wounds with the same methods that were used in antiquity, it is very probable that the main cause of fatality would be shock - haemorrhagic as well as neurogenic - ranking even higher than infection. It is therefore intriguing that there is so little mention in ancient literature concerning wound treatment of anything that

---

[48] *nam saepe in ipso opere vel profusione sanguinis vel animae defectione moriuntur.*
[49] *deficere tamen anima vel ipsa curatione vel postea pessimum omnium est.*
[50] λιποψυχία πολλὴ καὶ κίνδυνος ὀξὺς ἀπ' αὐτῆς
[51] ταῖς λιποθυμίαις ἔγγιστα θανάτου συνελαυνόμενος.
[52] λειποθυμία τοσαύτη ὡς μηκέτι ἀναληφθῆναι.

could be associated with what we would call shock. It goes without saying that it would be pointless to look for a concept of 'shock' similar to our own, but even individual symptoms that might be associated with it are rarely mentioned.

This general silence makes the two passages in which we find several of these symptoms all the more outstanding. In *How to Detect those who Feign an Illness* (*Quomodo simulantes morbum deprehendendi* [*Sim.*]), Galen speaks of the ways of distinguishing between those who are actually in pain and those who only pretend to be. Some of the symptoms by which to recognise those who are in severe pain are (XIX.7 K): distress, coldness and pallor of the extremities, sometimes cold sweat and an irregular pulse. In the next sentence (ib.) he also mentions vomiting, stomach upset and dizziness.

The second passage is in Oribasius,[53] who describes the state of those endangered by excessive haemorrhage (after an operation): "weakness, enervation [*atonia*], weak pulse, a dull voice, coldness of the extremities and some cold sweat".[54] Thus both passages read very much like a description of what we would call shock - in the Galen passage it is caused by pain, in Oribasius by loss of blood. We do not know if or from whom Oribasius copied his passage (although it is very likely that he did), but it is puzzling that he should be the only one except Galen to mention those symptoms.

We have already seen that fainting was not necessarily perceived as a natural consequence of wounding and surgical treatment to the degree we would expect, but as far as these other symptoms are concerned, it is possible that they were considered so natural and obvious that most authors did not take the trouble to describe them.

2.1.5. *Inflammation and suppuration*

In numerous cases our authors refer to inflammation casually, almost as to an unpleasant but necessary phase in the healing of a wound. Thus the author of *Fract.* (III.526 L) states: "In general the third and fourth day bring forth complications with most wounds, some of them turning towards inflammation and

---

[53] *Coll. Med.* L.50/IV.68.
[54] ἰσχνότης, ἀτονία, σφυγμὸς μικρὸς, φωνὴ ἀλαμπής, ἄκρων περίψυξις, ἰδρὼς ὀλίγος ὑπόψυχρος.

uncleanness [festering], some proceeding towards fever."[55] According to Celsus (V.26.26A/223.22f.), fever is dangerous if "it lasts beyond the inflammatory period"[56] and one should not induce vomiting "once inflammation has set in"[57] [ib.B/223.29]). Also, expressions in the form of "if there is inflammation, X, if not, Y" are fairly common (e.g. Paul, VI.88.4/II.132.8f.; Off. 11/III.310 L; Ulc., passim/ VI.400ff. L). These passages do not suggest that inflammation was considered a particularly alarming or abnormal occurrence.

One of the symptoms of inflammation would be the 'fever' prognosticated in the passage from *Fract.* cited in the preceding paragraph, i.e. a rise in body temperature accompanying the local inflammation of the tissues in and around the wound. It is mentioned by various authors, though never with much emphasis: "One does not have to fear fever", says Celsus (V.26.26A/223.20-3),

> when it persists in a large wound while there is inflammation. That is pernicious, which supervenes on a slight wound and either lasts beyond the inflammatory period or brings about delirium.[58]

He also says (ib.25A/223.10f.) that it is permissible to give cold water to drink - before inflammation sets in - "if it is summer and there is neither fever nor pain".[59]

Speaking of *good* signs following an operation, Oribasius (*Coll. Med.* L.50/IV.68) mentions strong pain in the wound on the first and second day and fever starting the first night or the second day or night. The author of *Fract.* (III.526 L, cited above) appears to see it as a negative consequence, but he does not elaborate his point (or suggest remedies).

Only the author of *Prorrh.* II (12/IX.36 L) appears to see fever as one of the dangerous consequences following a wound, when he says that one has to take in hand all but the obviously hopeless cases of fresh wounds, "taking heed that the people escape [the dangers of] fever, haemorrhage and spreading ulcers".[60] In

---

[55] τὸ ἐπίπαν γὰρ ἡ τρίτη καὶ τετάρτη ἡμέρη ἐπὶ τοῖσι πλείστοισι τῶν τρωμάτων τίκτει τὰς παλιγκοτήσιας, καὶ ὅσα ἐς φλεγμονὴν καὶ ἀκαθαρσίην ὁρμᾷ, καὶ ὅσα ἂν ἐς πυρετοὺς ἴῃ.
[56] *ultra tempus inflammationis durat.*
[57] *iam inflammatione orta ...*
[58] *Ac ne febris quidem terrere debet, si in magno vulnere, dum inflammatio est, permanet. Illa perniciosa est, quae vel levi vulneri supervenit, vel ultra tempus inflammationis durat, vel delirium movet.*
[59] *... si aestas est ac neque febris neque dolor est.*
[60] ὡς ἂν τούς τε πυρετοὺς διαφεύγωσιν οἱ ἄνθρωποι καὶ τὰς αἱμορραγίας τε καὶ τὰς νομὰς φυλασσόμενον.

general, however, fever with a wound is only mentioned in passing[61] – if at all - and seems not to have been considered a relevant symptom worth discussion.

To an even greater degree than inflammation, suppuration was something to be expected. The author of *Ulc.* speaks of inhibiting suppuration "except for the little quantity of pus that is necessary" (VI.400 L)[62] and many authors actually list remedies for inducing suppuration. This idea may seem surprising to the modern reader, but one has to keep in mind that on the one hand infection and hence suppuration was almost inevitable with the medication available and that on the other hand the idea of a 'cleansing' (*katharsis/purgatio*) of the wound by suppuration fitted in very well with the prevailing medical theories.

Any statement about 'medical theories' is, of course, a generalisation, since there was a great variety of mutually contradictory medical theories, but the process of selection in textual transmission leaves us with a majority of authors following theories showing some similarity to each other (or, in other words, we may be left with a distorted picture of ancient medicine).

The author of *Ulc.* claims that "wounds [or ulcers] which are not cleansed refuse to close when the sides of the wound are brought together" (8/VI.406 L)[63] and distinguishes (ib. 1/VI.402 L) between wounds that need suppuration (those in which the flesh is contused and crushed) and those that do not (cuts made by a sharp weapon). In the former case the crushed flesh has to be converted into pus to make room for new, healthy, flesh - a result which would be achieved by débridement in modern traumatology.

In the stages of wound healing, suppuration follows inflammation and several authors distinguish between 'good' and 'bad' pus - the same distinction being valid both for the suppuration of wounds and suppuration from other causes such as abscesses. Thus, according to *Aph.* VII.44. and 45/IV.590 L, Galen's *In Hipp. Aph.* I.XLI/XVIII.B.105 K and Celsus V.26.20/218.32-219.28, 'good pus' should be white, thick and not malodorous. (Celsus goes into much detail, quoting the Greek names for different types of pus.)

As for inflammation, although it was not a surprising consequence in a wound, it was nevertheless potentially dangerous. "One has to beware of two things, namely that neither

---

[61] E.g. in *Epid.* V.98/V.256 L and VII.33/V.402 L.
[62] ... πλὴν τοῦ ἀναγκαίου πύου ὀλιγίστου ...
[63] ἕλκεα οὐ κεκαθαρμένα οὐκ ἐθέλει ξυνιέναι ξυναγόμενα ...

bleeding nor inflammation kill [the patient]",[64] warns Celsus at V.26.21.A/219.29-31, and goes on to say (ib. 22/220.20-22) that inflammation is to be feared when the wound involves a bone, nerve, cartilage or muscle or when there has been only little bleeding in relation to the size or type of the wound. Inflammation was particularly feared in head wounds, where it would spread to the bone, the dura mater or the brain and would rapidly prove fatal. This appears to have been a well-known fact, as we can also find it mentioned in non-medical literature, e.g. the aforementioned passage from Procopius (*Goth.* VI.30-32).

Celsus' remark on inflammation following 'insufficient' haemorrhage can be understood only in the light of the theories on what caused inflammation. The author of *Ulc.* and Celsus agree that blood (or rather blood-clots in the latter) is transformed into pus, this transformation being accompanied by inflammation. While Celsus limits himself to saying (V.26.23.C/221.12) "it is changed into pus" (*in pus vertitur*), the Hippocratic author (*Ulc.* 1/VI.400f. L) provides a more theory-based explanation: "For it becomes feverish, then shivering sets in and throbbing; for wounds become inflamed when they are about to suppurate; they suppurate when the blood is modified and becomes hot, until it is corrupted and turns into pus."[65] (Other agents of inflammation are, according to Celsus (ibid. 221.13), lint left behind in the wound or the irritation caused by sutures [V.26.23D/221.20-22]). It is thus not surprising that both authors consider it beneficial to let the wound bleed in an attempt to control inflammation. According to *Ulc.* (2/VI.402 L) "with every fresh wound - except for those to the intestines - it is expedient to let more or less blood flow from the wound immediately, for [thus] both the wound and the area around it will become inflamed to a lesser degree".[66] Celsus echoes this advice in his statement (V.26.22.A/220.19f.) that the cure for inflammation lies in the bleeding itself.[67]

If one looks at these therapeutical guide-lines and at the large number of anti-inflammatory remedies to be found in the texts, one comes to the conclusion that inflammation was something that

---

[64] *Prospicienda duo sunt: ne sanguinis profusio neve inflammatio interemat.*
[65] πυρῶδες γὰρ γίνεται, ἐπὴν φρίκη ἐγγένεται καὶ σφυγμός· φλεγμαίνει γὰρ τὰ ἕλκεα τότε, ὁκόταν διαπυῆσαι μέλλῃ· διαπυεῖ δὲ, ἀλλοιουμένου τοῦ αἵματος καὶ θερμανθέντος, ἕως σαπὲν πῦον γένηται.
[66] ἕλκεϊ νεοτρώτῳ παντί, πλὴν ἐν κοιλίῃ, ξυμφέρει ἐκ τοῦ τρώματος αἷμα ῥυῆναι αὐτίκα πλέον ἢ ἔλασσον· φλεγμαίνει γὰρ ἧσσον τὸ ἕλκος καὶ τὰ περιέχοντα.
[67] *adversus inflammationem autem in ipso sanguinis cursu* [*sc. auxilium est*].

a Greek or Roman doctor felt able to control. At least it was seen as more easily controllable than some other complications.

2.1.6. Wounds made by poisoned weapons

Galen, Celsus, Rufus, Aetius and Paul of Aegina make mention of wounds made by poisoned arrows and the use of poisoned weapons is referred to by several non-medical authors (e.g. Homer, Pliny, Silius Italicus, Justin, Dio Cassius and Quintus Curtius) as well as in the mythological accounts of Heracles' poisoned arrows. The practice was obviously known at most stages in antiquity somewhere within the known world.

As for where and by whom these poisons were used, the information we have always shows 'barbarians' using them and one might suspect that this representation was biased by the attempt - wide-spread in antiquity - to depict non-Greeks or non-Romans as scheming and cowardly. However, the evidence of arrow poisons in the *Odyssey* (i.261f.: "... searching for man-killing poison, so that he could anoint bronze arrows")[68] and in the myths suggests that perhaps these means of fighting had not always been outlawed. According to Galen (*Ad Pisonem de Theriaca* [*Ther.*], XIV.244f. K) and Paul (VI.88.4/II.132.13-16) the Dacians and Dalmatians used substances called *helenion* and *ninon* to poison their arrows (neither source explains what these substances were), Silius Italicus speaks of "twice harmful missiles, arrows imbued with serpent's poison" (I.322)[69] used by North-Africans and of poisoned javelins used by the Nubians (III.272f.). According to the pseudo-Aristotelian *Mirabilia* (86), the Celts used an arrow poison (*pharmakon toxikon*) and in Curtius' history of Alexander it is the Indians who poison their weapons – swords in particular (IX.VIII.20). Justin (XII.X.3) also mentions a tribe using poisoned arrows, encountered by Alexander on the way back from India. In the passage from Dio Cassius mentioned in section 2.2.1.2 (XXXVI.5), the author also claims that the enemies whom Lucullus was fighting in Asia poisoned their arrows. A comment in Rufus (*Qu. Med.* 50ff.) reads as if arrow poisons had been fairly common in his period: "It is also necessary to ask in advance[70] about arrow poisons, because many have developed

---

[68] ... φάρμακον ἀνδροφόνον διζήμενος, ὄφρα οἱ εἴη / ἰοὺς χρίεσθαι χαλκήρεας.
[69] ... *hydro imbutas, bis noxia tela, sagittas* ...
[70] As he says a few lines further down, this is a question the doctor must ask prisoners or deserters.

poisons which they apply to their arrows, and they kill even if they make but a small wound."⁷¹

Even when used, the poisons may not have had the toxicity of, e.g., South American arrow poisons such as curare, as some authors seem fairly optimistic about possible cures. Rufus (loc. cit.) goes on to state: "If we know this beforehand, we may be able to provide a cure for every poison.'⁷² Celsus' not very helpful advice (VII.5.5/310.24f.) is to extract the arrow in the same way as an ordinary arrow, but to do so even faster if possible⁷³ - although he does not tell his audience how to recognise a poisoned arrow or the wound made by one before the extraction. After the removal of the missile, he continues, one should give the remedies normally used in cases of poisoning or snake-bite; i.e. he prescribes internal medication for dealing with the poison. Two examples of substances that would be used in such cases can be found in Pliny: *peplis*⁷⁴ and *galbanum*.⁷⁵ Aetius (XV, p.57 Z) writes of a compound drug which is also "for those wounded by poisoned arrows".⁷⁶

Paul, whose chapter on the extraction of missiles (VI.88/II.129-35) focuses on surgical treatment, recommends the excision of the affected tissues, being the only author to purvey a means of diagnosis. "This [sc. the affected flesh] stands out clearly", he writes (VI.88.4/II.132.11-13), "by being different from healthy flesh, for it is discoloured, blackish and looks as if necrosed."⁷⁷ (One can deduce from this that, very often, considerable time passed between the wounding and the surgical treatment, as this discolouring would not have occurred immediately.) He also explains that arrow poison is fatal only when assimilated into the blood stream, but harmless when eaten. The same is stated also in the aforementioned Galen passage (XIV.244 K), which may have been Paul's source for this piece of information. However, Paul

---

⁷¹ ἀναγκαῖον δέ που καὶ περὶ χρίσματος προπυνθάνεσθαι τῶν τοξευμάτων. πολλοὶ γὰρ ἐξευρόντες φάρμακα, οἷς τὰ βέλη χρίονται, κἂν πάνυ μικρὸν τρώσῃ, ἀποκτείνουσιν.

⁷² εἰ δὲ προειδείημεν, τάχα τι καὶ ὁρίσαιμεν ἂν ἑκάστου φαρμάκου ἴαμα.

⁷³ *At si venenato quoque telo quis ictus est, i[s]dem omnibus, si fieri potest, etiam festinantius actis, ...*

⁷⁴ *H.N.* XX.LXXXI: "... it counteracts the poisons of arrows and snakes ... when ingested, and extracts them when put on wounds" (*sagittarum venena et serpentium ... restingui pro cibo sumpta et plagis imposita extrahi*).

⁷⁵ *H.N.* XXIV.XIII: "... it also opposes poisons, most of all arrow poisons" (*adversatur et venenis, maxime toxicis*).

⁷⁶ πρὸς τοὺς ὑπὸ βελῶν πεφαρμαγμένων πληγέντας.

⁷⁷ δήλη δὲ καθέστηκεν ἐκ τοῦ διηλλάχθαι τῆς ὑγιοῦς σαρκός· ἔξωχρος γὰρ καὶ ὑποπέλιος καὶ οἷον νενεκρωμένη φαίνεται.

leaves this as a theoretical statement (he may have had the use of poisoned arrows for hunting in mind - and that is what Galen goes on to mention), and he does not suggest sucking out the wound. Lucan (IX.614f.) shows the same knowledge about snake venom, explaining that it its only dangerous when it mingles with the blood (*admixto sanguine*), but the more wide-spread belief was that only people with a particular gift for it, such as the North-African Psylli,[78] were able to suck out the poison and remain unharmed.

On the whole one could say that wounds made by poisoned weapons were considered more serious than wounds of the same type or size made by ordinary weapons, but they were not seen as hopeless or necessarily fatal.

2.1.7. *'Tetanus' and spasms*

At times these two terms are used as synonyms, while often there appears to be a differentiation between them, so for example "spasms and tetanus"[79] in *Aph*.V.20/IV.539 L, or Celsus, II.I.12/47.20-3: "Cold at times causes stretching out, at times stiffness, of the nerves; the former is called spasms, the latter tetanus, in Greek".[80]

The fact that we still use the term 'tetanus' in medical terminology complicates matters, making it particularly difficult to abstain from attempts to identify *tetanos* with the disease for which we use this word.[81] The concept of *tetanos* certainly encompassed a wider range of symptoms and pathological manifestations than the modern term: namely a variety of muscle contractions and convulsions triggered by various causes. This is quite obvious from the fact that wounds were not considered as the main cause for *tetanoi* by all authors: for example, Paul states at III.20.1/I.168.14-17 that the affliction can also be caused "although rarely, [by] fatigue, lying on the ground, lifting of heavy weights, or wounds, also heat, a blow or the other things that

---

[78] See Lucan, IX.923-37. Celsus also mentions them (V.27.3.C/232.5-8), but asserts that anyone can follow their example, provided he has no sore spot on his gums or palate. According to Vogel (1970), pp. 220ff., Native Americans were credited with the same skills.

[79] σπασμοὺς καὶ τετάνους; although the καὶ can sometimes be epexegetic, this does not appear to be the case here.

[80] *Frigus modo nervorum distentionem, modo rigorem infert; illud spasmos, hoc tetanos Graece nominatur.*

[81] On this pitfall, cf. Gourevitch (1982) who, however, does not mention tetanus.

can bring about the same harm to the nerves".[82] (One needs to keep in mind, though, that tetanus in the modern sense is frequently the result of trivial injuries, so it may often have been attributed to other causes.) All the causes are such as are capable of harming the *neura*, and the link between damage to the *neura* and *tetanoi* appears much earlier, in the Hippocratic *Places in Man* (*De locis in homine* [*Loc.Hom.*], 4/VI.285 L), where the author names the latter as one of the diseases which tend to become fixed in the *neura*.

In a wound, cold was seen as particularly harmful for the 'nerves' and therefore as the cause of 'tetanus' and spasms.[83] (Hence, as women's bodies were considered 'colder' than men, they were also said to be more susceptible to spasms.) Consequently, the treatment involved fomentations, hot baths, sweating, massage and the administration of hot melicrate (a mixture of honey and water).

Apparently a cure could be effected in some cases - which again suggests that not all the cases were what we would call tetanus (in which, even with modern medication, chances of survival are small once the spasms have set in, death occurring usually by asphyxia). According to *Aph.*V.6./IV.534 L, those afflicted by *tetanos* either die within four days or survive, so it appears that some did survive. Galen, *In Hipp. Aph.* VI/XVII.B.790 K, explains that, being a very acute (κάτοξυ) disease, it comes to a *krisis* at the first critical day. Some descriptions,[84] however, show much similarity with the disease in the modern sense.

There is a curious distinction between two or three types of tetanus (which is, however, not followed by all authors): according to the visible symptoms, the distinction is between ἐμπροσθότονος (*emprosthotonos*, in which the body is cramped forwards, with the knees pulled into the chest), ὀπισθότονος (*opisthotonos*, in which the body is arched backwards in the convulsions) and - according to some - τέτανος (when the body becomes stiff, but is not bent to either direction). Galen explains (loc. cit.) that *tetanos* is the

---

[82] ποιεῖ δὲ τὸ πάθος, εἰ καὶ σπανίως, καὶ κόπος καὶ χαμευνία καὶ βάρους ἄρσις καὶ τραῦμα, καὶ καῦσις καὶ πληγὴ καὶ τὰ ἄλλα τὰ τὴν αὐτὴν ἐπιφέρειν βλάβην τοῖς νεύροις δυνάμενα.

[83] E.g., *Aph.* V.20/IV.538 L: "In wounds, cold ... causes feverish chills, spasms and tetanus ..." (ἕλκεα τὸ μὲν ψυχρὸν ... ῥίγεα πυρετώδεα ποιέει, σπασμοὺς καὶ τετάνους); or ibid. 18, where it is said that cold is "hostile to the nerves" (πολέμιον νεύροισι).

[84] On *Internal Diseases* [*Int.*] 52/VII.293 L; Celsus, IV.6.1/156.10-16; Aret., I.VI/5.14-7.23.

generic term and that the two others are sub-categories of it.⁸⁵ Even more curious than the distinction itself is the fact that one can find remedies 'for tetanus' or 'for *opisthotonos*',⁸⁶ as though they were different diseases and not variations of symptoms of one and the same; this may be related to the strong front/back dualism, to which I shall return in Part II.

2.1.8. *Sepsis and gangrene*

There are many words in the Greek language designating the different stages of sepsis and mortification following a wound or other injury, such as σῆψις (*sêpsis*), different forms of the verb σαπῆναι (*sapênai*), σηπηδών (*sêpêdôn*), ἐρυσίπελας (*erysipelas*), γάγγραινα (*gangraina*), σφάκελος (*sphakelos*) or νέκρωσις (*nekrôsis*). Latin lacks this wealth of expression and the difficulty in rendering the Greek terminology is expressed by Celsus (V.26.31B/226.15): "This kind is divided into species by the Greeks, [but] in our language it is not."⁸⁷

Celsus himself uses the word *cancer* for a variety of pathological alterations of the tissues in and around a wound:⁸⁸ septic ulcerations, 'erysipelas' and 'gangrene'. Quite often wounds that were slow to heal would degenerate into ulcers, according to Celsus from exposure to moisture. At V.26.28.D/225.11-13 he warns that bathing can change a wound into a *cancer*, but (V.26.31.A/226.12-14) wounds can also become *cancers* through negligence, strong inflammation, excessive heat or cold, constriction by tight bandages, as well as old age or a bad constitution. Ulcers appear to have been very common, both spontaneous and as the long-term effects of poorly healed wounds, and one can find references to them throughout medical literature. The word *erysipelas* was used (by some of the Hippocratic authors) for different forms of redness of the skin, including the disease now called erysipelas (a form of streptococcal infection). Finally, "what the Greeks called gangrene" was the most advanced form of putrefaction and mortification of the tissues:

---

[85] κάτοξυ πάθος ὁ τέτανός ἐστιν ὡς ἂν ἐξ ὀπισθοτόνου τε καὶ ἐμπροσθοτόνου συγκείμενος ...
[86] Plato, *Ti.* 84e, also speaks of "tetanus and opisthotonos" (τέτανοί τε καὶ ὀπισθότονοι).
[87] *Id genus a Graecis diductum in species est, nostris vocabulis non est.*
[88] Cf. W. G. Spencer's Appendix I to the Loeb edition of Celsus, vol III, pp. 589-92.

The flesh in the wound is either black or livid, but dry and withered; the skin in its vicinity is mostly covered with blackish pustules, for the most part shrivelled, without sensation. Further away it [sc. the skin] is inflamed. (V.26.31.C/226.27-31)[89]

These symptoms were accompanied by fever, thirst and sometimes delirium and when thoroughly established, this condition was incurable.

In *In Hipp. Art.* Galen provides a detailed description of *gangraina*, which he distinguishes from the even more severe *sphakelos*. He himself points out a certain looseness in the terminology that he is discussing, saying (XVIII.A.688 K) that

> we sometimes use the name of the surrounding diseases .. thus we sometimes call a very strong inflammation, which has conserved neither its proper colouring nor its painfulness, gangrene, although it is not yet gangrene exactly, but will be in a little while if it is neglected.[90]

Earlier in the same paragraph Galen states that *gangraina* is a state which is more advanced than a strong inflammation, but not yet as advanced as *sphakelos*. The latter is incurable once it is established. At VII.726 K (*On Swellings against Nature / De tumoribus praeter naturam [Tum.]*), however, he explains that there is some similarity between the two diseases, but *sphakelos* befalls only the bones, while *gangraina* does not and is the result of strong inflammation.

The writers in the Hippocratic Corpus do not make these distinctions and the verb *sphakelizô* is used for mortification of the soft tissues as well as the bones.[91] Another word used by them and referred to by Celsus[92] is φαγέδαινα (*phagedaina*) - as its name (from the root φαγῶ, 'to eat/devour') suggests, a spreading 'gangrene' that can only be stopped by amputation of the limb.

The sources make it clear that these were life-threatening complications against which the doctors could offer little or no help, and the cure itself would often result in disablement. (One can get an idea of the frequency of septic ulcers, gangrene and other appalling complications in pre-antiseptic times by reading

---

[89] *Caro in ulcere vel nigra vel livida est, sed sicca et arida; proxumaque cutis plerumque subnigris pustulis impletur; deinde ei proxima vel pallida vel livida, fereque rugosa, sine sensu est; ulterior in inflammatione est.*

[90] καταχρώμεθα δ' οὖν ἐνίοτε τοῖς τῶν παρακειμένων παθῶν ὀνόμασι ... οὕτως οὖν καὶ τὴν μεγίστην φλεγμονὴν, ὅταν μήτε τὴν εὔχροιαν διασώζῃ τὴν ἑαυτῆς μήτε τὴν ὀδύνην, ἐνίοτε γάγγραιναν ὀνομάζομεν, μηδέπω μὲν οὖσαν ἀκριβῶς γάγγραιναν, εἰ δ' ἀμεληθείη, μικρὸν ὕστερον ἐσομένην.

[91] E.g., *Fract.* 11/III.545 L; *Art.* 69/IV.282 L; *Epid.* IV.39/V.180 L.

[92] E.g., V.28.3B/237.28-30 or VI.18.4/293.15-17.

the accounts written by surgeons in the Napoleonic army, for example the memoirs of Dominique Larrey.[93])

2.1.9. *Permanent disablement and disfigurement*

Depending on the part of the body that was involved, some wounds would result in permanent disablement, mainly lameness, loss of the use of a hand or arm and blindness, and facial wounds would sometimes leave disfiguring scars. Although these were not fatal consequences, they were certainly distressing and a severe practical as well as psychological handicap. In Rome disablement would also (cf. Plu., *Publ.* XVI.7) lead to exclusion from the consulship or, as well as in Greece, from priesthood.

Eye injuries would often lead to both loss of sight and disfigurement, and cases where the latter did not follow were given particular attention, as, for example the case of Arzes, struck in the face between the eye and the nose by an arrow.[94] The surgeon extracts the arrow through the back of the neck, leaving no mark on his face.[95] Pliny (*H.N.* VII.37.37) lists Critobulus among the most outstanding physicians for having extracted an arrow from the eye of Philip of Macedon, healing the wound "without disfigurement of the face".[96]

It is somewhat surprising that Tacitus (*Hist.* IV.XIII) and Aulus Gellius (II.27), in speaking about the general Sertorius who had lost an eye in battle - i.e. an honourable wound, one would think - call his injury a *dehonestamentum*, that is, a blemish with the added meaning of 'disgrace' and 'dishonour'. This conveys an idea of how disfigurement - whatever the cause - was conceived by the general public: the value attributed to physical perfection in antiquity may have made these consequences even harder to bear. (And it is worth pointing out that I am only speaking of men; for a woman the disaster of being disfigured would have been far worse.)

This concern about physical appearance is echoed, for example, in two passages in medical literature, one Greek and one Roman. In the instructions for cauterisation in the case of recurrent dislocation of the shoulder in *Art.*, the author warns against thick cauteries, because they could make the tissue between the eschars break down. This, he says (IV.106 L), will not bring any ill effects,

---

[93] *Mémoires de chirurgie militaire et campagnes.* 4 vols., Paris 1812-17.
[94] Proc., *Goth.* VI.II.14-33.
[95] οὐδὲ ἴχνος αὐτοῦ τῆς πληγῆς ἐς τὸ πρόσωπον ἀπελείπετο.
[96] *citra transformitatem oris.*

but it will be uglier and less skilful.⁹⁷ The surgical operations in Celsus' book VII include cosmetic surgery for remedying pierced ears (VII.8.3f./324.27-325.7) or mutilations of the ears, nose or lips (ib. 9.1-5/325.8-326.15). This suggests that not infrequently people were prepared to face the pain of unanaesthetized surgery, as well as other risks attending operations in antiquity, merely for the sake of their looks.

If we are to believe Plutarch (*Caes.* 45.2-4), it would appear that the fear of disfigurement could be taken for granted, to the point that Caesar was able to incorporate it into his strategy. According to Plutarch's story, Caesar tells his men facing Pompey's cavalry to aim at the face, (ib. 2) "hoping that men not much used to wars or wounds, young and glorying in their beauty and youth, would shrink most from such wounds and would not stand their ground, fearing the present danger as well as the later shame'.⁹⁸ The phrase "the later shame" is a surprisingly negative statement, considering that the author is speaking of honourable wounds sustained in a battle, and it would appear that, to fit the literary ideal of heroism, wounds not only had to be in front, but they also should not mar the young warrior's beauty.

As for those who were left so severely disabled that they were dependent on the help of others, presumably their families, one can assume that their situation varied considerably depending on the circumstances and on their families' attitude. There may be an echo of reality in the fears expressed by the Greek soldiers - mutilated by the Persians - in Quintus Curtius' *Historia Alexandri Magni* (V.V.10-16), when they at first refuse to return to Greece, because, as they say, their families will disown them and they will be a target of ridicule.

Loss of function as the result of wounds is also mentioned in a more matter-of-fact way in various passages, e.g.: Lucian, *Toxaris* 60 (lameness following a cut to the back of the leg), Procopius, *Vand.* III.XXII.18 (paralysis of the little finger after a hand wound), id., *Goth.* VI.IV.15 (a spear wound that severs the nerves in the hand and leaves the warrior unable to fight), ibid. VI.XXVII.14f. (loss of the use of a hand following an arrow wound) or Plutarch, *Publ.* XVI.7 (lameness). Celsus (V.26.28.A/224.22f.) also warns that in wounds in the joints "in

---

⁹⁷ The cosmetic results seem to be important although the cauterisation is done in the skin under the arm-pit and not in the face.

⁹⁸ ἐλπίζοντος ἄνδρας, οὐ πολλὰ πολέμοις οὐδὲ τραύμασιν ὡμιληκότας, νέους δὲ καὶ κομῶντας ἐπὶ κάλλει καὶ ὥρᾳ, μάλιστα τὰς τοιαύτας πληγὰς ὑπόψεσθαι καὶ μὴ μενεῖν, τὸν ἐν τῷ παρόντι κίνδυνον ἅμα καὶ τὴν αὖθις αἰσχύνην δεδοικότας.

which ... the sinews [nerves?] have been divided that held them together, weakness of the part follows".[99] It would seem that such consequences of war wounds, doubtless fairly frequent, were considered unpleasant but not as tragic as a disfigured face.

2.1.10. *Sympathetic reactions*

Beliefs about sympathetic or antipathetic connections between objects were wide-spread in antiquity, ranging from theories about the influence of the moon on human affairs, through the Stoic philosophical doctrine, to magical beliefs and explanations of the effects certain substances had on one another.[100] The concept appears to have been used on two levels - the popular one involving magic and amulets, and the 'scientific' level, dealing with theoretical considerations associated with theories current in natural philosophy. It has to be stressed right away not only that there is no satisfactory translation for the word *sympatheia*, but also that the concept itself is not clear and one cannot be confident in confining it to definite limits, although the context of the discourse sometimes provides clues to its use.

The same term can also be found in medical literature, in particular in Galen, Soranus, Aetius and Paul of Aegina. In the medical context, however, the term acquires an additional reference, covering two closely related concepts. The first, more faithful to the original usage (and the etymology of συμπαθεῖν [*sympathein*], i.e. 'suffering with'), refers to a system of connections between organs or parts of the body, according to which the diseased state of one of them would affect one or several others. In our extant material examples of sympathetic connection between the womb and other parts of the body (e.g. the stomach or the brain) are particularly common,[101] but *sympatheia* is in no way limited to gynaecology. Thus one can find it in a general statement by Galen (*In Hipp. Aph.* XIX/XVII.B.491 K) on acute diseases, claiming that some of them originate "through sympathy and without the place [itself] suffering".[102] The second reference of the term is a set of effects - never clearly defined - usually following inflammation (Sor., *Gyn.* II.49/88.22ff.; ib. III.22/107.17f.), injury (Sor., *Sign. Fract.* 24/

---

[99] ... *in quibus, si praecisi nervi sunt, qui continebant, debilitas eius partis sequitur.*
[100] See Lloyd (1983), pp. 178ff.
[101] Soranus, *Gyn.* III.22/107.17f.; Paul III.64.1/I.280.34, id. III.70.1/ I.288.8ff., etc.
[102] κατὰ συμπάθειαν καὶ χωρὶς τόπου πεπονθότος.

158.22-5 ; Paul VI.52.5/II.93.18ff.; id. VI.98.1/II.151.12-15) or violent modes of treatment (Sor., Gyn. II.11/58.19ff.: cutting of the navel-cord; ib. IV.9/140.6f.: extraction of the dead foetus; ib. IV.15/ 145.14ff.: pungent pessaries). The only qualification for *sympatheia* that Paul, Aetius and Soranus offer is νευρική (*neurikê*), which is not very clarifying either, but the term may be intentionally vague so as to make it more generally applicable.

Paul specifically mentions *sympatheia* in connection with the extraction of arrows at VI.88.3/II.131 1: "...it brings about risk of haemorrhage or sympathetic reaction".[103] He thus regards it as a danger on the same level as haemorrhage and we can find the same combination in Galen's *In Hipp. Art.*(XVIII.A.722f. K), where he says: "... for where there is danger of neither haemorrhage nor sympathetic reaction ...".[104] In speaking of the dangerous signs after an operation Oribasius (*Coll. Med.* L.51/IV.68) distinguishes between two dangers: "the one from the flow of blood, and the other from clotting and the sympathetic reactions resulting from it".[105] This, by the way, is the only passage to describe the symptoms of *sympatheia*, which in this case are: pain in the abdomen, the temples, the sinews and the spine, tension in the epigastrium and fever, sleeplessness, loss of appetite, heaviness in the head, etc., from the second or third day onwards. It may well be that these symptoms apply only in this particular case, but it is also possible that Oribasius is giving a list of what he considers to be the general symptoms of *sympatheia*.

In *Gyn.*(IV.15/145.14ff.), Soranus explicitly says what is implicit in the passage from Oribasius: the immediate danger is haemorrhage, νευρικὴ συμπάθεια (*neurikê sympatheia*) following later. Are we to understand the passage from Paul in the same way - i.e. *sympatheia* not being an immediate consequence? In *Sign. Fract.* (24/158.22-5), Soranus lists *sympatheia*, blackening (presumably necrosis), loss of voice and chills as the dangerous complications of open fractures; the second and third in particular would not be simultaneous with the moment of injury, but can one judge from this information that *sympatheia*, too, is a later consequence? Concerning our most relevant passage, Paul VI.88.3/II.131.1, we are only left to guess, given the lack of definition. It may even be the case that plain *sympatheia* and *neurikê sympatheia* are not the same thing.

---

[103] ἐξ αἱμορραγίας ἢ συμπαθείας ἐπάγει κίνδυνον.
[104] ὅπου γὰρ οὔθ' αἱμορραγίας ἐστὶ κίνδυνος οὔτε συμπαθείας.
[105] τὸν μὲν ἐκ τῆς ῥύσεως τοῦ αἵματος, τὸν δ' ἐκ τῆς θρομβώσεως καὶ τῶν ἐξακολουθουσῶν συμπαθειῶν.

One is tempted to suggest inflammation as a meaning, but Paul speaks of this in his next paragraph, using the usual term, φλεγμονή (*phlegmonê*), which he uses throughout his work. Not only is there no reason for him to use a different word for the same reference, but inflammation is also not considered as particularly dangerous, so it would seem an unlikely explanation. Furthermore, in the aforementioned passage from Galen the list of dangerous complications reads: "neither [of] haemorrhage ... nor [of] sympathy nor [of] inflammation",[106] and Soranus (*Gyn.* II.41/120.13) has "sympathetic reactions *and* inflammations".[107] It seems improbable from these passages that the two words were synonyms.

In some passages[108] *sympatheia* is linked to spasms, and Aetius (XII and XV) writes that a certain remedy is good for "those suffering from opisthotonos and for any sympathetic reaction of the nerves".[109] In his list of symptoms Oribasius also mentions - in hopeless cases - inability to open the jaws or to swallow, which reads very much like descriptions of 'tetanus'. As we have seen, convulsions were symptoms related to the *neura* and this is obviously the link between these and *sympatheia*. The connection is made very obvious by Galen in *Comp. Med. Gen.* (XIII.598 K), where he is speaking of those wounded in the nerves (*neurotrôtoi*):

> It has been said before that the tendons, in which most of the muscles terminate, also bring about considerable sympathetic reactions, first generating spasms and later becoming corrupted themselves and utterly destroying all the neighbouring parts with them as well.[110]

The examples show that *sympatheia* is (as said initially) a very general concept and covers a wide range of references, and we cannot even be certain that it means the same for Paul as it does, e.g., for Galen. What we can tell from the scarce material is that *sympatheia* - apart from its more obvious meaning of a causal link between symptoms or even diseases in different parts of the body - was also the effect of this link, a group of dangerous consequences following a wound or other injury, transmitted by the nerves.

---

[106] οὔθ' αἱμορραγίας ... οὔτε συμπαθείας οὔτε φλεγμονῆς.
[107] συμπαθείας ... καὶ φλεγμονάς ...
[108] E.g. Galen XVII.B.884 K; id. XVIII.B.782 K; Sor., *Gyn.* IV.15 /145. 14ff.
[109] ὀπισθοτονικοῖς καὶ πρὸς πᾶσαν νευρικὴν συμπάθειαν.
[110] εἴρηται γὰρ ἔμπροσθεν ὅτι καὶ οἱ τένοντες, εἰς οὓς οἱ πλεῖστοι τῶν μυῶν τελευτῶσι, συμπαθείας οὐ μικρὰς ἐπιφέρουσι, πρῶτον μὲν τοὺς σπασμοὺς γεννῶντες, ὕστερον δὲ σηπόμενοί τε αὐτοὶ καὶ τὰ πλησιάζοντα πάντα συνδιαφθείροντες.

2.2. Problems concerning the doctor's diagnosis and treatment

The main problem that a Greek or Roman doctor facing a battle casualty would have in common with any other doctor of his times, would be to make a correct diagnosis and - based on this - an accurate prognosis. The lists of fatal and life-threatening points (already cited in Section 2.1.3)[111] that can be found in numerous authors show the great concern with this problem and the importance attributed to it. This was vital knowledge if the surgeon wanted to avoid disrepute and abuse (or worse) and one can already find this idea expressed in the Hippocratics. The author of *Prorrh.* (II.12/IX.34f. L) gives the advice to avoid treating casualties with no hope of recovery, and so does Celsus at V.26.1.C/215.17-20:

> But in these things [sc. wounds] above all the doctor has to know which ones are incurable, for which the cure is difficult and for which it is more practicable. For it becomes a prudent man first not to touch a patient whom he cannot save, and not to risk the appearance ..... of having killed one whom his own fate has destroyed.[112]

The same thought can also be found in Paul (VI.88.5/II.132.27f.), who makes the motives for refusing to undertake treatment sufficiently clear: "... so that we do not, in addition to being of no help, offer the laymen an excuse for reproach."[113]

This knowledge is based mainly on experience and the different authors are furthermore following medical traditions similar to each other. It is therefore not surprising that they agree largely on the fatal and dangerous wounds as well as on the symptoms by which to recognise these wounds (cf. Celsus and Paul).

Armed with this knowledge, the doctor was well equipped to keep out of trouble, but some authors agree that, unless a case was totally hopeless, one ought to attempt a cure[114] - having first

---

[111] *Prorrh.* II.12/IX.34 L; *Aph.* VI.18/IV.566f. L; *Coac.* IV.XXIX.499/ V.698 L; *Morb.* I.3/VI.142f. L; Galen, *In Hipp. Aph.* XVIII.A.27-30 K; Celsus V.26.2-3/215.28-216.16; Paul VI.88.6-7/II.133.10-134.5.

[112] *In his autem omnia scire medicus debet, quae insanabilia sint, quae difficilem curationem habeant, quae promptiorem. Est enim prudentis hominis primum eum, qui servari non potest, non attingere, nec subire speciem* ...[here the text is corrupt] ... *eius , ut occisi, quem sors ipsius interemit.* The state of the text makes an exact translation impossible.

[113] ἵνα μὴ πρὸς τῷ μηδὲν ὠφελῆσαι καὶ λοιδορίας πρόφασιν τοῖς ἰδιώταις παρέσχομεν.

[114] *Prorrh.* II.12/IX.35 L: "with all the others one must perform treatment" (τοῖσι δ' ἄλλοισι πᾶσιν ἐπιχερέειν).

warned the patient or his friends or relatives of the danger: "having stated the danger beforehand, one must put hand to",[115] as Paul says, or, as Celsus puts it more eloquently (loc. cit., 21-3):

> Then, where there is severe fear, without, however, [reason for] certain despair, to disclose to the kinsmen of the person who is in danger that there is hope with reservations [lit.: hope is difficult], so that he [sc. the doctor] may not appear to have been ignorant or to have deceived [them], if the art be overcome by misfortune.[116]

The author of *VC* (19/III.252 L) makes essentially the same suggestion with regards to head injury: "... from these signs one needs to make the diagnosis that [the patient] is going to die, and [one needs to] say in advance that which is going to be."[117]

Prognosis was important not only for fatal wounds, but also for those wounds which would result in disablement, as in these cases, too, the surgeon would need a safeguard against having the blame put on his treatment.

And indeed, this is precisely what people will do, according to the author of *Morb.*, when he states (I.8/VI.156 L) that "for what misfortunes happen by necessity on top of misfortunes, in diseases as well as wounds, they usually put the blame on the physician when they happen, and do not know the necessity that forces those things to happen".[118]

In *De Anat. Admin.* (II.228f. K) Galen explicitly refers to disablement when he stresses the importance of knowing the action of all muscles, so that in the case of a large wound, where a muscle is severed, one will be able to predict the loss of function. In doing so one will be safe from the accusations of those who would usually attribute the result to faulty treatment.[119]

It would not only be invaluable for the doctor's reputation and safety to predict a fatal outcome and refuse any such case, but it could actually be inevitable to do so in the aftermath of a battle. When there was a large number of casualties and only an

---

[115] ... προειπόντας τὸν κίνδυνον ἐγχερεῖν δεῖ.

[116] *deinde ubi gravis metus sine certa tamen desperatione est, indicare necessariis periclitantis in difficili spem esse, ne, si victa ars malo fuerit, vel ignorasse vel fefelisse videatur.*

[117] ἐκ τῶνδε τῶν σημείων χρὴ τὴν διάγνωσιν ποιέεσθαι τοῦ μέλλοντος ἀποθνήσκειν, καὶ προλέγειν τὸ μέλλον ἔσεσθαι.

[118] σχεδὸν δέ, ὅσα ἀνάγκας ἔχει ὥστε γίνεσθαι ἐν τοῖσι νοσήμασι καὶ τρώμασι κακὰ ἐπὶ κακοῖσι, τὸν ἰητρὸν αἰτιῶνται τούτων γινομένων, καὶ τὴν ἀνάγκην τὴν τοιαῦτα ἀναγκάζουσαν γίνεσθαι οὐ γινώσκουσιν.

[119] References to prognosis of disablement can also be found at *Prorrh.* II.15/IX.40f. L, *Art.* 9/IV.100 L and ib. 12/IV.112f. L. On the doctor's liability in Roman law, see Below (1953); Amundsen (1973); Kislinger (1986); Gómez-Royo and Buigues-Oliver (1990).

insufficient number of surgeons available, it would be vital to know who had a chance of survival and treat them as soon as possible, as delays created by attempts to treat hopeless cases would risk the lives of others.

Another obvious problem was the occasional lack of resources. Evidently in a war, on an expedition into enemy territory in particular, a doctor would not have all the supplies that he could normally count on and he would have to make do with a smaller number of instruments and drugs and perhaps unskilled assistants, not to speak of his place of work. Paul, whose stated purpose was to provide a work of reference for those practising in the country or on ships,[120] repeatedly suggests substitutes in case certain remedies were not available, e.g. III.22.5/I.174.3f. or III.22.24/I.181.19f.

A passage in Galen's *In Hipp. Off.* (XVIII.B.686f. K) sheds some light on another problem faced by the surgeon, an aspect particularly relevant for surgical treatment, but which would not immediately spring to mind. He describes how the doctor can deceive patients who are afraid of the treatment, a situation which must have been fairly common. Persuading the patient is mentioned frequently, although few doctors would have enlisted professional help like the physician Herodicus who, according to Plato (*Gorg.* 456b), took his brother, the sophist Gorgias, along to his patients:

> Often already have I gone with my brother and with the other doctors to visit some patient who did not want to drink a remedy or allow himself to be cut or cauterised by the doctor; when the doctor could not persuade him, I persuaded him, by no other art than rhetoric.[121]

In the aforementioned passage, Galen is speaking of surgery in general, but with the surgical treatment of war wounds, especially the extraction of arrows, the doctor may often have found himself in the same situation. In explicating 'Hippocrates' in his *In Hipp. Off.* (I/XVIII.B.707 K), Galen comments on another problem, that of patients (not surprisingly) moving during surgery:

> These things happen to those who are being bound,[122] sometimes also to those being operated upon who, when the operation is on the stomach, raise themselves as far as their spine is concerned,[123]

---

[120] Prooem./I.3.18ff.
[121] πολλάκις γὰρ ἤδη ἔγωγε μετὰ τοῦ ἀδελφοῦ καὶ μετὰ τῶν ἄλλων ἰατρῶν εἰσελθὼν παρά τινα τῶν καμνόντων οὐχὶ ἐθέλοντα ἢ φάρμακον πιεῖν ἢ τεμεῖν ἢ καῦσαι παρασχεῖν τῷ ἰατρῷ, οὐ δυναμένου τοῦ ἰατροῦ πεῖσαι, ἐγὼ ἔπεισα, οὐκ ἄλλῃ τέχνῃ ἢ τῇ ῥητορικῇ.
[122] This could mean either bandaged or tied down.
[123] I.e. push themselves upwards along their spine?

twisting towards the side, ... Sometimes, doing none of these things, they tighten the muscles strongly ...[124]

A few lines further down he becomes more specific:

> It is obvious to everyone how bad it is when, during *parakentêsis* of the eye [i.e. couching for cataract], the patient does not preserve the form and shape, either by shifting or by straining so strongly that the face is covered with blood. Similarly, also [sc. how bad it is] when the doctor excises the bone of the head and, either by lifting some of it a little or by lowering it or turning it to the side, he who is being operated upon spoils the accuracy of the operation.[125]

What makes these glimpses of everyday medical practice particularly fascinating is that they demonstrate just how far removed from realism or reality certain aspects of the descriptions of wound treatment in non-medical literature are.

After this outline of the preliminaries we can now pass on to a description of the modes of treatment themselves.

3. *Surgical treatment*

3.1. *Control of haemorrhage*

Given that haemorrhage is recognised as one of the greatest dangers, with most wounds haemostasis would be the surgeon's most immediate concern and from experience with bleeding wounds the distinction between arterial and venous haemorrhage was made as follows, at least in late antiquity (very much the way we make it):

> You will know whether it is a vein or an artery that is bleeding by the fact that the blood of the arteries is more yellowish and thinner, and it is expelled [lit.: emptied] with a pulsating movement, that of the veins is blacker and without pulsation (Paul V.53.2/I.374.22-5).[126]

---

[124] γίνεται δὲ ταῦτα καταδεδεμένων, ἐνίοτε δὲ τῶν χειριζομένων, οἷον ὅταν μὲν ἐπὶ γαστρὶ χειρίζοντος καὶ κατὰ τὴν ῥάχιν ἑαυτοὺς ὑψομένων πρὸς τὸ πλάγιον ἐκτρεπομένων, ... ἐνίοτε δὲ τούτων μὲν οὐδὲν πραττόντων, τεινόντων δὲ σφοδρῶς τὰς μύας ...

[125] πηλίκον δὲ κακόν ἐστιν ὀφθαλμοῦ παρακεντουμένου τὸν κάμνοντα μὴ φυλάξαι τὸ σχῆμα καὶ εἶδος ἢ μετακινούμενον ἢ ἐντεινόμενον οὕτως σφοδρῶς, ὡς αἵματος πληροῦσθαι τὸ πρόσωπον εὔδηλον παντί. παραπλήσιον δέ, κἀπειδὰν ἐκκόπτοντος ἰατροῦ τῆς κεφαλῆς ὀστοῦν ἢ ὑψώσας βραχύ τι ταύτης χειριζόμενος ἢ ταπεινώσας ἢ πρὸς τὸν πλάγιον ἐκτρέψας διαφθείρειν τὴν ἀκρίβειαν τῆς χειρουργίας.

[126] διαγνώσῃ δέ, πότερα φλὲψ ἢ ἀρτηρία ἐστὶν ἡ αἱμορραγοῦσα τῷ τῆς μὲν ἀρτερίας ξανθότερόν τε καὶ λεπτότερον εἶναι τὸ αἷμα καὶ σφυγματωδῶς κενούμενον, τῆς δὲ φλεβὸς μελάντερόν τε καὶ χωρὶς σφυγμοῦ.

We have detailed accounts of the different methods to stop bleeding from a wound both in Greek (Galen, *De methodo medendi* [*MM*] II.1-7/X.318f. K, partly copied by Oribasius, both in *Syn.* VII.20.1-7/223.16-224.10 and *Ad Eun.* III.36.1-3/416.23-31 and by Paul, IV.53/I.373.20-376.15) and in Latin (Celsus V.26.21/219.21-220.18), but only scattered remarks in the Hippocratics.[127] The first attempt to staunch the bleeding would be by raising the limb and applying pressure (with a dry dressing) or cold water to the wound - according to the author of *Aph.* V, cold water was applied around the wound and not on it: "[apply cold] from where there is or is about to be haemorrhage; not on the parts from where it flows, but around them".[128] Galen (loc. cit.) recommends gentle and painless pressure[129] with one finger directly on the haemorrhaging blood-vessel, if it was sufficiently near the surface, otherwise pulling it up with a hook and twisting it. Paul (IV.53.1/I.373.24-374.9) prescribes the same:

> ... immediately put your finger on the mouth of the blood-vessel, pressing gently and squeezing painlessly [Galen verbatim]; for [thus] you will stop the bleeding at the same time as making a blood-clot coagulate on the lesion ... If it is large, pierce the blood-vessel with a hook, pull it up and twist it with moderation ...[130]

If the bleeding continued, the doctor would then have the choice between a range of styptic substances (see Ch. 3) - Galen (*MM* V/X.323 K) explains how these were used when he suggests holding the blood-vessel with the left hand while applying a compound remedy of one's choice and then holding it steady until the blood begins to coagulate - and forming an eschar either by using caustics or by cauterising with a red-hot cautery. One can get an idea of how wide-spread and well known the use of cauterisation was for haemostasis from its use in the myth of Heracles and the Lernian Hydra. As Diodorus Siculus tells it (IV.II.6): "[Heracles] ordered Iolaus to cauterise the surface of the cut-off part with a burning torch in order to stop the flow of blood."[131] However, Galen points out the danger of secondary

---

[127] *Art.* (IV.282 L), *Mochl.* (IV.376 L), *Aph.* V.23/IV.540 L.
[128] ὁκόθεν αἱμορραγεῖ, ἢ μέλλει, μὴ ἐπ' αὐτά, ἀλλὰ περὶ αὐτά, ὁκόθεν ἐπιρρεῖ.
[129] ἐρείδων πρᾴεως καὶ πιέζων ἀνωδύνως.
[130] ... αὐτίκα μὲν ἐπίβαλλε τὸν δάκτυλον ἐπὶ τὸ στόμα τοῦ κατὰ τὸ ἀγγεῖον ἕλκους ἐρείδων πρᾴως καὶ πιέζων ἀνωδύνως· ἅμα τε γὰρ ἐφέξεις τὸ αἷμα καὶ θρόμβον ἐπιπήξεις τῇ τρώσει· ... μεγάλου δὲ ὄντος αὐτοῦ διαπείρας ἀγκίστρῳ τὸ ἀγγεῖον ἀνάτεινε τε καὶ περίστρεφε μετρίως.
[131] ... προσέταξεν Ἰολάῳ λαμπάδι καομένῃ τὸ ἀποτμηθὲν μέρος ἐπικάειν, ἵνα τὴν ῥύσιν ἐπίσχῃ τοῦ αἵματος.

haemorrhage which was imminent if the eschars dropped off: "And in many cases a bleeding which is hard to check has followed when the eschars dropped off" (*MM*, X.324 K).[132] If all these methods failed, there were still other possibilities left: the doctor could tie ligatures around the vein or artery and then cut it between the ligatures, as this would cause the ends to retract and coalesce. In *On the Use of Pulses* (*De Usu Pulsuum* [*U.Puls.*]), V.160 K, Galen mentions ligatures as a very common measure for wounds: "It has already happened often to many gladiators, soldiers and hunters to be wounded in such a way to the veins or arteries that the doctors were forced to tie these with a ligature."[133] He could also do the same to the blood-vessel at its 'root', i.e. between the wound and the heart or liver. (Celsus does not mention this method.)

While most of these methods appear very plausible even today, it may be more difficult to understand the reasoning behind the use of venesection or cupping to counteract bleeding as it was recommended by some, e.g. Celsus V.26.21C/220.15-18: "... it is nevertheless most convenient to apply a cup to a different part, so that the flow of the blood is called back there".[134] The idea was to deflect the course of the blood, so that it would flow to unaffected parts of the body.

There was also general consensus that loss of consciousness would make the bleeding stop, the two phenomena thus being elements of a reversible relationship of cause and effect. We can find this fact depicted in the Hippocratics (*Epid.* VI.VII.2/V.336f. L), Galen (*MM*/X.327 K), a fragment of Erasistratus in Caelius Aurelianus (*Tard. Pass.* IX.186) and Paul (VI.40.5/II.80.25f.), but also in non-medical writers, e.g. Arrian, *An.*VI.11.2.

In *Epidemics* II.14 (V.114.f. L) we find the remark that during phlebotomy a loose tie around the limb made the bleeding stronger while a tight one made it stop, but the reason that this idea was not followed up for the use of a tourniquet is presumably the high risk of 'gangrene' that it entailed. Arterial ligature was not

---

[132] καὶ πολλοῖς αἱμορραγία δυσεπίσχετος ἐπηκολούθησεν ἐπὶ ταῖς τῶν ἐσχαρῶν ἀποπτώσεσιν.

[133] πολλοὺς οὖν ἤδη πολλάκις μονομάχους τε καὶ στρατιώτας καὶ κυνηγέτας οὕτω τρωθῆναι συνέβη φλέβας καὶ ἀρτηρίας, ὥστε ἀναγκασθῆναι τοὺς ἰατροὺς βρόχῳ διαλαβεῖν αὐτάς. I have left out the word μονάρχους, which does not make sense (unless there was a type of gladiator of this name) and looks like either a misread diplography of μονομάχους or an alternative reading, perhaps by Kühn, that has somehow found its way into the printed edition.

[134] ... *commodissimum tamen est cucurbitulam admovere a diversa parte, ut illuc sanguinis cursus revocetur.*

used in pre-Alexandrian times and without it the doctor would have been faced with the choice between taking off the tourniquet after some time (and causing a fresh haemorrhage) or leaving it on and risking mortification of the limb.

It is likely that, at least before the development of ligatures, an arterial haemorrhage would often have been fatal, but even with this technique it would have been difficult to deal with bleeding from wounds other than those of the extremities.

3.2. Treatment of head wounds

Because of the specific nature of head wounds (with the exception of very shallow superficial wounds not touching the bone), their treatment is also described separately in the different authors, or even, as in the Hippocratic *VC* (III.182-261 L), in a separate treatise. In book VIII, concerned entirely with bones, Celsus discusses head injuries in considerable detail (VIII.4/377.14-382.16) as does Oribasius (XLVI.7-21/III.26-32), and Paul's work also contains a chapter on skull fractures, with or without wounds, and their effects on the membrane (VI.90/II.136.4-143.6), some of which follows Galen, *MM* VI 6 (X.448ff. K). The passage 55-62 in Rufus' *Quaest. Med.* also deals with head injuries.

First, writes Celsus (VIII.4/377.14-18), one needs to ask "whether the man vomited bile, whether his sight was obscured, he became speechless, blood flowed from his nostrils or ears, he fell down or lay senseless as if asleep; for these things do not happen unless the bone is broken."[135] All authors suggest baring the skull by incising the wound where this is not sufficiently large to allow for an examination of the bone. However, according to *VC* 13.42-7/III.234 L, this should not be done at the temples or above them, "for spasm seizes the one who has been cut".[136] The day following the incision (having plugged the wound with lint in the meantime), if it is not clear to what extent the bone has been injured, it should be scraped with a raspatory: "for rasping ascertains the ill clearly, even if the injuries in the bone themselves are not otherwise visible" (*VC* XIV.25-7).[137]

---

[135] ... *num bilem homo is vomuerit, num oculi eius occaecati sint, num obmutuerit, num per nares auresve sanguis ei fluxerit, num conciderit, num sine sensu quasi dormiens iacuerit: haec enim non nisi osse fracto eveniunt.* Cf. *VC* 14.43-7/III.238 L; Rufus, *Quaest. Med.* 55.

[136] σπασμὸς γὰρ ἐπιλαμβάνει τὸν τμηθέντα.

[137] ἐξελέγχει γὰρ ἡ ξύσις μάλα τὸ κακόν, ἢν μὴ καὶ ἄλλως καταφανέες ἔωσιν αὐταὶ αἱ πάθαι αἱ ἐοῦσαι ἐν τῷ ὀστέῳ.

If the doctor suspected a fracture (from the symptoms mentioned above) but could not distinguish it, the suggested solution was to pour "the very black solution"[138] or, according to Paul (VI.90.3/II.138.5) even writing ink,[139] onto the skull and scrape the bone on the following days. (The fracture would then be visible as a black line.) If the crack was deep and did not disappear with scraping, the case called for trepanning. (According to VC 9/III.210, both contusions and fractures, whether visible or not, needed to be trepanned.[140]) This part of the treatment appears to have been the object of changing fashions over time, for Galen writes in his *Introduction* (*Introductio seu Medicus* [*Intr.*]):

> Every kind of skull fracture is subjected to excision, removing that [part] of the bone which is broken by means of chisels. The ancients excised them sawing with a [crown] trepan by twisting it. Those after them with trepans,[141] submitting *hedrai* to chisels.[142] Those [who live] now are satisfied with chisels alone (XIV.783 K).[143]

Nevertheless, in *MM* (VI.6/X.447 K), he mentions drilling rather than chisels where the bone is strong. Paul, who quotes Galen, adds the detail (VI.90.5/II.139.11f.) of plugging the patient's ears with wool because of the noise made by the chisels or the trepan. The authors also advise cooling the trepan often so as not to burn the bone with the heat caused by the friction.[144] Thus fractured or contused parts of the bone were removed as far as this was possible, often using a specialised instrument, the μηνιγγοφύλαξ (*mēningophylax*; 'membrane-protector'),[145] a metal plate inserted between the bone and the dura mater.

3.3. *Removal of missiles or other foreign bodies*

---

[138] τὸ τηκτὸν τὸ μελάντατον (*VC* 14.47f./III.240 L).

[139] τὸ γραφικόν.

[140] τούτων τῶν τρόπων τῆς κατήξιος ἐς πρίσιν ἀφήκει, ἥ τε ἡ φλάσις ἡ ἀφανὴς ἰδεῖν, καὶ ἢν πως τύχῃ φανερὴ γενομένη, καὶ ἡ ῥωγμὴ ἡ ἀφανὴς ἰδεῖν, καὶ ἢν φανερὴ ᾖ.

[141] Galen appears to be making a distinction between the crown trepan, a metal cylinder with a serrated edge, and the drill.

[142] *Pace* Kühn, who translates ἕδρα as a 'seat' for the patient.

[143] πᾶν δὲ εἶδος τῶν ἐν κεφαλῇ καταγμάτων τῇ ἐκκοπῇ ὑπάγεται διὰ ἐκκοπέων περιαιρουμένων τὸ κατεαγὸς τῶν ὀστῶν. οἱ μὲν οὖν παλαιοὶ χοινικίοις πρίοντες ταῖς διὰ τῆς περιστρεφομένης ἐξέκοπτον αὐτά· οἱ δὲ μετὰ ταῦτα κεφαλοτρυπάνοις, ἕδρας παρέχοντες τοῖς ἐκκοπεῦσιν. οἱ δὲ νῦν μόνοις τοῖς ἐκκοπεῦσιν ἀρκοῦνται.

[144] *VC* 21/III.258 L; Celsus VIII.3.7/376.6f.

[145] E.g. Celsus VIII.3/376.17; Galen, *De Anat. Admin.* VIII/II.686 K; Alex. Trallianus I.14.

In the extant medical writings there are two complete step-by-step instructions how to remove a missile from a wound - Celsus VII.5/308.6-310.28. and Paul VI.88.3-9/II.130.25-135.5 - but they were certainly not the only ones written in antiquity, given the importance of the topic. Thus the Hippocratic work about "arrows and wounds", which has not come down to us, must have contained a description of how to remove an arrow from a wound.[146] In *De Anat. Admin.* II and III (II,283f., 394f. K) Galen stresses the importance of anatomical knowledge specifically for the treatment of war wounds, in particular for the extraction of arrows,[147] so apparently these cases were not infrequent. (He does not explain the extraction of arrows anywhere, nor does he describe any cases of arrow wounds.)

As mentioned before, this was the domain of the expert, requiring particular skills and training as well as equipment, while other areas of wound healing were far more open to those who had had no formal training. Those who were trained in these skills, on the other hand, would have had a predominantly practical training involving little or no book learning. It is quite clear from a study of the relevant chapters in Celsus and Paul that they would not have enabled a person without practical training to extract an arrow. On the other hand, they would not have been necessary for anyone who had been trained as a surgeon. In the light of this consideration it is therefore not surprising that treatises of this kind did not fare well in textual transmission, and it may be for this reason that only two descriptions have survived.

The first impulse of a man hit by an arrow was either to pull it out himself or to ask one of the other soldiers to do so on the spot: we can see this reaction reflected in Ammianus Marcellinus (XVIII.8.11), where a soldier with an arrow stuck in his thigh asks the author to pull it out, and also in Aeneas Tacticus (XXXI.16): an arrow carrying a secret message strikes the shoulder of a man "around whom a crowd ran together, as it often happens in war, immediately taking hold of the arrow...".[148] The dangers of doing so are spelt out in Rufus (*Quaest. Med.* 51), who stresses the need to avoid this. The soldiers must be told, he writes, "to put up with the arrows until they can have them removed by a person who can

---

[146] Galen is presumably thinking of the same treatise when (XVIII.A.28 K) he speaks of a work about dangerous wounds (Περὶ τῶν ὀλεθρίων τραυμάτων).

[147] βελῶν ἐξαιρέσεις.

[148] ... πρὸς ὃν βληθέντα περιέδραμεν ὄχλος, οἷα φιλεῖ γίνεσθαι ἐν τῷ πολέμῳ, αὐτίκα δὲ τὸ τόξευμα λαβόντες ...

do so properly".¹⁴⁹ Apart from other complications, such as haemorrhage or unnecessary tearing of the wound, the main danger was that only the shaft would be pulled out, leaving the arrowhead behind. This would both cause inflammation and make the later extraction more difficult and painful. According to Rufus, "it can escape even an altogether experienced man that the point is concealed".¹⁵⁰ This statement is also borne out by *Epid.* V.95/V.254 L (=VII.121/V.466 L). Describing the symptoms - and eventual death - of a man wounded in the chest with a catapult bolt, the author writes: "It appeared to me that in taking out the wood[en shaft] the doctor left something of the missile [literally: 'spear'] in the diaphragm, and it seemed so to him, too."¹⁵¹

The essential skill for obtaining more information about the wound and the missile itself was probing (μηλώσις / *mêlôsis*), by which the surgeon could determine the depth and direction of the wound, the shape and size of the missile, whether it had struck a bone or, if it was an arrow, whether it had barbs and - if the shaft was not attached - whether the arrowhead ended in a tail or in a hollow socket. Paul stresses the use of this technique when he says (VI.88.4/II.131.23f.): "And if the arrow has a tang (this is known to us from probing)...".¹⁵² When Curtius writes in his history of Alexander (IX.V.23) that, before the extraction, "they discovered that the arrow had barbs",¹⁵³ he can only be thinking of probing, which shows how common the practice and how popular the notion was.

When an arrow was entirely embedded in the soft tissues, there were two ways of removing it : either from the side from where it had entered (ἐφελκυσμός / *ephelkysmos*) or by making a counter-opening on the opposite side (διωσμός / *diôsmos*). The first was appropriate either when the wound was shallow or when a large

---

¹⁴⁹ [διόπερ καλῶς παρακελεύονται τοῖς στρατιώταις οἱ ἰατροὶ] φέρειν τὰ τοξεύματα ἐμπεπηγότα, ὡς ἂν εἰδεῖεν αὐτοὶ κομιζόμενοι μή τι ἐγκαταλειφθείη τῷ ἕλκει, καὶ ἅμα ἐμπείρως κομίζοιντο.
¹⁵⁰ λάθοι γὰρ ἂν καὶ τὸν πάνυ ἔμπειρον ὑποῦσα ἡ ἀκίς.
¹⁵¹ ἐδόκει δέ μοι ὁ ἰητρὸς ἐξαίρων τὸ ξύλον ἐγκαταλιπεῖν τι τοῦ δόρατος κατὰ τὸ διάφραγμα, δοκέοντος δὲ αὐτοῦ. W. D. Smith, *Hippocrates*, vol VII (Loeb Classical Library), Cambridge, Mass./London 1994, p. 213, takes the 'him' to refer to the patient. However, I find it more probable that - given the use of αὐτοῦ rather than ἐκείνου - it refers to the last person mentioned, hence the other doctor. It may well be that he discussed the case with the author. Although Robert's (1989) suggestion of a 'medical team' touring the north of Greece is anachronistic, it is not unlikely that there were several doctors present at the time.
¹⁵² καὶ εἰ μὲν οὐραχὸν ἔχοι τὸ βέλος (τοῦτο δὲ ἐκ τῆς μηλώσεως ἡμῖν γινώσκεται), ...
¹⁵³ ... *animadvertunt hamos inesse telo* ...

blood-vessel, nerve or tendon was likely to be affected in the case of *diôsmos*. If the point had no barbs, it could often be pulled out without a preliminary incision - either by the shaft or by grasping the point with the fingers or with a forceps, but a barbed arrowhead (used frequently for precisely the purpose of complicating the extraction) necessitated some precautions. If pulled out, it would lacerate the tissues on its way, therefore the wound would have to be enlarged by incision. Both authors suggest covering the barbs with reeds and Celsus also recommends clipping them off with a forceps "if they are short and fine". With any type of extraction, if a large artery, sinew, etc. was in danger of being injured, it was pulled away from the arrow or the scalpel with hooks.

Celsus is the only author to mention a specialised instrument for the extraction of large arrowheads - the *Diocleus cyathiscus*, i.e "spoon of Diocles", supposedly invented by Diocles of Carystus. According to Celsus' description, this was a flat spoon with a perforation in the curved end, which is pushed along, and then under, the arrowhead. It is then twisted to make the point rest in the hole and both the arrow and the instrument are pulled out together. From the description of its use it appears to have been a highly impractical instrument, as it would only fit a certain size of arrowhead and would presumably involve more manoeuvering inside the wound than the use of forceps. There is one instrument fitting the description exactly, found in Asia Minor, in the Meyer-Steineg collection at Jena,[154] but it has since been revealed to be a fake.[155] Even so, it is unlikely that whoever made the imitation, presumably some blacksmith in rural Turkey, based its shape on Celsus' text, and it is hard to imagine that by sheer coincidence he thought up something that corresponded so perfectly to Celsus' description. It is far more probable that the fake is the copy of a real "spoon of Diocles" which may have been lost, or may still be lying in a dusty drawer in some museum. The fact that it existed suggests that someone had at least intended to use it at some point in time. It is very unlikely that its use was very wide-spread. Celsus may have been describing it for its novelty value and it will have been acquired by some physicians for this very reason.

The method of *diôsmos* would usually be practised when the wound was in an arm or leg and the already existing wound was deeper than the remaining distance to the opposite side. The

---

[154] See Meyer-Steinegg (1912) and Künzl (1988).
[155] E. Künzl in: *Theodor Meyer-Steineg (1873-1936) - Arzt, Historiker, Sammler* (catalogue of the exhibition, Jena, 18 June - 4 August 1991), pp. 26f.

counter-opening was made by the scalpel and the arrow pushed out - either by using the shaft to propel it or by using an instrument called διωστήρ (*diôstêr*), mentioned only by Paul (VI.88.3/II.131.20). This was a metal (?) rod with a pointed or 'male' end, used when the arrowhead had a socket, and a hollow or 'female' end, for use if it had a tail.

When the arrow was firmly stuck in a bone and would not move even with strong traction or when struck with an instrument, the bone around the point had to be scraped or excised or even removed by drilling.

At VI.88.4/II.131.25-132.1, Paul again refers to the composite arrowheads described by him earlier, as their extraction presents specific problems:

> If, after the removal, the arrowhead appears to have grooves as though other thin pieces of metal could have been inserted into them, we again make use of probing and, if we find any, we remove those as well by the same methods.[156]

As mentioned in Section 1, arrow and spear points were not the only missiles that had to be removed from wounds: the lead bullets, pebbles or shells used by the slingers would sometimes penetrate as deeply as other missiles and would be more difficult to locate than arrowheads. Depending on their depth, these wounds would have to be enlarged by incision and then the missile would be lifted out with the fingers, a spoon-probe, forceps or a lever.

Within the perimeter of wound treatment, the extraction of the arrow (or other missile) was probably the most ideology-laden aspect - both for the doctor and for the patient. With its Homeric connotations - the verse about the "physician who cuts out arrows" being "worth many another man" was well known throughout antiquity - it implied an archaic ideal of medical practice for the doctor as well as heroic ideals for the wounded man himself.[157]

3.4. *Wound closure and dressing*

Large wounds were usually united by sutures (ῥαφαί /*sutura*) to help agglutination and also, according to Celsus

---

[156] τὸ δὲ βέλος ἐξαιρεθὲν εἰ φανείη γλυφίδας ἔχον τινὰς ὡς ἐν αὐταῖς ἐντεθῆναι δυναμένων λεπτῶν σιδηρίων, πάλιν τῇ μηλώσει χρησάμενοι εἴπερ εὑρίσκομεν, κἀκεῖνα κατὰ τὰς αὐτὰς μεθόδους κομισόμεθα.

[157] This aspect will be discussed in Part II.

(V.26.23B/221.7f.), for cosmetic effects - "so that later the scar will be less wide".[158] The material for sutures would be flax or linen thread, which may explain why we hardly ever read about the removal of stitches - the material would rot before the wound was completely healed. So, for example, Galen writes in *MM* V (X.320 K) that one has to make the wound heal as quickly as possible before the thread rots.[159]

Celsus (V.26.23B/221.2-8) distinguishes between *sutura* (using a needle and thread) and *fibulae*. The meaning of the latter has been a topic of some controversy among medical historians for some time, but it must mean something different from a normal suture. The original reference of the word - a kind of safety-pin/brooch used on clothes - suggests some type of metal pin, perhaps a pin fixed by a thread wound round it in a figure of eight.[160] Paul's injunction (VI.88.4 /II.132.f.) not to stitch a wound when there is inflammation again suggests that some time would have passed between the moment of wounding and treatment, as one would hardly expect inflammation in a fresh wound.

In *MM* VI, Galen writes about the problems particular to the suturing of abdominal wounds: "... first one needs to put away the prolapsed intestines into their proper place, second after that [one needs to] suture the wound, ..."[161]

> The reposition of the intestines to their proper place, when it is done on a large wound, needs a dexterous assistant. For, grasping the entire wound with his hands from the outside, he needs to push it inwards and press it together and present it to the one who is suturing little by little, and then also compress moderately that which has ben sutured, until it has all been sutured accurately.[162]

This is followed by instructions for abdominal suture (γαστρορραφία/ *gastrorrhaphia*), the needle piercing first the skin and the muscle going inwards (but not the peritonaeum), then the peritonaeum, muscle and skin of the opposite edge of the wound

---

[158] ... *quo minus lata postea cicatrix sit.*
[159] Or literally 'runs off' - ἀπορρυῆναι.
[160] Cf. W. G. Spencer's Introduction to vol II of the Loeb edn. of Celsus, p. lxi.
[161] προηγεῖσθαι μὲν χρὴ ἐς τὴν οἰκείαν χώραν ἀποτίθεσθαι τὰ προπεπτωκότα ἔντερα, δεύτερον δὲ ἐπὶ τόδε ῥάψαι τὸ ἕλκος, ... (X.413f. K).
[162] αἱ δ' ἀποθέσεις τῶν ἐντέρων εἰς τὴν οἰκείαν χώραν, ὅταν ἐπὶ τοῖς μεγάλοις γίγνωνται τραύμασιν, ὑπηρέτου δέονται δεξιοῦ. χρὴ γὰρ αὐτὸν ὅλον ἔξωθεν καταλάβοντα τὸ τραῦμα ταῖς ἑαυτοῦ χερσὶν εἴσω προστέλλειν τε καὶ σφίγγειν, ὀλίγον ἑκάστοτε τῷ ῥάπτοντι προγυμνοῦντα· καὶ μέντοι καὶ τὸ ῥαφὲν αὐτὸ μετρίως προστέλλειν, ἄχρι περ ἂν ὅλον ἀκριβῶς ῥαφῇ (X.415f. K).

going outwards, then piercing the skin and muscle of that same edge (inwards) and all three layers of the opposite edge (outwards), i.e the side from which one started, etc. (X.416 K). Celsus (VII.16.4.f./333.24-334.7) describes a two-handed suture, with a threaded needle in each hand, for abdominal wounds (this will be quoted below, in Chapter 5.2; both this and the Galen passage are good examples of how difficult it is to describe even a relatively simple surgical procedure in a written text).

It appears that not all wounds were dressed, and the author of *Ulc*. (3/VI.404 L) states that one should only purge wounds "where one wants to bandage".[163] In most cases, however, wounds were covered with one or several of a variety of dressings. These could be dry linen bandages or sponges (or μότοι [*motoi*], tents inserted into the wound), sponges or cloths soaked in water, vinegar, wine, oil or some liquid remedy, or wool (either greasy or washed, the former being particularly valued for its capacity of keeping the wound warm). In *On Bandages* (*De fasciis* [*Fasc*.]), Galen makes a distinction between different types of bandages for different kinds of wounds (XVIII.A.773 K): " We use linen ones on whatever has need of pressure, but for what does not need constriction because of some inflammation counter-indicating it, and needs only coherence and protection, woollen ones."[164] Occasionally the dressing was covered with a layer of fresh leaves, especially when it was moist, so as to avoid evaporation, and we can find this practice referred to even in Aeneas Tacticus (XXXI.4), who speaks of a secret letter written on leaves "bound on to a wound ... in the thigh",[165] thus apparently not arousing suspicion.

Judging from warnings in the Hippocratic Corpus against unnecessarily elaborate bandaging styles (*Medic*. 4/IX.210 L; *Art*. 35/IV.158 L), it seems that many doctors saw bandaging as an occasion to show off their dexterity. Two works devoted entirely to different types of dressings and bandages have come down to us - Soranus' *De fasciis* and Galen's work of the same title, mentioned above. Oribasius, quoting from the lost works of Heliodorus, (*Coll. Med.* XLVIII.20-69/III.273-91) also describes an astonishing number of ways of bandaging. Presumably in order to help memorisation, the various kinds of bandages were given names, some descriptive - e.g. 'the eye' (ὀφθαλμός) or 'four-

---

[163] ὅκη ἂν μέλλῃ ἐπιδεῖν.
[164] ὅσα γοῦν σφίγξεως δεῖται λινοῖς ἐπ' αὐτῶν χρώμεθα, ὅσα δὲ οὐ σφίγξεως διὰ τὸ ἐναντιοῦσθαι τισι φλεγμοναῖς, συνεχείας δὲ δεῖται μόνης ἢ σκέπης ἐρεοῖς.
[165] ἐφ' ἕλκει καταδεδεμένα ... ἐπὶ κνήμην.

legged' (τετρασκελής) (XVIII.A.774ff. K) - and others more fanciful - e.g. the 'royal' (βασιλικός), 'pastoral' (βουκολίσκος) and, most memorably, the 'hare with ears' (λαγωὸς μετ' ὤτων; ibid. 777).[166] As far as our topic is concerned, the work-load of a surgeon in an army at war may have discouraged aspirations towards excessive elegance in bandaging, and often it may have been left to assistants.

---

[166] Oribasius, *Coll. Med.* XLVIII.27/III.276, also knows a 'hare without ears'.

CHAPTER THREE

PHARMAKA

The Greek word φάρμακα (*pharmaka*) is more appropriate here than the English 'drugs', as *pharmaka* include a wider range of substances than those which we would consider as drugs. Thus the texts list, e.g., wine, oil, vinegar and substances such as sheep's dung, none of which we would call a drug. This can be understood if we consider that, in the words of the author of *Loc. Hom.* (45/VI.340 L), "anything which modifies the present state is a *pharmakon*."[1] One also has to remember that the highly charged word *pharmakon* - with its extended use for poisons and magical potions - has a network of related ideas regarding efficacy and potential danger which cannot easily be captured by any modern term.[2]

Pharmacological treatment was certainly more common than surgical treatment, for while many wounds did not require any form of surgical intervention, most would necessitate the application of some sort of pharmacological substance (or rather, would have been considered to necessitate it). Also, knowledge of *pharmaka* would be open to a far greater number of people - many of whom would not have had any form of medical training - than that of surgery, the successful practice of which was based on a high level of skill and training and thus limited to a small number of practitioners.

A large number of medical and scientific writers deal with materia medica for wound treatment, considerably more than those describing trauma surgery. The wider applicability of pharmacological treatment, and hence also a greater interest for it among the lay public, may be one reason for this proportional relation, but perhaps not the only one. It may also be that this type of material was both easier to put into writing and actually called for written records, its extent making it difficult to memorise, while surgery would mostly be taught by demonstration and resisted textual representation - even more so in the absence of a universally accepted medical terminology.

---

[1] πάντα φάρμακά εἰσι τὰ μετακινέοντα τὸ παρεόν.
[2] On this ambiguity, see Artelt (1968). Cf. Schmiedeberg (1918) on *pharmaka* in the Homeric epics.

Whereas the works of some authors such as Aetius, Scribonius Largus, Theodorus Priscianus and Paul contain mainly composite remedies, some authors have left us with lists of single plants and substances, enumerating their properties and medical uses: namely Theophrastus (to a very limited extent), Dioscorides, Galen, Pliny and Oribasius. As for wound remedies in the Hippocratic Corpus, there is only the list in *Ulc.* (11/VI.410-26 L) and a paragraph on anti-inflammatory preparations in *Aff.* (38/VI.246f. L), unless one counts the fairly frequent mentions of pitch and cerate (e.g. III.428, 486, 496, 510 L; IV.100, ib. 170 L) in the surgical treatises.[3] Book V of Celsus' *De medicina* also contains wound remedies, and he follows the approach of classifying substances by their effects (e.g. *sanguinem supprimunt*, etc.).

As one might expect, the description of a drug and its effects was influenced by the medical theories to which the writer subscribed. An exhaustive account of ancient medical theories would fill several books, so a brief outline has to suffice here: Dioscorides, our richest source of information about pharmacological material, developed his own system of classification, independent of rival schools of medicine.[4] He usually arranged drugs by affinities of effect - i.e. by how they worked - classifying them by a fairly large number of powers or faculties (δυνάμεις; *dynameis*) - e.g. styptic (στυπτικός; *styptikos*), dispersing (διαφορητικός; *diaphorêtikos*) or detergent (ῥυπτικός; *ryptikos*) - on a purely empirical basis, and criticised earlier writers (*praef.* 2) for allowing disputes to prejudice their observations. However, Riddle[5] argues that, by not giving a detailed theoretical explanation of his scheme he doomed its chances of survival.

Galen ignored Dioscorides' system - although he refers to him frequently and calls his work "the most perfect of all treatises on materia medica"[6] - and (perhaps for that very reason) so did the later authors. As Riddle[7] puts it, Galen's treatises were harmful to Dioscorides' work, "because Galen supplied a theory as an explanation for pharmaceutical behavior". Galen, following his own interpretation of 'Hippocrates', worked on the basis of four

---

[3] For medicinal plants and substances in the Hippocratic Corpus, see Stannard (1961); Dierbach (1969); Harig (1980); Rehounek (1981); Scarborough (1981).
[4] Cf. Riddle (1985) for a detailed analysis of the system.
[5] (1985), p.42f.
[6] XI.794 K.: καὶ μοι δοκεῖ τελεώτατε πάντων οὗτος τὴν περὶ τῆς ὕλης τῶν φαρμάκων πραγματείαν ποιήσασθαι.
[7] (1985), p. 169.

primary faculties only (namely warm, cold, dry and wet), related to the four humours, which were related in their turn to the four elements. As every element was seen as a combination (κράσις; *krasis*) of an active faculty (warm/cold) and a passive faculty (dry/wet), and drugs were seen as mixtures of elements, it follows logically that every drug had to have an active and a passive property. According to Galen, these properties were graded in four increasing degrees of intensity[8] - e.g. cooling to the third degree - and were accompanied, for the sake of therapeutical precision, by secondary properties, such as 'cutting' (τμητικός / *tmêtikos*) or 'thinning of humours' (λεπτυντικός / *leptyntikos*). These properties were obviously the result of a purely theoretical elaboration and often unrelated to the mere physical effects: one can see this from Galen's mention of the dispute whether vinegar was 'hot' or 'cold' (XI.415f. K). Galen also claimed different *kraseis* according to sex and age and even according to individual temperament. While this might suggest a wide scope for experience, he nevertheless rejected knowledge based merely on experience.[9]

Many of the medical writers coming after Galen appear to be following theories similar to his and, as far as other 'schools' (Empiricists, Dogmatists or Methodists) are concerned, we have too little by self-proclaimed followers of any of them to go by. To a great extent we have to rely on Galen's testimony for information on most of these schools or sects, biased as it is by his intention to prove the excellence of his own and 'Hippocratic' theory.

In the verbs and adjectives used for the expected effects of remedies we can discern a small number of major categories, mirroring the main areas of concern in wound healing, along with unspecific remarks, such as 'heals wounds',[10] etc. Three groups are particularly common, namely styptics, agglutinants and anti-inflammatory remedies. (There is, however, no overall agreement among ancient writers on the action of certain *pharmaka* and some appear in different categories depending on the author.) In the case of the first category we are again faced with the problem of technical vocabulary: whereas στυπτικόν (*styptikon*) is often used for substances which would staunch a bleeding when applied externally, it can also mean that the remedy in question checks

---

[8] See Harig (1974) for an extremely detailed discussion of the idea of intensity in Galen's pharmacology.
[9] Cf. XII.208 K.
[10] Expressions such as τραύματα ἰᾶται, τραυματικόν or ἐπὶ τῶν νεοτρώτων ἁρμόζει.

internal haemorrhage, excessive menstrual flow or - by analogy - diarrhoea. Thus with many *pharmaka* in Dioscorides, Galen or Oribasius we cannot be certain whether they were applied to bleeding wounds, or were meant for the other uses or both. ἴσχαιμον (*ischaimon*; haemostatic), αἱμορραγίαν ἵστησιν (*haimorrhagian histêsin*; stops bleeding) and other expressions of this kind present similar problems, as again, unless wounds are explicitly mentioned, the nature of the haemorrhage is not clear. The same is true for anti-inflammatories, which could be meant to heal the inflammation of a wound as well as, e.g., an inflamed spleen.

The following are some of the styptics: κηκίς (oak-gall), charred on hot coals and extinguished with vinegar or vinegar with brine;[11] ἀράχνης τὸ ὕφος (spider's web);[12] *tus* (frankincense) or *aloe* (*Aloe vera*);[13] ἀρνόγλωσσον (plantain; *Plantago major*).[14]

It may well be, of course, that the distinction was never meant to be that clear and that we are looking for a subdivision into categories which was not made in Greek medicine. It is possible that the affinity between different types of inflammation or haemorrhage was seen as stronger than the disparity between, e.g., bleeding from a wound and internal bleeding from an ulcer.

The second category of drugs, which may at times overlap with the first, contains any substance which can be said to τραύματα κολλᾶν (*traumata kollan*; or in Latin *glutinant vulnus*; agglutinate wounds) or to be κολλητικόν (*kollêtikon*; agglutinant). Examples of these are: ἄσφαλτος (asphalt, bitumen);[15] δρυὸς φύλλα (oak leaves) as a cataplasm;[16] *cummi* (gum, especially of bearsfoot; *Acanthus mollis*);[17] *ovi album* (egg-white);[18] κισσός (ivy), boiled in wine.[19] While the effect of *kollêtika* may involve some haemostatic action, the main purpose in using these drugs is the closing of the wound. Thus, opposed to the immediate action of the first group, the *kollêtika* have a slightly more delayed, more long-term effect.

As has been said in Chapter 2, presumably the most inevitable consequence of wounding was inflammation and it is therefore

---

[11] Diosc. I.107; Galen, *Simpl.*, XII.25 K
[12] Diosc. II.63.
[13] Celsus V.I/190.25.
[14] Galen, *Simpl.* XI.838 K.
[15] Diosc. I.73. It is also an anti-inflammatory.
[16] Paul IV.37.1/I.358.2.
[17] Celsus V.II/191.1.
[18] Ibid. 191.3.
[19] Galen XII.30 K.

not astonishing that this was what the third major category of *pharmaka* was aimed at. These were said to be ἀφλέγμαντα (*aphlegmanta*; anti-inflammatory), to have a δύναμις ἀφλέγμαντος (*dynamis aphlegmantos*; anti-inflammatory faculty) or described by similar expressions such as πρὸς φλεγμονὰς ἁρμόζουσι (*pros phlegmonas harmozousi*; they are suitable against inflammation). Substances of this group include: ἀναγαλλὶς (pimpernel; *Anagallis arvensis*);[20] ἰός (rust or verdigris);[21] 'Αχίλλειος (Achilles' woundwort; *Achillea tomentosa*);[22] σέλινον (celery; *Apium graveolens*) raw as a poultice.[23] The number of anti-inflammatory preparations corroborates the hypothesis that inflammation was seen not as a consequence that could be avoided altogether, but as one that should not be allowed to get out of hand, as excessive inflammation was seen as leading to sympathetic reactions or even gangrene.

Other wound complications, too, find their repercussion in the expected properties of remedies: thus we find drugs supposed to cure a 'septic' condition,[24] gangrene,[25] tetanus or *opisthotonos*.[26] We also find a type of drug for which there is no modern equivalent- the πυοποικά (*pyopoïka*; pus-makers) or καθαρτικά (*kathartika*; cleansers). As we have already seen, suppuration was considered a cleansing process, necessary and beneficial for the wound - especially in post-Hippocratic medicine - and it would therefore be natural to promote it in order to achieve the right amount and type of suppuration at the right time. Some of the drugs used for producing pus were: στέαρ ὕειον (pig fat);[27] πίσσα (pitch);[28] εἴρια (wool) boiled in water and wine;[29]

---

[20] Diosc. II.178..
[21] Diosc. V.80.
[22] Diosc. IV.36 (it is also *enaimon* and *kollêtikê*).
[23] *Aff.* 38/VI.248 L.
[24] E.g. Theophrastus, *HP* IX.XVI.5: ἀκόνιτον (wolf's-bane; *Aconitum Anthora*); Galen, *Simpl.*, XI.829 K: ἀναγαλλίς again.
[25] Galen, *Simpl.*, XI.885 K: θέρμος (lupine; *Lupinus albus*).
[26] Note again the differentiation: Dioscorides lists seven drugs for *opisthotonos* - e.g., III.128, σατύριον (man orchis; *Acera anthropophora*) drunk in astringent red wine (also in Galen, XII.118 K) - against only one for both conditions, namely (III.80.5) σίλφιον (laserwort; *Ferula tingitana*) given as a pill covered in wax.
[27] Paul IV.39/I.359.18.
[28] Ibid.; Diosc. I.72.5; Celsus V.II/191.11; Galen, *Comp. Med. Gen.* IV.4./XIII.759.
[29] *Ulc.* 12/VI.414 L.

κρόκινον ἔλαιον (saffron oil; *Crocus sativus*);[30] *tincta in melle linamenta* (dressings soaked in honey).[31]

Other types of drugs which we can find in our sources are (along with the aforementioned) those that stop wounds from suppurating (e.g. *Ulc.* 13/ VI.416 L)[32] and sarcotics, i.e. preparations which are supposed to promote the growth of sound flesh.[33] Caustic remedies also feature in the texts: they were used as a slower, safer and supposedly less painful alternative to the actual cautery, although it seems that the more powerful ones were strong enough irritants to raise blisters. Celsus distinguishes between drugs with increasing degrees of intensity, namely those which *rodunt* (gnaw),[34] *exedunt* (consume) [35] and *adurunt* (burn),[36] but several of the substances appear in more than one category.

Among the less frequently mentioned remedies Galen (*De naturalibus facultatibus* [*Nat.Fac.*] II.53 K) speaks of those which he calls ἑλκτικὰ φάρμακα (*helktika pharmaka*; 'drawing' remedies) and which are supposed to draw poison, or even arrowheads, from the flesh. Theophrastus, *H.P.* IX.XVI.1, and Pliny, *H.N.* XXVI.LXXXVII.142, both mention the plant δίκταμνον/*dictamnum* (dittany; *Origanum dictamnus*) for that purpose.

However, one cannot fail to notice the almost total absence of two categories which one would expect in the context of wound healing, namely febrifuges and analgesics. As for the former category, this is not so surprising, given that - as noted above - fever following a wound is mentioned only in passing in the medical texts. Since the raised temperature accompanying inflammation and infection of the wound was not seen as a 'fever' like, e.g., the recurrent fevers, it would not have been treated with one of the many preparations normally used to dispel fever, but it would have been allowed to take its course - avoiding wine and baths in the meantime - until eventually (in the case of a

---

[30] Diosc. I.54.
[31] Celsus V.29/225.16.
[32] στυπτηρίη (alum or ferrous sulphate).
[33] E.g. *Ulc.*15/VI.418 L: λαγώπυρος (hare's foot trefoil; *Trifolium arvense*); Celsus V.14/193.15f.; *cera* (wax); Diosc.V.85 μολύβδαινα (probably galena).
[34] E.g. *alumen liquidum* (liquid alum): V.VI/192.1; *resina* (resin): ibid./192.9.
[35] E.g. *spuma argenti* (litharge or lead monoxide): V.VII/192.13; *auripigmentum* (orpiment or trisulphide of arsenic): ibid./192.14.
[36] E.g. *chalcitis* (copper pyrites): V.VIII/192.20; *charta combusta* (burnt papyrus): ibid./192.21.

favourable outcome) it disappeared together with the infection that had caused it.

The case is more puzzling if we look at analgesics: while there are several drugs repeatedly referred to as ἀνώδυνα (*anôdyna*; pain-killers) and ὑπνοποιά (*hypnopoia*; sleeping-drugs), they are hardly ever related to the pain caused by a wound. Whenever they are mentioned in relation to any particular conditions,[37] these tend to be internal diseases such as colic, pleurisy, dysentery or painful coughs. There are four passages speaking of remedies meant to alleviate the pain of wounds, but in reality this amounts to only two independent passages: one used twice by Oribasius (*Syn.* VII.1.12/212.19-24 and *Eun.* III.14/407.20-4) and copied by Paul (IV.38/I.359.7-10), suggesting a decoction of pomegranate in wine,[38] and one in Pliny (*H.N.* XX.LXXXI), recommending a type of *porcillaca* (purslane?), called *peplis*, with oil and pearl barley. Both are external applications.

In the descriptions of war wounds in *Epid.* VII (and their parallels in *Epid.* V) the only measure taken against the pain is a purge in V.95/V.254 L (=VII.121/V.466 L), and the accounts dealing with injuries other than war wounds do not mention analgesics either. Neither do the extant Hippocratic treatises dealing with trauma, but it may be argued that the pharmacological treatment lies beyond their scope. The same argument can be used regarding the passages in the *Epidemics*, as they do not necessarily represent a full therapeutical record, but the silence on the topic of analgesics remains remarkable.

The most commonly mentioned analgesic and soporific drugs, most of them taken orally for a variety of painful conditions, are:[39] ἀγρία θρίδαξ (wild lettuce; *Lactuca scariola*), ἄνησσον (anise; *Pimpinella anisum*), στρύχνον ὑπνωτικόν or ἀλικάκκαβον (sleepy nightshade; *Withania somnifera*), ὑοσκύαμος (henbane; *Hyoscyamus niger*), μανδραγόρα (mandrake; *Mandragora officinalis*) and several types of μήκων (various kinds of poppy, in particular opium poppy, *Papaver somniferum*). Of these only mandrake is mentioned in connection with surgery, namely as an anaesthetic to be used for surgical operations, e.g. by Dioscorides, IV.75.7: "The doctors make use

---

[37] E.g. in Galen, On the Composition of Remdies according to Place (*De compositione medicamentorum secundum locos* [*Comp. Med. Loc.*]) 9/XIII.267ff. K; Paul VII.11.14/II.300.16-19 or Oribasius, *Eun.* IV.135/496.18-20.

[38] ῥοιὰν γλυκεῖαν ἐψήσας ἐν οἴνῳ καὶ τρίψας κατάπλασσε.

[39] For most of these plants identification appears to be less controversial than for some others.

of this, too, when they are about to [treat by] cut[ting] and burn[ing]".[40]

In mandrake and the other two most effective drugs (henbane and opium), however, there is a strong presence of the negative aspects of the word *pharmakon* and the medical texts abound in warnings about their dangers.[41] Poppy is mentioned as a poison, e.g. in Galen's *De Antidotis* [*Ant.*] II (XIV.138 K) and Pliny, *H.N.* XXI.CV.180, calls *halicaccabon* (which may or may not be the equivalent of the Greek homonym) "more swiftly fatal than opium".[42] Of opium he says at *H.N.* XX.LXXVI.200 that "Diagoras and Erasistratus condemned it altogether as being lethal".[43] Although this cannot be taken as a historical statement - Pliny admittedly not being one of our most reliable sources - these passages show a general consent regarding the dangers of the strong narcotic drugs.

Celsus (V.25.1/212.10-13) also warns against the use of analgesics because of the powerful drugs they contain and because of their effect on the stomach:

> They call those [drugs] anodynes which relieve pain by sleep. It is unsuitable to make use of them, unless the utmost necessity press [us to do so], for they consist of drugs which are violent as well as hurtful to the stomach.[44]

Different authors also agree, even if their medical theories differ, that the potential danger of these substances lies in their excessive cooling effect. This conviction is not based on sensory perception, but what makes them cooling is the ensuing loss of consciousness and eventually - if the dose is too large - of life. As one would expect, the idea of a measurable degree of coolness is developed in particular by Galen as part of his quantitative system of drug properties.[45]

While the diffidence regarding analgesics displayed by some authors may have been a deliberate show of conscientiousness in

---

[40] Χρῶνται δὲ καὶ ταύτῃ οἱ ἰατροί, ὅταν τέμνειν ἢ καίειν μέλλωσι. Cf. also id. IV.75.5, Pliny, *H.N.* XXXV.94 and, according to Ellis (1946), later authors such as Pseudo-Apuleius, Lucius Apuleus Barbarus and Isidore of Seville.

[41] E.g. Dioscorides IV.64.3, Celsus V.25.1/212.10-13 (see below); Oribasius, *Coll. Med.* XV.12.19f./II.264.31f.; Pliny, *H.N.* XX.LXXVI.

[42] *opio velocius ad mortem.*

[43] *Diagoras et Erasistratus in totum damnavere ut mortiferum.*

[44] *Anodyna vocant, quae somno dolorem levant; quibus uti, nisi nimia necesitas urget, alienum est: sunt enim e vehementibus medicamentis et stomacho alienis.*

[45] Oribasius (*Coll. Med.* XIV.22/II.199.13) takes up the idea when he lists opium as the only drug that "cools to the fourth degree": τῆς δὲ τετάρτης τάξεως ψύχει.

some cases, their scruples were certainly justified and based on therapeutical experience with the drugs in question, the main problem being their safe dosage. (Their active substances, e.g. scopolamine or hyoscyamine, are potentially lethal poisons.[46]) Given fluctuations in the purity of the drugs and a variety of other factors (environmental, chemical, etc.) influencing the grade of toxicity, as well as the absence of means of accurate measurement, it was certainly easier, to put it simply, to use them as poisons than to make safe use of them in therapy. As Galen phrases it in *Glauc.* II (XI.114 K), however, in certain cases a well-calculated risk was worthwile:

> If the pain continues in these cases, [you must] venture to use the remedies made from opium such as that of Philo of Tarsus, known to all doctors, [whilst being] aware that by necessity there will be some damage to the affected parts from that kind of remedies, but by counteracting the urgent symptom, you will choose to save, with some small harm, the person fainting from the intensity of the pain.[47]

Although there are no similar passages concerning the treatment of wounds, one can assume that the decision on the amount and type of analgesic used was left to the individual doctor.

Although analgesics for internal use are not mentioned in connection with wounds, it can hardly have been the case that surgeons were not aware of the need for them - witness the remark in *Prorrh.* (II.12/IX.34 L) that in some cases "the wound hurt[s] so much that they cannot breathe".[48] There would have been two main scenarios for the use of pain-killing drugs in relation to war wounds: on the one hand the case of strong pain from a wound, either after surgical treatment or when there was no need for surgery, and, on the other hand, the case of a wound necessitating, e.g., the removal of an arrow. It is obvious that the amount of drugs needed in the first case is much lower than in the second (i.e. the difference between an analgesic and an anaesthetic) and therefore the danger of inadvertently giving a lethal dose is less acute. One could thus cautiously deduce from these facts that in the first case the doctor was more likely to administer an analgesic. We have no written evidence for how the situation

---

[46] Cf. Lewis/Elvin-Lewis (1977), pp. 54f.

[47] εἰ δ' ἐπὶ τούτοις ἐπιμένοιεν αἱ ὀδύναι, τολμήσεις χρήσασθαι τοῖς δι' ὀπίου φαρμάκοις, ὁποῖόν ἐστι καὶ τὸ τοῦ Ταρσέως Φίλωνος ἅπασι τοῖς ἰατροῖς γινωσκόμενον, εἰδὼς μὲν ἐξ ἀνάγκης τινὰ βλάβην τοῖς πεπονθόσι μορίοις ἐκ τῶν τοιύτων φαρμάκων ἐσομένην, ἀλλὰ πρὸς τὸ κατεπεῖγον ἐνιστάμενος αἱρήσῃ μετὰ μικρᾶς βλάβης σῶσαι τὸν ἄνθρωπον ὑπὸ τοῦ τῆς ὀδύνης μεγέθους συγκοπτόμενον.

[48] οὕτως ὠδύνησεν ἡ πληγὴ ὥστε μὴ δύνασθαι ἀναπνεῦσθαι.

would have been handled in the case of an obviously fatal wound. Having pronounced an unfavourable prognosis (and thus safe from blame), would not at least some doctors risk speeding a death for which they would not be blamed, to avoid unnecessary suffering? There is no definitive answer to this question, but it may well be that strong drugs were used more readily in such cases.

From a purely practical point of view it seems highly improbable that every casualty was given strong anodynes in a war-time situation, with an army on the march in particular (such as the army of Alexander the Great, for example), as this would have necessitated large quantities of potentially lethal drugs to be held by the army's doctors. (We do not know how the logistics of medical supplies worked, but in particular on a long and far-flung expedition like Alexander's, doctors will have had to acquire drugs locally.)

It may seem surprising at first sight that wine is never mentioned in the context of wound treatment for its analgesic and soporific qualities, although these were well known. Pure wine would certainly have had those qualities - although not to the point of making it an anaesthetic - for men used to drinking it diluted. It would also have been easily available most of the time, even to an army on campaign. However, when one looks at the diet generally considered good for the wounded - scarce food, if any, and water to drink - it appears that wine was seen as counter-indicated.[49] The drinking of wine to alleviate the pain of a wound would therefore not have been recommended by the surgeons, but rather, as Majno[50] puts it, "they left tipsiness to private initiative".

As for Dioscorides' extravagant claims concerning anaesthetics,[51] the silence of other writers on this topic makes one wonder how widespread the practice was. There is no doubt that mandrake, taken in large quantities, could produce a sufficient degree of unconsciousness, but the unconsciousness had to be reversible and here the dosage was even more problematic than in administering analgesics, involving not only the correct quantity of the drug, but also the patient's tolerance. Referring to sleep-inducing drugs, Celsus (III.18 15/125.15-17) advocates moderation. "lest we are afterwards unable to rouse the man whom

---

[49] E.g. Celsus V.26.30B/225.29-31.
[50] (1975), p. 295.
[51] He is more cautious when speaking of the 'Memphis stone' (λίθος Μεμφίτης) and its use as a local anaesthetic (V.140), quoting it only as something that "people tell" (ἱστορεῖται).

we want to put to sleep".[52] In one passage regarding mandrake (*Loc. Hom.* 39/VI.328 L), the author speaks of the correct dosage and appears to be rather optimistic on his ability to measure the correct amount, although this may be a mere show of self-confidence not based on fact. One is to give root of mandrake to drink, he says, "less than the quantity which would lead to frenzy".[53] .

However, nowhere in the treatises dealing with surgery is there any mention of anaesthesia and there is even stronger evidence than an *argumentum ex silentio* in the instructions given by several authors on how to have one's patient bound or held by one's assistants (e.g. *Off.* 6/III.288 L; *On Haemorrhoids* (*De Haemorrhoidibus* [*Haem.*]) 2/VI.438 L; Aetius, XV, p.19 Z).This evidence is corroborated by the two Galen passages about patients who are frightened or move under the knife, quoted in 2.2.2., not to speak of Celsus' famous description of the ideal surgeon.[54] As for non-medical literature (where anaesthetics are never mentioned), stories like those describing the courage and endurance of Alexander or Marius[55] would become pointless if there was no pain associated with wounds or surgical treatment.

It has to be stressed again, though, that all we have are small surviving fragments of ancient literature - medical or otherwise - and that even if we had all the written sources that ever existed, it is still doubtful whether that would enable us to reconstruct everyday practice from them. Consequently, we are in no position to give definitive answers to all the questions concerning ancient medical practice and we can only make judgements on a hypothetical situation as we see it in our sources. For the problem of anaesthesia this means that all we can say is the following: it looks as if the use of mandrake as an anaesthetic had been regarded as an interesting possibility in theory, worth mentioning, but had not been applied much, if at all, in practice. Considering the importance of success and reputation for the ancient doctor and

---

[52] *..ne, quem obdormire uolumus, excitare postea non possimus.*
[53] ἔλασσον ἢ ὡς μαίνεσθαι.
[54] VII.prooem. 4/302.2-5: along with other characteristics, the surgeon also needs to be "compassionate to the extent that he wants to heal the person whom he has taken on [as a patient], but not [to the extent] that, moved by the latter's cries, he either hurries more than is required or cuts less than necessary, but he must do everything just as if no sympathy were aroused in him by the other's screams" (*misericors sic, ut sanari velit eum , quem accepit, non ut clamore eius motus vel magis quam res desiderat properet, vel minus quam necesse est secet; sed perinde faciat omnia, ac si nullus ex vagitibus alterius adfectus oriatur*).
[55] These will be discussed in Part II.

the resulting reluctance to take risks,[55] it seems very questionable whether many doctors would have taken chances with an unpredictable drug.

There is also another point to be considered: research into pain perception[57] has shown that there are considerable differences in the way pain is perceived between cultures as well as, within one and the same culture, in different situation. Thus Beecher[58] discovered during World War II (in a case study particularly relevant for this topic) that wounded soldiers with otherwise normal levels of pain tolerance perceived far less need for pain relief than patients with comparable wounds after general surgery in peace-time. On the one hand, given the choice, a wounded soldier may well have preferred bearing the pain of, say, the extraction of an arrow to risking his life for the sake of painlessness. On the other, a battle wound would be perceived as honourable and an emblem of manliness, and a feeling of pride (as well as relief at still being alive) may well have modified the psychological and emotional impact of the pain. (I also believe that it is practically impossible for us to know what it was like to be wounded or submit to surgery in a world in which anaesthesia or reliable and safe analgesics had never existed and would therefore not be expected.)

When it comes to the question which plants and other substances were actually used for medication, we are faced with the almost insurmountable problem of identification - of plants in particular - and more often than not the translation of a name is highly arbitrary. It has to be added that plant names were by no means universally agreed upon in antiquity as we can see, for example, from the synonyms Dioscorides often provides for the name of a plant. Furthermore, even when a Roman author, e.g. Celsus, quotes the Greek name, this is no guarantee that he is actually talking about the same plant as the one to which Greek authors would refer by that name. This fluctuation in terminology is but one of the many variables which make it almost impossible to determine the efficacy of ancient drugs.

Other factors (apart from errors in MSS) are our lack of knowledge about harvesting and preparation methods, chemical variations within plant species or between individual plants,

---

[56] The modes of treatment that appear risky to us, such as the administration of hellebore, succussion or phlebotomy, may have been perceived as safe by a Greek or Roman doctor.

[57] See especially Melzack (1961) and (1973), pp. 22 and 29f.; Beecher (1959) and Morris (1991), in particular pp. 38-56.

[58] (1959), pp.164f.

varying degrees of purity of a drug, variations in the method of administration and individual patient variable factors affecting drug metabolism.[59]

There is, however, a standard set of 'solvents' (to use a modern term) common to all authors, on which the remedies were based or in which they were diluted, the most important ones being vinegar, wine, oil and honey. These substances on their own would have had some therapeutical effect on a wound,[60] especially vinegar being both haemostatic and what we would call antiseptic in its action, and thus even combined with pharmacologically useless plants they would have influenced wound healing positively.

It is not my intention to investigate whether remedies 'worked' or not in comparison with modern drugs, and this would be a questionable approach to historical research, but the problem of efficacy is an interesting one where it pertains to the question why certain substances were used if they could be proved to be ineffective. This question cannot be treated in depth here, but in some cases substances appear to have been chosen by analogy. This may be the case with the sap of fig leaves,[61] which makes milk curdle but does not make blood coagulate. In other instances symbolic associations may well be at work, e.g. the use of blood[62] or other reddish substances (rust, cinnabar, haematite, etc).[63]

In post-Hellenistic authors compound remedies become increasingly frequent[64] and so do mineral substances in relation to plants. Whereas it seems that writers extolling the virtues of past simplicity[65] exaggerate them in their nostalgia for some imaginary good old times, the development of compound medicines and mineral remedies may be influenced by the increase of a wealthy urban population and hence the necessity of keeping drugs in store rather than gathering fresh plants as the need arose. The

---

[59] For a more detailed discussion, see Riddle (1985), p. xxiv.
[60] See Majno (1975), pp. 186ff., for chemical analyses.
[61] *Ulc.* 11/VI.410 L; Theophr., *HP* IX.VIII.2.
[62] E.g. the blood of turtle-doves used to treat head wounds: Galen, *Simpl.* X/XII.256; Dioscorides I.160.
[63] Diosc. V.80 : rust (ἰός); id. V.96.: red ochre (μίλτος Σινωπική); id. V.94: cinnabar (κιννάβαρι).
[64] Riddle (1985), p. 175, suggests that this was the result of Galen's method, but the trend appears to have set in before Galen: cf., for example, the compound remedy quoted by Galen in *Comp. Med. Loc.* (XIII.267ff. K). See Calame (1984), the recipe of a compound wound remedy on a first-century AD papyrus.
[65] E.g. Seneca, *Epist. Mor.* XCV.15: "Medicine was once the knowledge of a few herbs by which bleeding was stopped and wounds closed; then little by little it came to such manyfold variety." (*Medicina paucarum quondam fuit scientia herbarum, quibus sisteretur sanguis, vulnera coirent; paulatim deinde in hanc pervenit tam multiplicem varietatem.*)

higher prestige of complex and exotic drugs and costly mineral substances must not be underestimated either, since our sources contain mainly information on those rich enough to pay for doctors and drugs. The prescription and administration of exotic drugs would not only have enabled the doctor to impress his patients but also to charge more for his remedies.

When faced with a multiplicity of *pharmaka* and complicated prescriptions one has to keep in mind that the extant sources are presenting an ideal situation, that of the sedentary city physician, and that on campaign or after a battle many remedies would probably not have been available. As was the case with surgical instruments, here too, the army surgeon would have had to make do with what was at hand. This fact was obvious to the authors themselves and some of them speak of means of improvisation. Thus, after a list of anti-inflammatory poultices, the author of *Aff.* (38/VI.248 L) advises: "If you have none of these nor any other poultices, mix flour with water or wine and plaster it on."[66] Similarly, Paul repeatedly suggests alternatives to remedies, e.g. at III.22.5/I.174 and III.22.24/I.181.

There is one last point to be made: unlike surgery, pharmacological treatment is hardly ever mentioned in purely literary descriptions of wound treatment and when it is described, this is done in very vague and generic terms, such as *pharmaka*, φύλλα (leaves), ῥίζα (roots), *herba* or *medicamenta*. The only exceptions to this rule are the *dictamnum* in Virgil (*Aen.* XII.412) and Nonnos' *Dionysiaca*: κενταυρίς (the plant *kentauris*, perhaps centaury; *Centaurea salonitana*: XVII.359), myrtle (XXIX.270), ivy (XXIX.155), honey (XVII.371), chalk (XXIX.274), and wine (in all quoted passages). This scarcity of information might be caused less by the authors' lack of knowledge regarding pharmacology than by a lack of interest on the part of the readers. As we shall see in Part II, descriptions of wounds and their surgical treatment held certain functions in literature and the treatment using *pharmaka* may not have fulfilled the same criteria.

---

[66] ἢν δὲ μηδὲν τούτων ἔχῃς μήτε ἄλλο τι μηδὲν κατάπλασμα, ἄλφιτον φυρήσας ὕδατι ἢ οἴνῳ κατάπλασαι.

CHAPTER FOUR

MEDICAL SERVICES IN ARMIES

1. *Greece*

Discussions of medical services in ancient armies usually focus on Imperial Rome, with only a small number of articles concerning the Greek world.[1] This is not surprising, given that we have almost no detailed information on the extent to which medical treatment was available in a Greek army in any given period. It seems quite unlikely that there was ever an organised army medical service as part of the various military systems. However, throughout Greek literature historians, poets and other authors mention *iatroi* treating the wounded. Their presence is never explained as an extraordinary occurrence would be, so one can assume that these authors did not expect their readers to be surprised by this fact. Thus one can say that for most Greeks the presence of doctors in an army would have been an expected thing.

Among the general silence on these topics one sentence in Xenophon (*Anab*. III.IV.30f.) stands out all the more. It could shed some light on these problems, although it is debatable whether the implications of his account are valid beyond the specific situation in question. On their retreat the Greek troops reached some villages in the hills west of the Tigris "and appointed eight doctors, because the wounded were numerous".[2] Xenophon does not explain whether these *iatroi* were appointed from among the Greeks - which would imply that either some doctors had joined the army as mercenaries or that some of the soldiers had sufficient medical knowledge to be called ἰατροί - or from among the villagers. In the latter case this would mean that local healers, working with a medical system totally different from the Greeks', were accepted as doctors. As Xenophon specifically mentions the large number of casualties as the reason for appointing doctors, it is likely that their job was limited to the treatment of wounds. Therefore the criteria for deciding who had enough knowledge and experience to be called an *iatros* may have differed from the ones generally in use. Even keeping in mind that

---

[1] Mollière (1888); a part of Sudhoff (1929); Jacob (1932). For a detailed discussion, see Salazar (1998a).
[2] ... καὶ ἰατροὺς κατέστησαν ὀκτώ· πολλοὶ γὰρ ἦσαν οἱ τετρωμένοι.

the situation represented here is the very specific one of a defeated army in retreat through enemy terrritory, this may still be true for a war-time situation in general, when the minimum requirement for being considered a physician would have been lower than in time of peace.

The choice of the word 'appointed' (κατέστησαν) suggests that the appointment of the eight doctors was a decision taken by the commanders and that therefore the eight men would have been paid by them - if they were paid at all. Provisions and horses appear to have been taken by the Greeks without payment, so we need not necessarily expect them to pay for services either.

The situation would obviously be different with an army fighting on their own territory or in the vicinity of an allied city, or again in the case of a town under siege. In these cases one could expect a certain number of trained doctors to be at hand and the treatment of casualties would presumably be a task for the town-physician.[3] Two (possibly three) inscriptions support this hypothesis. One is the text of a letter to the Coans from the city of Gortyne in Crete, praising their town-physician Hermias - sent from Cos[4] upon their request - for having saved many of those wounded in a civil war (221-219 BC).[5] The second,[6] dated variously between 449 and 386 BC, is from Cyprus and expresses the city's gratitude towards a medical family - Onasilos and his brothers - for the treatment of battle casualties. It is possible that two fragments (*IG* II2 304 + 604) apparently belonging to one and the same Attic inscription of 337/6 BC were also part of a similar public statement of gratitude. Although the names of the honorands and the reasons are missing, C. J. Schwenk[7] suggests that, given the date and the connection with the temple of Asclepius, the inscription could be a decree honouring two physicians for treating the Athenian wounded after the battle of Chaeronea in 338 BC. It is tempting to accept this conjecture, but unless further fragments are found, the evidence is insufficient.

As far as most mentions of *iatroi* in non-medical sources are concerned, one of the obvious problems is that these sources are usually concerned almost exclusively with kings and generals and we hardly ever hear about the fate of the common soldier. Thus we often

---

[3] This is Jacob's (1932) opinion.
[4] Epigraphical evidence suggests that Cos managed to establish itself as a valued source of physicians for the rest of the Greek world.
[5] *I. Cret*. IV.168; published in Herzog (1903), p. 11. The same man is also honoured in *I. Cret*. I.8.7.
[6] Solmsen (19304), p. 11, and Jacob (1932).
[7] (1985), pp. 68-71. I am obliged to Dr Reinhard Selinger, Vienna, for this reference.

read about 'the doctors' examining and treating the commander's wounds as soon as he is carried back from the battle-line,[8] but the sources do not mention ordinary soldiers in the same situation. From the accounts we have we can judge what was considered the normal situation for the leader of an army, and one might also suggest that being attended by several doctors was something of a status symbol. For the ordinary soldier, i.e. the majority of those in need of treatment, the situation would be quite different. Some comments by medical authors, mentioned in Chapter 2,[9] appear to indicate that in most cases considerable time passed between the wounding and the treatment, a fact which will have led to chances of survival varying according to a man's rank.

Where Greek armies are concerned, we also have to admit that we cannot be certain where casualties were treated - again, except for the commanders. It appears that the latter were taken back to their own tents and that their wounds were treated there, but we do not know what happened to those who did not have tents of their own. Occasionally our sources speak of the king or general visiting the wounded,[10] but these statements are never accompanied by more detailed information. Presumably it meant that the commander went from tent to tent, but even this would only prove that the wounded were taken back to the tents where they usually slept after treatment. It seems unlikely that the surgeons actually went out on the battlefield, either during or after the battle - hence the references to wounded men being carried back - but it is not clear whether the wounded were all taken to one place in the army camp or whether the doctors moved about. From the point of view of practicality the former would seem far more plausible, as in the latter case not only the doctors would have to move about constantly, but their assistants would have to follow them about as well, carrying their instruments, bandages and remedies. Having one particular place, e.g. one tent, reserved for medical treatment would also enable the doctors to set up their place of work in a way convenient for themselves - for example benches and chairs of the right height.[11] This, however, is only conjecture for which there is no evidence, and a Greek doctor's idea of practicality may have been different from our own.

---

[8] For some examples, see Arrian, *An*. VI.11.1 (Alexander) and D. S. XV.87.5 (Epaminondas).

[9] E.g. Paul VI.88.4/II.132.7-9 (about not stitching inflamed wounds) and ibid. II.132.11-13 (about the discolouring caused by arrow poison).

[10] E.g. Xen., *Cyrop*. V.IV.17f.; Arrian, *An*. II.12.1.

[11] The operating table appears to be a more recent idea; ancient authors usually write of making patients sit or lie on chairs and benches. At V.26.25A/223.8 Celsus remarks that the patient is to be put to bed after treatment, so he was obviously not treated in his bed.

Xenophon, who obviously had a keen interest in questions concerning the organisation of an army, also provides us with the only other piece of fairly concrete information. In the *Constitution of the Lacedaemonians* (XIII.7) he speaks of the Spartan army on the march, with its "soothsayers, doctors and flute-players and those commanding the army"[12] following after the first three *morai*, including the one led by the king. This would suggest that it was current practice for the Spartan army to take several surgeons[13] along with them in times of war. Xenophon does not specify who those doctors were, but if it is true that Spartans were not allowed to learn a trade,[14] it is unlikely that it was possible for them to train as doctors. If it was not, their doctors must have been helots or foreigners.

The casualties listed in *Epid*.V and VII[15] are further evidence for medical treatment given to wounded soldiers, but they furnish no details as to where this was done. In these cases the doctors may have been based in a nearby town, but we do not know by which side the author was employed. (It may not have been choice or formal employment so much as a question of where he happened to be at the outbreak of hostilities.) For V.95/V.254 L (=VII.121/V.466 L) - the case of Tychon being wounded at the siege of Daton - there are two possibilities. The surgeon who treated the wound could have been in the Macedonian army camp or in the besieged town, as Tychon appears to have been treated on the day he was wounded and there were no other large towns in the vicinity. Where an army used a town as its base, the doctors would presumably be stationed in that town. This is the situation reflected in Procopius (*Goth*. VI.II.25): "When they all arrived in the town [i.e. after nightfall], they looked after their wounds."[16]

Even from our scarce material it appears legitimate to deduce that in most Greek armies at war more than one or two doctors were available for the treatment of those wounded in battle (and presumably also of the sick). It is highly probable that when there was a camp they worked there, presumably in a fixed place - to enable the casualties to find them. The latter were carried back from

---

[12] μάντεις καὶ ἰατροὶ καὶ αὐληταὶ καὶ οἱ τοῦ στρατοῦ ἄρχοντες.

[13] In the same passage Xenophon uses the dual (δυοῖν μόραιν), so the plural form ἰατροί suggests three or more doctors.

[14] Plu., *Ages*. XXVI.5.

[15] V.21/V.220 L, 46,47/V.234 L, 49/V.236 L; VII.29,30, 31, 32, 33, 34/V.400f. L and 121/V.466 L. Some of these are the only cases in the *Epidemics*, and indeed the only passages in the Hippocratic Corpus, that can be dated with some confidence: they belong to the years around 356 BC when Philip of Macedon attacked Thrace in the course of his expansion to the east.

[16] ἐπεὶ δὲ ἅπαντες ἐν τῇ πόλει ἐγένοντο, τῶν τραυμάτων ἐπεμελοῦντο. (A few lines further down in the same passage 'doctors' in the plural are mentioned.)

the battlefield by their comrades, slaves, or, if they were officers, by their men - either on the other men's arms or on their own shields (as it was done with the dead).

It is again Xenophon (*An.* III.IV.32) who points out the problems which arise from having to evacuate casualties. The Greeks encamp in a village, "because there were many who were *hors de combat*, the wounded, and those carrying them, and those who had taken over the weapons of those carrying [the wounded]".[17] Thus even a moderate number of casualties could deplete the ranks very quickly.

It is not clear whether the *iatroi* treating the commanders were the same as those treating the soldiers, but it is probable that they often were. It appears, though, that even when this was the case, they were more readily available for the generals and officers than for the mass of the soldiers. It is beyond doubt that kings such as Alexander had their own personal physicians,[18] who upon their command might treat the king's friends, but would not be available for the common soldier. In general, various authors describe how commanders are carried back to the camp, where they are examined and treated by anonymous surgeons (usually in the plural). The death of Epaminondas provides one of the examples (D. S. XV.87.5): "Epaminondas was carried, still living, to the encampment, and when the doctors who had been summoned declared ...".[19]

An army doctor who is at the general's command is mentioned in Achilles Tatius' novel *Cleitophon and Leucippe* (IV.10: "... to summon the doctor of the army.."[20]). Although the novel does not claim to be anything but fiction, one can expect some reflection of everyday life in the author's time in it. Thus the fact that there is a doctor in the camp is not presented as something out of the ordinary which would capture the audience's attention, but is only mentioned in a matter-of-fact way, as something that is taken for granted would be. One can therefore assume that, at least by the second century AD it was not unusual to provide the services of a doctor for an army. (Since the text has "of the army" [τοῦ στρατοπέδου], he is obviously not meant to be the general's personal physician.) The

---

[17] πολλοὶ γὰρ ἦσαν οἱ ἀπόμαχοι, (οἵ τε) τετρωμένοι καὶ οἱ ἐκείνους φέροντες καὶ οἱ τῶν φερόντων τὰ ὅπλα δεξάμενοι.

[18] In a few cases they are mentioned by name, such as Alexander's doctors Philippos (Curtius III.V.16-VI.16 and IV.VI.17) and Kritodemos (Arr., *An*. VI.11.1; he is called Critobulus in Curtius IX.V.25).

[19] 'Επαμεινώνδας δ' ἔτι ζῶν εἰς τὴν παρεμβολὴν ἀπηνέχθη, καὶ τῶν συγκληθέντων ἰατρῶν ἀποφηναμένων ... The 'called together' need not be taken to mean that the doctors had to be gathered from throughout the camp, merely that they were assembled by Epaminondas' side.

[20] ... τὸν τοῦ στρατοπέδου ἰατρὸν μετακαλέσασθαι.

Antigonos mentioned by Galen (XII.557) as "practising successfully in the army"[21] may have been in a similar position.

In mercenary armies the presence of a doctor or several doctors may have been expected. Thus in the discussion of siege engines and of measures to be taken by those about to sustain a siege, the fifth book of the *Mechanical Syntax* by Philo of Byzantium contains two passages regarding medical treatment for the mercenaries employed by the city. At V.94.12-24[22] he says that the wounded merceraries must be provided with whatever they need and that those who have nobody to care for them should be billeted on citizens.

The first passage seems to be concerned mainly with the nursing of the wounded, but at V.96.15-19 (VII.96.72 Diels--Schramm) Philo is more specific as to who will actually perform the treatment: "There need to be very accomplished doctors in the town," he says, "who are experienced in the treatment of wounds and in the extraction of arrows, possessing the necessary drugs and instruments; and the city must provide cerate, honey, dressings and bandages."[23] Philo is quite obviously speaking of experts in 'army surgery' (rather than just any doctor), who would come with their own specialist equipment - instruments and *pharmaka* - whereas the basic dressings would be provided by the city. These measures must not be mistaken for humanitarianism, and at ib. 21-26 Philo leaves no doubt about the motives: the idea is to make the soldiers fit for the next battle as soon as possible and also to make them fight more bravely out of gratitude for the good treatment bestowed on them.

While a city or army may have wanted to hire an experienced surgeon, we can find the doctor's idea of a similar situation reflected in the suggestion made by the author of the Hippocratic *Medic*. From his point of view war is a good occasion to hone one's surgical skills (14/IX.220 L): "He who wants to practise surgery must join the military and follow mercenary armies; for thus he will be[come] experienced for this necessity."[24] Although there may be a clash of interests between doctors on the one hand and prospective employers or patients on the other, both passages suggest that medical treatment

---

[21] ἐν στρατοπέδῳ ἐπισήμως ἰατρεύσαντος.

[22] In Schoene's 1893 edition. According to H. Diels and E. Schramm (1970), the passage is VII.94.45 in the book *Paraskeuastika*.

[23] Δεῖ δὲ καὶ ἰατροὺς χαριεστάτους ἔνδον εἶναι ἐμπείρους τραυμάτων καὶ βελῶν ἐξαιρέσεως ἔχοντας φάρμακα καὶ ὄργανα τὰ προσήκοντα, καὶ τὴν πόλιν χορεγεῖν κηρωτὴν καὶ μέλι καὶ ἐπιδέσμους καὶ σπληνία. (I am following Haase's and Miller's emendation of the meaningless ἐξαιρέ-ως to ἐξαιρέσεως.)

[24] τὸν μὲν οὖν μέλλοντα χειρουργεῖν στρατεύεσθαι δεῖ καὶ παρηκολουθηκέναι στρατεύμασι ξενικοῖς· οὕτω γὰρ ἂν εἴη γεγυμνασμένος πρὸς ταύτην τὴν χρείαν.

was provided at least for mercenary armies from Hellenistic times onwards.[25]

One can assume that quite often the soldiers would turn to each other for help (as the warriors of the *Iliad* do) - hence Rufus' warning (*Qu. Med.* 55) that the soldiers had to be enjoined to leave the arrow in the wound until they found a surgeon to remove it, so that it would be done properly. However, this passage only shows that it would often be a wounded man's first reaction to attempt to rid himself of the missile, either by drawing it out himself or by asking a friend to do so,[26] but it gives us no further evidence on whether or not doctors were present or whether their number was sufficient. It can be used - cautiously - to corroborate the hypothesis, suggested by other texts, that there were no doctors present on the battlefield, but that the casualties had to be taken back to where the doctors were, which was presumably the camp.

The sources leave many questions unanswered. How many doctors would the Athenian or the Spartan army have - in the Persian Wars, for example - and how many were there in a large army such as Alexander's? Who paid them, and was there a standard pay, one varying according to the work-load, or a share in the booty? Would an army on the march bring all their doctors from their home town or country or would they appoint local doctors - or healers? For example, did Alexander's army eventually have Persian and Indian surgeons?[27] We can assume that army surgeons brought their own instruments along, but did they have to supply their own drugs as well (as Philo recommends)? Who provided the bandages? The extant material contains no answers to these questions.

2. *Rome*

The situation for Rome differs strongly from the one we have seen for Greece. There is far more evidence - literary, epigraphical and archaeological - for the existence of something that we would call a medical service in the Roman army, but, perhaps as a natural consequence of the amount of material, there is far more controversy

---

[25] *Iatroi* are mentioned, without further explanations, as being among the non-combatants by two writers on tactics, Asclepiodotus (I.1) and Aelianus (II.2), as well as by Onasander (I.13-15).
[26] Cf. Ammianus Marcellinus XVIII.8.11: the passage will be discussed in Ch. 5.
[27] On the subject of possible interaction between Greek and Persian or Indian medicine, see Adamson (1968).

over its significance.[28] Furthermore, the difference between the situation in the Republic and that under the Empire appears to be greater than differences between Greek armies of various regions and periods. As one can observe major changes in the status and practice of medicine in general on the one hand, and in the organisation of the army on the other, it seems only logical that the attitude towards the availability of medical treatment in the army should also be subject to changes.

We have no evidence for an organised medical service in the armies of Republican times, but for this period the material is too scanty and undefined to draw any definite conclusions. Hence it is not possible to exclude the possibility of some kind of medical personnel at that stage. One also has to keep in mind that our literary sources describing earlier Roman history (Livy, Dionysius of Halicarnassus, Tacitus) are not contemporary with it and thus what we have is at best a second-hand view.

Speaking of the war against the Etruscans in 480 BC, Livy (II.47.12) describes how the wounded were billeted on patrician families.[29] This in itself does not prove the absence of other medical treatment, as one would assume that the families were only expected to nurse the wounded and not, e.g., to extract arrows or set broken bones.[30] Even if the soldiers needed surgical treatment of any kind, the quoted passage does not imply that this had to be done by the *patres*. It may well mean that the latter would take on the responsibility and expense of calling in somebody who was an 'expert' in treating war wounds. Although we have no evidence for what one could call professional doctors in the early Republic and although historians - Roman as well as modern - stress the importance of a 'family medicine' in the style of the Elder Cato, it is highly improbable that specialised techniques, such as surgical treatment of wounds or the setting of fractures and dislocations, were left to the ordinary *paterfamilias*. Common sense would make one expect the existence of some type of local healer specialised in these

---

[28] The following articles and monographs contain (sometimes conflicting) information about different aspects of medicine in the Roman army: Brau (1866) and (1874); Callies (1968); Casarini (1929); Davies (1969), (1970) and (1972); Frölich (1880); Haberling (1909); Harig (1971); Jacob (1933); Jetter (1966), vol. I; Mollière (1888); Nutton (1968) and (1969); Penn (1964); Rossi (1966) and (1969); Scarborough (1968); Schultze (1934); Simpson (1872); Sudhoff (1929) and in particular Wilmanns (1995).

[29] *saucios milites curandos dividit patribus*.

[30] Livy does not mention treatment, but it can be argued that for him this was not an interesting aspect of the story. He goes on to say that the family that particularly excelled in their care for the wounded were the Fabii, and it may be relevant that they were the ancestors of the tribe in which the citizens of his home town Patavium were enrolled when it became a Roman municipality.

skills - similar to, e.g., the Marsi and Psylli, considered experts for snake-bite, or the Scythian healers following Mithridates (Appian XIII.88). One can find similar examples of specialists outside the established systems in later centuries, such as the itinerant lithotomists of mediaeval and Renaissance Italy, the *rebouteurs* of the Vosges region in eighteenth-century France or the Japanese bone-setters, who still co-exist with Western medicine - not to mention the various branches of alternative medicine in present-day Europe.

Another account of wounded soldiers - the Etruscans in this case - being looked after by private Roman citizens can be found in Dionysius of Halicarnassus (V.36.3). He writes that the Romans received them "with nourishment and care",[31] but again there is no explicit mention of medical treatment, let alone surgery. Doctors are mentioned by Tacitus (*Ann.* IV.63), who admittedly describes an event as late as 27 AD, but compares it to the earlier days of Rome. This time it is not a battle, but the collapse of the theatre of Fidena near Rome, which causes a large number of casualties:

> ... the houses of the leading citizens stood open under the influence of the recent misfortune; medication and doctors were offered repeatedly, and in these days the city - although with a sad aspect - resembled the state of the ancients, who, after large battles, supported the wounded by their liberality and care.[32]

Certainly in Tacitus' days it was normal to call in a doctor (or perhaps to have a slave who was one), so we cannot draw any conclusions on earlier Roman history from his statement, except that in his times that was what people believed would have happened in the Republic. This may form part of a nostalgic concept of medical treatment in the past, as we have seen in Seneca's remark (*Epist. Mor.* XCV.15, quoted in Ch. 3) on the small number of drugs used in earlier times.

It appears very plausible that in the times when wars were limited to a small part of the Italian peninsula it was possible to either take the wounded back to Rome or leave them in other towns or villages. We have seen the same situation in Greece when the army was near their own or an allied town. It was only with the growth of the empire - and of the army - that a more elaborate system of medical assistance became necessary.

The development of an army medical service also has to be seen in connection with the situation of medical practitioners in Rome in

---

[31] τροφαῖς τε καὶ θεραπείαις.
[32] ... *sub recentem cladem patuere procerum domus, fomenta et medici passim praebiti, fuitque Urbs per illos dies, quamquam maesta facie, veterum institutis similis, qui magna post proelia saucios largitione et cura sustentabant.*

general and the great turning-point for this may have been the years around Aemilius Paulus' victory at Pydna, in 168 BC, and 146 BC, when Greece became a Roman province. With these events Greek goods and slaves, as well as all aspects of Greek culture became available to the Roman upper classes - and soon acquired a position as fashion and status symbols. While there is not much one can say about Roman medicine before this period, given the scantiness of information, any later material clearly shows Greek influence - or rather, it is Greek medicine that is described. However, there is one earlier date, 219 BC for the first Greek doctor in Rome - Archagathus, supposedly a 'wound specialist' (*vulnerarius*), although a similar specialisation cannot be found in contemporary Greek sources. It is difficult to decide how much, if any, of the information furnished by Pliny (*H.N.* XXIX.VI) is historical, as the continuation of the story - that Archagathus soon came to be feared by the Romans because of his cruel methods of treatment: "... soon, because of his cruelty in cutting and burning, his name was changed into 'tormenter'"[33] - may well be no more than xenophobic slander. If it is indeed true that the Romans were taken aback by the Greek methods, the proverbial "cutting and burning", this might suggest that surgery had not been practised in Rome before that time,[34] although it is hard to imagine how arrow wounds would have been treated without recourse to at least as much surgery as it takes to cut out an arrow.

In his war commentaries Julius Caesar often mentions casualties, e.g. their large or small number, or having to give the army a rest of several days because of them, but he never speaks of medical treatment. One example is. *B. Gall.* I.26.5: "... since our men could not follow them, having tarried three days both on account of the men's wounds and because of the burial of the fallen, ...".[35] This is not particularly surprising as he has no reason to do so and his silence on this topic is no sufficient proof for the total absence of a medical service. The combination of burying the dead and caring for the wounded is often mentioned as standard procedure both in Greek and Roman authors.[36] and one can assume that the latter involved more than just resting the soldiers.

It is likely that the wounded rested in (their own?) tents and Nutton[37] points out that the earliest known Roman army hospital,

---

[33] *mox a saevitia secandi urendique transisse nomen in carneficem.*

[34] For the clash in expectations between Roman patients and Greek doctors, see Marasco (1995) and Nijhuis (1995).

[35] *... cum et propter vulnera hominum et propter sepulturam occisorum nostri triduum morati eos sequi non potuissent..*

[36] E.g. Dion. Hal. II.42.1; Proc., *Goth.* .V.XXIII.27, ib.VII.XXIV.15.

[37] (1969), p. 266, n. 1.

Haltern, shows a plan that obviously derives from a collection of tents, *tentoria*, so one might deduce from this that there were special 'hospital' tents for the sick and wounded.

Livy (VIII.XXXVI.6-8) provides some evidence for the wounded lying in tents in the army camp - although what he is describing is more likely to be the situation as it was in his own life-time than that of the fourth century BC, in which the account is set. He describes the general L. Papirius visiting casualties after a battle (in an effort to make himself more popular with his men): "... he himself made the round of the wounded, sticking his head into the[ir] tents".[38] Here again a description of medical treatment would be beside the point, and Livy goes on to describe how much the soldiers appreciate their general's attention. Tacitus (*Hist.* II.45.3) describes how, after the battle of Bedriacum in AD 69, the soldiers apparently treated each other's wounds.[39] Although he does not mention any doctors, the passage does not prove that there were none, but it may show merely that their number was insufficient after a major battle.

The first author to mention *medici* in a military context is Cicero in his *Tusculan Disputations*, (II.XVI.38), emphasising the difference between a recruit in his first battle and a hardened veteran: while the former is totally dismayed by the slightest wound, the latter, "well trained and old, and therefore more steadfast, is merely asking for a doctor by whom he would have his wounds bandaged".[40] As the aim of the text is a discussion of courage and fortitude and not one of the availability of medical treatment in the army, Cicero does not go into any detail on the status and rank of the *medicus*, but it is quite obvious that he is not expecting his reader to be astonished at the mention of a doctor in connection with the military.[41] One may therefore draw the conclusion that by Cicero's time doctors in the army were a commonly accepted fact and there is no basis in the text for Scarborough's suggestion[42] that the *medicus* was just another soldier with some experience in wound dressing. In fact, elsewhere (e.g. *Fam.* XVI.IX) Cicero uses the word *medicus* only for what we would call a doctor, and there is no reason why he should use it any differently in the passage in question.

---

[38] ... *ipse circuit saucios milites, inserens in tentoria caput.*
[39] *isdem tentoriis alii fratrum, alii propinquorum vulnera fovebant.*
[40] *exercitatus et vetus ob eamque rem fortior medicum modo requirens a quo obligetur.*
[41] Wilmanns (1995), p. 16, n. 32, argues that Cicero is thinking of a dialogue between Patroklos and the wounded Eurypylos in a tragedy by Ennius, but the setting for his hypothetical veteran is distinctly Roman.
[42] (1968), p. 256.

Polybius' account (III.66.9) that the general Publius "at the same time treated himself and the other wounded"[43] has given rise to speculations on the generals dispensing medical treatment,[44] but nothing in the text makes it necessary to translate θεραπεύω as anything more than 'to look after' or perhaps 'to cause to be treated' or 'to care for' - in particular if one considers that the general was himself wounded.

The earliest epigraphical evidence for the presence of doctors in the army is a votive tablet by Sextus Titius Alexander, *medicus* of the fifth Praetorian cohort, dedicated to "Asclepius and the health of his comrades"[45] in AD 82 (*CIL* VI.20=ILS 2092).[46] The *cognomen* Alexander points to Greek origin, which is evident with many other of the *medici*, e.g. C. Terentius Symphorus, Claudius Thamyras, Aurelius Hegumenus or Claudius Hymnus, to name but a few. The majority may have been Roman citizens, as service in the legions was limited to those, while service in the auxiliary units was open to non-Romans as well. However, we do not know whether these regulations extended to the medical staff and to other non-combatant units, such as veterinary surgeons or engineers.

The word used in the epigraphical sources is *medicus*, often accompanied by varying epithets. Some of these indicate the unit (*medicus legionis / cohortis / alae*) or a particular speciality (*medicus clinicus / medicus chirurgus*), but others are of more difficult interpretation. The *medicus castrorum* or *castrensis*, mentioned only on three inscriptions, was presumably in charge of the medical services within the *castra*,[47] while the *medicus duplicarius* - meaning that he received double pay[48] - appears to have been limited to the fleet. There are two examples of a *miles medicus*, a doctor of the *legio XXII Primigenia* and another of *legio I Minervia*, the addition of *miles* suggesting that the two men were not officers. Similar structures of titles can be found, e.g., in *ILS* 2424: *miles librarius*.

The title *medicus ordinarius* occurs on five inscriptions - *ILS* 2432,9182; *CIL* III 4279,5959; *RIB* 1618 - all dated later than AD 150, perhaps even later than AD 200. Scarborough[49] suggests that

---

[43] ἅμα μὲν αὐτὸν ἐθεράπευε καὶ τοὺς ἄλλους τραυματίας.
[44] See especially Scarborough (1968), p. 256: "Roman consuls were often skilled wound dressers in their own right."
[45] *Asclepio et saluti commilitonum*. The word *commilitones* makes it obvious that this *medicus* considered himself a member of the Roman army.
[46] Most of of the epigraphical evidence can be found in Davies (1969) and (1972), but these lists have been superseded by J. C. Wilmanns' excellent monograph (1995).
[47] As Nutton (1969), p. 267, very plausibly assumes.
[48] On the *duplicarius* in general, see Sanders (1959).
[49] (1968), p. 258.

ordinarius indicates a soldier in the ranks, following Domaszewski's[50] argument, but to quote all the opinions in the controversy over this term would be pointless here. Sander's[51] and Nutton's[52] interpretation that the *medicus ordinarius* had the rank of a centurion appears more convincing, as the *medicus* - upon taking the military oath - remained a *miles* until his promotion to the rank of a centurion, and thus the epithet *ordinarius* would set him off against the *medicus* of lower rank.

Other titles - for which we only have literary evidence - are *optio valetudinarii* and *capsarius*, both listed in the *Digest* (L 6,7), with the *medici*, among the *immunes*, i.e. soldiers exempt from fatigues. We read in Vegetius (II.10) that the *praefectus castrorum* was responsible for "sick comrades and the doctors by whom they were treated"[53] (the 'sick' would presumably include the wounded), thus one can assume that he was in control of the *valetudinarium*, or hospital, and the *optio* was in charge of its administration. The word *capsarius* is said to have derived from the *capsa* in which the *capsarii* kept the bandages, and they may have been dressers or medical orderlies of lower rank than the *medicus*.

An inscription found in Lambaesis in North Africa (*CIL* 2438), mentioning apprentice orderlies (*discentes capsariorum*), makes it clear that - at least in some cases - medical instruction was available for men who presumably had entered the army without any previous medical training. It is conceivable that there was also some form of instruction enabling *capsarii* to become *medici*, as the 'on-the-job-training' with a senior *medicus* would follow the pattern of medical instruction in a civilian context.

One need not therefore assume that all doctors in the Roman army only started their training after they had been drafted and it is highly likely that many of them had had at least some form of medical training in civilian life. There is some material which supports this claim. V. Nutton[54] brings up an example of comparative evidence, namely a trained architect joining the legion at Aquincum, and Pedanius Dioscorides as well as Scribonius Largus appear to have been trained doctors by the time they enlisted. Callies[55] suggests that such 'experts' may have been enrolled with the higher rank of a *medicus ordinarius* in the first place. He cites the example of Anicius Ingenuus, *medicus ordinarius* of the first cohort of the Tungrians at

---

[50] (1967).
[51] (1959), pp. 240f.
[52] (1968), p. 268.
[53] *aegri contubernales et medici, a quibus curabantur.*
[54] (1968), p. 265.
[55] (1968), p. 24.

Housesteads (*CIL* VII.690=*RIB* 1618), who died at the age of twenty-five and (so Callies claims) could therefore hardly have been in the forces long enough for being promoted to a rank corresponding to that of a centurion.

It also seems obvious to make the connection between the frequency of names of Greek origin among the army doctors and the large number of Greeks in the medical profession in civilian society, and to suggest that some Greek doctors joined the army as medical staff. It is possible that this was a means of obtaining the status of a Roman citizen - a way open to non-Romans serving in the *alae*.

The concept of the *valetudinaria*, or military hospitals, deserves further elaboration, as this is an entirely Roman idea, apparently without precedents in the ancient world. There is no evidence for military hospitals before the Augustan period, but with the growth of the empire and the resulting distances separating the military units from Rome it had become impossible to send the sick and wounded back and the need for camp-based medical facilities arose. All the *valetudinaria* that have been found are near the frontiers of the empire, in Britain and near the Rhine and the Danube, both in legionary fortresses and auxiliary forts, and present a distinctive architectural pattern, with an entrance hall, a relatively large room behind it and two rows of small rooms, separated by a corridor, on either side of the rectangular courtyard. The small rooms would guarantee the sick and wounded sufficient quiet, a concern already expressed by Hyginus in his manual on fortifications and the building of army camps (*Mun. Castr.* 4), where he specifies the position of the *valetudinarium* within the camp "so that it will be quiet for the convalescents".[56]

Schultze,[57] the first to publish the finds of Vetera (the present-day Xanten), appears to be the first to suggest an interpretation for the room behind the large entrance hall of the building. According to him it is an operating theatre, the hearths found there in some hospitals having served to "sterilise instruments and dressings". There is no literary evidence for either an operating theatre or for sterilising instruments and there is no reason why a doctor with a Graeco-Roman concept of medicine should want to 'sterilise' instruments or dressings, yet this myth has been repeated uncritically as an established fact by most authors since.[58] Nevertheless, it is not inconceivable that the casualties were first treated near the entrance

---

[56] *ut valetudinarium quietum esse convalescentibus posset.*
[57] (1934).
[58] With the exception of Jetter (1966), who (p. 4) calls this idea a "questionable conjecture' and argues for the remains of an altar.

hall and then carried to their individual rooms or, if they were able to walk, sent back to their barracks. For the reasons already mentioned in the section on Greece, it would have been more practical to have one central area for treatment than to make the doctors walk from room to room. If the hearths were at all related to medical treatment, they may have been used to heat water or cauteries.

One part of the relief on Trajan's Column[59] has been used to corroborate the evidence for or against the existence of an army medical service, depending on the respective scholar's theory. The scene[60] shows two men wearing the uniform of auxiliaries, attending two soldiers, one of them a legionary wearing the *lorica segmentata*, the other belonging to a unit of *auxilia*. In the same way as the 'operating theatre', the identification of this scene as a field dressing-station appears to have been generally accepted despite the absence of literary references to anything of the kind.

It is obvious from the relief that the two soldiers are wounded or injured and it is very unlikely that the two other men are anything other than medical personnel of some kind, for one appears to be examining the legionary's arm, while the other is treating the auxiliary's (perhaps cavalryman's?) thigh. It would be unwise, though, to assume that the scene is a realistic representation of the medical assistance that Roman soldiers would receive in the second century A. D. Rossi[61] is alone in pointing out the symbolic value of, e.g., the difference in armour, although even he attempts to identify one of the men with a *medicus* and the other with a *capsarius*. Even if this should have been the artist's intention, we have no conclusive evidence for it. Rossi[62] also explains scenes showing Dacians carrying their dead off the battlefield as "specialised personnel for the treatment of the wounded", but this interpretation amounts to wishful thinking.

By the same token, the fact that the scene is situated more or less on the battlefield should not be overestimated, as this may be an artistic convention contrived to express simultaneity between the treatment of the wounded and the battle. So far our sources describe only casualties being taken back to the camp (Caes., *B. Gall*. VIII.48; Dio Cassius, LXVIII.14; Dion. Hal. XI.26.1), the town (Dion. Hal. VIII.86.1) or, at any rate, away from the battle-line (Polyb. XV.14.3) and unless further evidence for field dressing-stations is found, the

---

[59] Cichorius (1896), Pls.XXX and XXXI.
[60] See Fig. 2.
[61] (1969).
[62] (1977).

scene on Trajan's Column alone will not be enough to prove their existence.

Two accounts of some relevance to medical treatment in the army are written by men describing their own experiences. Velleius Paterculus, of the first century AD, describes (II.114.2) how the emperor Tiberius puts at the disposal of the author and his fellow-soldiers "now his doctors, now his cooking equipment and the bathtub brought for him alone".[63] This passage shows that the emperors obviously took along their private physicians - as Greek kings did - but cannot be used as evidence for the absence of a medical service. The way these physicians are listed together with the kitchen equipment and the bath may be indicative of their status seen through the eyes of a Roman officer.

The second source, Ammianus Marcellinus writing in the fourth century AD, in particular appears to suggest that, while there was a medical service, the doctors were not available on the battlefield and, at least after a battle, they were numerically insufficient. At XVIII.8.11, a soldier of the guard asks the author to pull out an arrow that has struck his thigh (which is precisely what Rufus [*Quaest. Med.* 55] warns against). At XIX.2.9 and XIX.2.15, Ammianus describes the suffering of those wounded by the Parthian arrows. In both of the latter cases he mentions men who were "experts in extracting [arrows]" or "experts in healing"[64] without, however, stating whether these were Roman army surgeons, local doctors, or perhaps laymen with some experience in treating wounds.

From an examination of the present evidence it is possible to say the following: we can be certain that some kind of medical service existed in the army of Imperial Rome, although we do not have enough evidence to draw definite conclusions regarding the rank, status and number of doctors.[65] The exact extent, structure and organisation of this medical service may have been in constant change as were the structure and organisation of the army itself, of which the medical service was an integrated part.

---

[63] *iam medici, iam apparatus cibi, iam in hoc solum uni portatum instrumentum balnei.* Although he writes that these commodities were offered to all "of higher and lower rank than ourselves alike", it is unlikely that this includes common soldiers.

[64] *vellendi periti* and *medendi periti.*

[65] Willmans (1995) calculates that in the mid second century AD the *c.* 400,000 soldiers in the Roman army would have needed a minimum of 500 to 600, up to about 800, doctors. She suggests an average of 10 per legion.

CHAPTER FIVE

EXPERT AND LAYMAN

Before I go on to examine the use of scenes of wounding by lay authors, some other questions have to be investigated, in particular: What was a 'lay' author? Did the Greeks or Romans have the concept of a sharp division between layman and expert? Was there something that one might call technical terminology? And finally: did the description of surgical techniques involve any particular problems as opposed to other fields of medicine?

1. *Medical knowledge*

> Every sensible man who realises that health is the most valuable thing for humans must know how to receive succour from his own understanding in the case of diseases; he has to be able also to know and understand what is said by the doctors and what is administered [by them] to his own body; [and] to know all these things to the extent to which it becomes a layman.[1]

Thus reads the opening sentence of *Aff.* (VI.208 L), and the author repeats the idea some lines further down: "... what is appropriate for the layman to know".[2] Two facts are obvious from these sentences: first, that the author makes a clear distinction between the *iatros* (or, at 45/VI.254 L, the *cheirotechnês*) on the one hand and the layman or *idiôtês* on the other, and second, that according to the author's opinion, the *idiôtês*, too, should have a certain amount of medical knowledge. Despite the author's promise at the end of the first paragraph, "I shall say what the layman needs to know about each of these",[3] it is not quite clear whom he is addressing. He always mentions the *idiôtês* in the third person, so the audience addressed by "if you want to learn something"[4] at *Aff.* 45/VI.254 L may or may not be identical with

---

[1] ἄνδρα χρὴ, ὅστις ἐστὶ συνετὸς, λογισάμενον ὅτι τοῖσιν ἀνθρώποισι πλείστου ἄξιον ἐστιν ἡ ὑγιείη, ἐπίστασθαι ἀπὸ τῆς ἑωυτοῦ γνώμης ἐν τῇσι νούσοισιν ὠφελέεσθαι· ἐπίστασθαι δὲ τὰ ὑπὸ τῶν ἰητρῶν καὶ λεγόμενα καὶ προσφερόμενα πρὸς τὸ σῶμα τὸ ἑωυτοῦ καὶ διαγινώσκειν· ἐπίστασθαι δὲ τούτων ἕκαστα, ἐς ὅσον εἰκὸς ἰδιώτην.

[2] ὀκόσα εἰκὸς γινώσκειν ἰδιώτην.

[3] ἤδη οὖν τούτων ὁπόθεν ἕκαστα δεῖ τὸν ἰδιώτην ἐπίστασθαι, ἐγὼ φράσω.

[4] ἢν τι θέλῃς μανθάνειν ...

the *idiôtês*. It is conceivable that the treatise was intended for physicians, telling them what to teach laymen.[5]

One can find the notion of the *idiôtês* - or of the *dêmotês* in *VM* 2 (I.572 L) - as opposed to the expert quite frequently and the examples are not limited to medicine. Thus, e.g., Aeschines (*In Timarch.*, 7) distinguishes between the *idiôtês* and the *rhêtôr*, Plato's *Republic* (525c) contains the injunction that arithmetics and geometry should be known "not after a layman's fashion",[6] and his *Statesman* (298c) also refers to those who are not experts in navigation as *idiôtai*.

One should, however, be wary of seeing a clear distinction between expert and layman in our sense when it comes to medicine. While it is fairly obvious in most situations who is a ship's pilot and who is not, the situation is less straightforward in the case of an *iatros*. The problem is usually obscured by the necessity of translating ἰατρός/*medicus* as 'doctor' or 'physician' for lack of a more appropriate expression, whereby the word takes on our connotations of the term. but we can catch a glimpse of the difficulty in Plato's *Laws* (720a): the Athenian distinguishes between doctors and their assistants (ὑπηρέται) who, as he says, are also in a way called doctors.[7] This statement is followed by a discussion (ibid. b) of the difference between slave doctors,[8] who learn their craft by watching their masters, "by experience" (κατ' ἐμπειρίαν) and the free doctors, who have learnt it "naturally" (κατὰ φύσιν). The Athenian refers to these two groups as "two types of those called doctors".[9]

The criteria for the decision of who was to be considered a doctor may have varied from situation to situation or from audience to audience. Thus it is unlikely that the eight doctors appointed by Xenophon's officers on their retreat[10] were the same type of practitioner who would have been referred to by that name in Athens by citizens of a certain standing. By the same token, the ἰατροί or *medici* following the armies were not necessarily the kind of men called thus by the Hippocratic authors or by Celsus.

---

[5] Kollesch (1991), p. 179, argues that it was written for lay people.
[6] μὴ ἰδιωτικῶς.
[7] ἰατροὺς δὲ καλοῦμεν δή που καὶ τούτους.
[8] One of these is mentioned in an Athenian inscription regarding manumission, cited in Lewis (1968), p. 370 (1.11). On doctors and patients in Plato, see Langholf (1996). Cf. also Joly (1969). According to Kudlien (1970), p. 8, Athenian law did not allow slaves to become doctors, only *hypêretai*, i.e. assistants.
[9] δύο γένη τῶν καλουμένων ἰατρῶν. The absence of the definite article could be taken to suggest that there are more than two categories.
[10] *An.* III.IV.30f., quoted in Ch. 4.1.

The aforementoined injunction - *Medic.* XIV/IX.220 L - to follow mercenary armies in order to gather experience in surgical skills should not lead us to believe that all those who treated the wounded after a battle were men who had had a theoretical medical education comparable to that of the doctors portrayed by the authors in the Hippocratic Corpus - or even shared their beliefs.

The words were probably used for a wide range of people who claimed to heal wounds, injuries or illness in vastly differing ways. Given that our written sources[11] only represent one particular type of medical treatment, it is only too easy to assume that this was 'orthodox' medicine and everything else was the ancient equivalent of - at best - alternative medicine, if it was not discarded as 'magic' altogether. It appears, however, that, although this may reflect the self-image of many medical authors, it was not the general attitude among the potential patients. In Plato's *Republic* (426b), for example, incantations and amulets are mentioned in one breath with remedies, cauterisation and incisions as possible therapeutic means. In the *Charmides* (155b) Critias introduces Socrates to Charmides as a doctor who will know a remedy for the latter's headaches. Although Charmides is aware of Socrates' identity, he shows as little surprise at this introduction as he does when Socrates explains (155e) that the remedy consists in the administration of a herb (φύλλον τι), accompanied by an incantation (ἐπῳδή). Rather, Charmides' eager reply that he would copy down the incantation suggests that it was common practice to use them. The story is obviously not to be taken at face value and the exchange between Socrates and Charmides about the treatment is slightly jocular, but it can still be used as an indicator for what was considered as the possible range of the term *iatros*.

In the same passage (ib.156d) Socrates claims to have learned the use of the remedy from "one of the Thracian physicians of Zalmoxis, who are said even to aim at immortality".[12] Not only are the men in question barbarians, who are unlikely to be trained in the same way as Greek doctors, but the mention of the cult of Zalmoxis and of immortality clearly suggests magical practices - and yet Socrates uses the term *iatros*. As for the Latin term *medicus,* we have already encountered the problem in relation to medical treatment in the army. The fact that some of the men

---

[11] Apart from very few examples such as the Epidaurus inscriptions - the official story - or Aelius Aristides' account of temple medicine from the patient's point of view.

[12] ... τινος τῶν Θρᾳκῶν τῶν Ζαλμόξιδος ἰατρῶν, οἵ λέγονται καὶ ἀπαθανατίζειν.

treating the sick and wounded soldiers were called *medici* does not prove that they had necessarily had the same type of training as the *medici* referred to in medical literature. It is quite conceivable that some of them were common soldiers who had acquired some surgical skills, or local village healers.

The problem is complicated further by the fact that - in the absence of legally agreed standards - the main criterion in the decision who was a doctor was the individual's claim to be one. Although there is a clear definition of who can be accepted as a doctor in Ulpian's *Digest* (L.13.3.), it is a relatively late source[13] and - as V. Nutton[14] points out - the definition serves a purely legal purpose. It is concerned with problems of status and taxation from the viewpoint of the Roman administration, not of the consumer, and may be no indication of the latter's opinion.

According to one definition in Xenophon's *Memorabilia* (III.1), which may only reflect his own point of view, the difference between a person who is an expert and one who is not lies in the knowledge of the field and in having learned about it. Thus, according to him, "one who has learned to heal, even if he is not practising, is a doctor all the same",[15] while the man who does not have knowledge[16] is not a doctor, even if he is held to be one by all the world. As we shall see, at least the first part of Xenophon's reasoning does not correspond to the distinction between expert and layman as it was made in reality, where medical knowledge without professional practice (for payment) did not make a man an *iatros*.

In general it is possible to make the distinction between the two ends of the scale, i.e. between the person who would be acknowledged as a doctor by anyone at any given time on the one hand and the absolute layman on the other. However, between those two extremes lies the large grey area of people involved in healing in one way or the other. These include root-cutters, masseurs, midwives, the *Marsii* who cured snake-bite, gymnastic trainers, etc., and even Galen does not hesitate to quote people belonging to this group as his authorities for pharmacological material in *Comp. Med. Loc.*: e.g. Diogas the *iatraleiptes*, or masseur, (XIII.104 K), Pharnaces the root-cutter (ib. 204), a Bithynian barber (ib. 259f.) and even a boxer (ib. 294). Again, when he speaks of "those practicing medicine in rural areas

---

[13] Early third century AD.
[14] (1988a), pp. 29f.
[15] ὁ μαθὼν ἰᾶσθαι, κἂν μὴ ἰατρεύῃ, ὅμως ἰατρός ἐστιν.
[16] μὴ ἐπιστάμενος.

(literally 'the field')",[17] it is not quite clear whether these are physicians like himself, who find themselves working in rural areas, or whether they belong to a different class of practitioners altogether. Galen's use of these sources is in accordance with a remark about the knowledge of remedies in *Aff.* (45/VI.254 L): "People do not find these things by reason, but rather through chance, and the experts no more [often] than the lay people."[18]

In this context Philostratus' claim[19] concerning gymnastics is worth mentioning, in particular as it is contrary to what one tends to expect from a discipline involving physical exercise:

> As for diseases such as those which we call catarrhs, dropsy and consumption, and for sacred diseases, the doctors stay them by pouring something on or by giving something to drink or by spreading on something; gymnastics stops diseases of that kind by diet and massage. However, if a man has something broken or is wounded or his eyesight is obfuscated or he has sprained one of his joints, one has to take him to the doctors, as for these gymnastics is of no avail.[20]

One would expect an expert on gymnastic training to claim experience in the treatment of such injuries as are likely to occur during sports, namely sprains, dislocations and even fractures, as well as minor wounds - if he were to make any claims regarding medical knowledge at all. However, Philostratus challenges medicine on its own ground and claims to achieve the same success as doctors in healing internal diseases. The methods he proposes to use are different, though: diet and massage as opposed to the pharmacological treatment, internal as well as external, used by the doctors. Unfortunately no other similar writings have come down to us and we have no point of comparison, but it is conceivable that others in the same position, i.e those in what we would call the para-medical professions, would construct their arguments in a similar way.

However, it is not only these professions that lie in the overlap zone between the expert and the layman, but also the large group of laymen with varying degrees of medical knowledge - and even medical experience. The obvious interest in medicine taken by

---

[17] οἱ κατὰ ἀγρὸν ἰατρεύοντες.
[18] οὐ γὰρ ἀπὸ γνώμης ταῦτα εὑρίσκουσιν οἱ ἄνθρωποι, ἀλλὰ μᾶλλον ἀπὸ τύχης, οὐδέ τι οἱ χειροτέχναι μᾶλλον ἢ οἱ ἰδιῶται.
[19] *On Gymnastics*, ch. 14 (late second / early third century AD).
[20] νοσήματα ὁπόσα κατάρρους καὶ ὑδέρους καὶ φθόας ὀνομάζομεν καὶ ὁπόσαι ἱεραὶ νόσοι, ἰατροὶ μὲν παύουσιν ἐπαντλοῦντές τι ἢ ποτίζοντες ἢ ἐπιπλάττοντες, γυμναστικὴ δὲ τὰ τοιαῦτα διαίταις ἴσχει καὶ τρίψει· ῥήξαντά τι δὲ ἢ τρωθέντα ἢ θολωθέντα τὸ ἐν ὀφθαλμοῖς φῶς ἢ ὀλισθήσαντά τι τῶν ἄρθρων ἐς ἰατροὺς χρὴ φέρειν, ὡς οὐδὲν ἡ γυμναστικὴ πρὸς τὰ τοιαῦτα.

people who had no intention of becoming professional doctors is a phenomenon peculiar to both Greek and Roman antiquity. Stanford[21] compares Aeschylus' use of medical language to the modern writer's turning towards psychology and one could see the same analogy in the widespread interest in medical matters. The theory as well as the practice of medicine were obviously matters of great interest to lay writers and their audiences, and a man who claimed to have had a good education was expected to have some idea of medicine: one could indeed compare this to the way in which psychology has entered popular awareness nowadays. Galen's statement, in *De Anat. Admin.* (II.280 K), that in the past "not only the doctors, but the philosophers, too, studied dissection adequately"[22] may be a typical exaggeration concerning a lost golden age of higher knowledge, but it is a fact that one can observe a pronounced interest in medical topics from the fifth century BC onwards.[23]

It has to be stressed that in this case 'medicine' means the brand of medical teaching which makes its appearance in the Hippocratic writings. It would appear that Hippocratic medicine held a peculiar appeal even for people who had no intention of ever making it their profession, and the reason for this could hardly have been the novelty value, as the interest continued unabated for several centuries, but the underlying theoretical structure appears to be a likely candidate for the cause of this attraction. By its theoretical framework medicine appealed to those who were accustomed to philosophical modes of thought,[24] and Plato in particular appears to have found medicine a useful model for philosophical similes.[25] (The *Timaeus* in itself would be

---

[21] (1942), p. 57.

[22] ἱκανῶς γὰρ ἐσπουδάκασιν οἱ παλαιοὶ τὴν ἀνατομὴν, οὐκ ἰατροὶ μόνον, ἀλλὰ καὶ φιλόσοφοι.

[23] As this coincides with the spread of literacy on a larger scale, it can of course not be excluded that this interest was present in a pre-literate era as well, but it is more likely to be related to the availability of written material. On the impact of literacy, see Fantuzzi (1981); Havelock (1982); Easterling (1985); Knox (1985); Pigeaud (1988); Usener (1990); Thomas (1991) and (1992); Nieddu (1993). Cf. also Jouanna (1984) and Kollesch (1991) on the orality of some of the Hippocratic writings. The importance of literacy for the development of a specialised literature was not limited to medicine: to cite just one example, theoretical mechanics also came to be established from *c.* 400 BC (Krafft [1967]).

[24] See, e.g., Kudlien (1974) and Demand (1993).

[25] E.g. *R.* 426a-b, ib. 564c-d; *Amat.* 135c, ib. 138d; *Phdr.* 268b-c, to cite only a few examples. Wehrli (1951b) discusses medical similes in Plato. For Aristotle's use of medicine in his ethics, see Jaeger (1957), and Hernández Muñoz (1992) for medical metaphors and expressions in Demosthenes' orations.

sufficient proof of Plato's interest in medicine and his medical knowledge.)

Jaeger[26] goes as far as calling Greek medicine a "preliminary stage, in the history of thought, of Socratic, Platonic and Aristotelian philosophy" and claims that the "ethical science" of Socrates is unthinkable without the model of medicine.[27] While this is an overly bold claim, the strong presence of medical thought in philosophical writings is undeniable. The influence obviously worked both ways, and medicine gained the style of the medical *epideixis* or *logos*, following the example of the sophists.[28]

A similar interrelation existed, according to Momigliano,[29] between Hippocratic medicine and Herodotean historiography, both being contemporary novelties sharing the descriptive approach, the observation of sequences and the search for natural causes. This may have prompted doctors like Ktesias (Xen., *An.* I.VIII.26; Plut., *Art.* VI.6) or Kallimorphos (Lucian, *Hist. Conscr.*,16) to try their hand as historians and it may also have been an incentive for Thucydides to write his famous description of the plague (II.XLVII.-LI)[30] - discussions of its value for retrospective diagnosis being quite beside the point. There is, however, an important difference between the two disciplines. While both history and medicine have the use of literacy in common, history is not a *technê* [31]- or indeed a profession - in the way medicine is. Therefore the distinction between *technitai* and *idiôtai* is not an issue in historiography.

The frequent allusions to medical practice and theory in philosophical and historical writings as well as in tragedy, comedy and even poetry make it obvious that a certain degree of medical knowledge had quickly become general and could and would be expected among the educated.[32] Plutarch (*Alex.* VIII.1) notes Alexander the Great's penchant for medicine (φιλιατρεῖν) and (ib. XLI) his active interest in the treatment of his friends' wounds

---

[26] (1947), vol. III, p. 11.
[27] The most in-depth discussion of the use of medicine in Plato's philosophy is Vegetti (1965-9), but cf. also Wichmann (1960) and Herter (1963).
[28] Cf. Jaeger (1947), vol. III, p. 21.
[29] (1987), pp. 13f.
[30] Cf. also Wunderer (1989) on medical language in the historian Polybius.
[31] A notoriously untranslatable word, *technê* can be 'art', 'craft', 'skill', 'cunning' or 'method', to mention just a few meanings. On the use of the term in Aristotle, see Bartels (1965).
[32] Hadot (1984), p. 94, explains the interest philosophers took in medicine as a facet of the attitude favouring universal knowledge as far as possible, which stretched from Plato to Plutarch and Apuleius.

or illnesses, but in this particular case it is not clear whether this interest can be regarded as following the general Greek trend or whether it is rather a manifestation of Alexander's emulation of Achilles - or of the historiographical mythology thereof.

The amateur interest in medicine was by no means limited to Greece: it would seem that much of the Greek layman's attitude towards medicine was taken over together with the medicine itself and many of the philhellene Romans were also *philiatroi*. However, it was not mere imitation. For the Roman upper class - for this would be the group where Greek ideas were most easily accepted - Greek medicine, like Greek philosophy, had the added flavour of the foreign and the different, but this was not the only reason for its attraction. It also touched the right chord with the conservative landowner who believed, or claimed to believe, in the myth of a past in which every *paterfamilias* had been in charge of his family's health, in the way represented by Cato, without a need for professional medical experts.[33]

This practical element in the layman's involvement in medicine is occasionally made explicit in the Greek world,[34] but it is more pronounced in Roman times. Pliny the Younger explicitly states in the prolegomena to his *De Medicina* (and here even the author himself is a layman) that it is meant as a handbook (*velut breviario*) to be taken along when travelling. The purpose is to avoid being defrauded by dishonest doctors - as Pliny claims it happened both to himself and to his friends.

Celsus, who may have been a non-professional with medical experience,[35] thought of laymen as at least part of his audience. This becomes clear from a sentence in VI.18.1./290.19f., where, introducing the section on diseases of the genitals, he justifies his writing about them by explaining that it is "because their treatment particularly has to be known among the people".[36] This statement only makes sense if Celsus expects lay people to read his book and also to attempt the cures he suggests. Wellmann[37] claims that Celsus' work is not a compilation but the translation of a Greek handbook for laymen, with brief interpolations by Celsus himself, but his evidence is not sufficiently convincing. (Wellmann's bias

---

[33] Cf. Mudry (1980).
[34] For example Socrates' pretended treatment for heaviness of the head in the *Charmides*, the example of a man administering a *pharmakon* to his son in Xen., *Mem.* IV.2.17, and Alexander supposedly inspecting his soldiers' wounds (Arr., *An.* I.16.5).
[35] On the question of the extent of Celsus' knowledge and experience of medicine, see Meinecke (1941).
[36] *quia in volgus eorum curatio etiam praecipue cognoscenda est.*
[37] (1913), p. 4.

becomes evident in his statement[38] that all medical works written by Romans are nothing otherthan translations of Greek works.)

The same interest in the practical use of medicine can be seen in Scribonius Largus' dedication of his work to C. Iulius Callistus, who, it would appear, had been asking him for the compositions of some remedies (12): "But what further need is there to prove that the use of remedies is necessary, in particular to you who, since you understood their usefulness, asked me for some writings about this matter?"[39] It is obvious that Iulius Callistus' interest lies not so much in medicine as an intellectual pursuit as in the practical side of pharmacology. A similar interest may lie behind Oribasius' dedication of the *Eclogae Medicamentorum* to the emperor Julian.

Another example for (presumably) practical medical knowledge is the passage in Ammianus Marcellinus (XVIII.8.11.), which has already been mentioned in Ch. 4.2. The text in full is:

> While I looked about what to do, having strayed from the march of my comrades, Verennianus, a body-guard of the (emperor's) household, came up to me, his thigh pierced by an arrow. When I attempted to extract it upon my companion's entreaties, I was surrounded on all sides by the advancing Persians and made for the town.[40]

The relevant factors are that a soldier of the body-guard, apparently acquainted with the author, urges the latter to extract an arrow that has struck him in the thigh, and that Ammianus actually sets about doing so. This would suggest that the author was known to have given medical help in similar cases before. Unfortunately for our research, Ammianus' attempts are interrupted by the advance of the enemy and he does not mention how he would have gone about it. (Neither do we know what happened to the unfortunate Verennianus, but the very inconclusiveness of this story gives it a touch of authenticity, as does the fact that the author is not cast as a hero.) As mentioned before, it was quite likely that soldiers would turn to each other for help and some of them may have acquired considerable expertise - such as the veteran Marus in Silius Italicus' *Punica* (VI.74-100) -

---

[38] Ibid., p. 5.

[39] *sed quid ultra opus est probare necessarium usum esse medicamentorum, praecipue tibi, qui quia percepisti utilitatem eorum, idcirco a me conpositiones quasdam petisti*? On the prooemium of Scribonius Largus, see Deichgräber (1950).

[40] *Mihi dum avius ab itinere comitum quid agerem circumspicio, Verennianus domesticus protector occurrit, femur sagitta confixus, quam dum avellere* [one would expect *evellere* here] *obtestante collega conarer, cinctus undique antecedentibus Persis, civitatem petebam.*

but this is the only time that we see an officer and magistrate involved in treating another man's wounds.

This passage is not the only one in which Ammianus Marcellinus displays a knowledge of medicine and an interest in medical matters: after reporting (XVI.8.2.) that Constantius had decreed the death penalty for anyone using incantations for the purpose of alleviating pain, he comments that this is even permitted by medical authority.[41] One could deduce from this that he was familiar with the medicine of his day, possibly with medical writings.[42] While his descriptions of the sufferings of those wounded by Persian arrows (XIX.2.9. and ib.15.) may have been inserted merely to make for a more vivid eye-witness report, or, as I shall discuss in Part II, because it was a topos based on literary models, the accounts of the deaths of Julian (XXV.3.6-23) and of Valentinian (XXX.6.3-6) seem to linger on medical details: the spear lodged in the liver (XXV.3.6.: *in ima iecoris fibra*), the swelling of the veins hindering breathing (ib. 23) or the minute description of Valentinian's condition (loc. cit.).

The non-medical authors, both Greek and Roman, displaying varying degrees of medical knowledge are far too numerous to be quoted here - including, e.g., Seneca.[43] Although, as I intend to show in Part II, much of the material concerning wounds and wound treatment in non-medical literature is governed by the use of stock motifs, there is much anatomical and therapeutical detail, e.g. in Ovid's descriptions of wounds in the *Metamorphoses*: for example, the piece of lung adhering to the barbs as the arrow is pulled out (VI.252f.), the attempt to stop the bleeding with bandages (VII.848f.) or the statement that an incurable wound has to be excised to prevent the sore from spreading to the sound parts,[44] to cite but a few. The interest in the therapeutic aspect is even more pronounced in the *Dionysiaca* by the fifth-century (AD) poet Nonnos, who lists the remedies used[45] and, e.g., describes the excision of contaminated flesh around a wound (XVII.367ff.). Even if we assume that descriptions of wounds have become standing literary topoi by the time those passages

---

[41] *quod medicinae quoque admittit auctoritas.*

[42] For example with Soranus' remark (*Gyn.* III.42/121.29-31) that although amulets are useless, doctors should allow patients to use them if this makes the latter happier.

[43] *Q. M.* L.IV.13.11; *Ep.* L.I.6, etc. Cf. also Dutoit (1948) on Livy; Lehmann (1982) on Varro and Boscherini (1993) on medical terms in Cato.

[44] *immedicabile vulnus ense recidendum est, ne pars sincera trahatur* (I.190f.).

[45] See above, Ch. 3.

were written, the amount of medical detail expressed in them still remains surprising.

One has to distinguish, though, between the interest in medical theories and the knowledge of basic facts on wounds and their treatment. As we shall see in Part II, scenes of wounding and wound treatment appear to have a particular metaphorical value, which other topics related to medicine do not have. What links the two spheres of interest is the fact that men who did not make a living in these fields knew something about them and expected their audiences to understand them.

In the case of practical skills in treating wounds one can assume that a large number of people possessed them, mostly among those who had served in armies for a long time and among the rural population. Literary vestiges regarding these groups are practically non-existent, although in Silius Italicus (VI.74-100, cited above) and Menander's *Farmer* (60ff.) we can catch a glimpse of non-professionals treating wounds. Both approaches to medicine - the theoretical and the practical - are of equal interest for our research, but the reconstruction of everyday practices can only be based on conjectures and we must therefore concentrate on the theoretical interest as expressed in literature.

Medical knowledge of any kind could be acquired by laymen in different ways, for example by personal contact with doctors, through public talks given in the style of a sophistic *epideixis*,[46] or through book-learning. In his *Memorabilia* (IV.2.10), Xenophon speaks of Euthydemos and his large collection of medical books, and in the *Phaedrus* (268c) Socrates' interlocutor suggests that a man claiming to understand how to apply drugs may have come by this knowledge by having a book read to him.[47] These examples would suggest that medical books were in circulation as early as the fifth century BC - and that their audience was not limited to medical experts.

When reading the works in the Hippocratic Corpus, it is very important to take account of the heterogeneity of audiences envisaged by the single authors. As G. E. R. Lloyd[48] suggests, the differing degrees of self-confidence displayed in different treatises may serve as a guide: apparent self-confidence could be the sign of a book written for a lay public, while those intended mainly for a professional audience would more readily admit to

---

[46] Cf. v. Staden (1995), pp. 53ff., on Galen's anatomical displays as a form of rhetoric.
[47] ἐκ βιβλίου ποθὲν ἀκούσας. (Literally "having heard it from a book", that is, somebody else, perhaps the author or a slave, would have read it out.)
[48] (1987), p. 131.

hesitation or even helplessness. Although any of the treatises could theoretically have been read by laymen, some - such as *Morb.* or *VM* - will have had more appeal than others. While the surgical treatises contain fewer complicated theories and present less difficulties for the reader's understanding than some of the other, more theoretical, treatises (although, of course, some of the techniques are fairly complicated), their contents and, in particular, their practical tone may have made them an item of low priority on the layman's reading list. *Airs, Waters, Places* (*De aëre, aquis et locis* [*Aër.*]) may have been another treatise with great appeal for the layman, and one of the fragments of Euripides (973, quoted by Clement of Alexandria) reads very much as if Euripides had known it, when he speaks of "the diseases ... in relation to the diet of the inhabitants and the nature of the soil."[49]

The *Aphorisms* are to be considered as a case apart, their condensed form making them of little use without further, perhaps oral, explanations.[50] They may have been intended either as *aides-mémoire* for students (perhaps for oral memorising?) or as guidelines for lectures - either way intelligible only to those who had had prior training. This is not as strange a situation for a written treatise as it would seem, for, e.g., Galen claims in *De Captionibus*[51] that Aristotle's *Sophistici Elenchi* was written for "those who have already heard it",[52] and Plutarch (*Alex.* VII.9) says the same of Aristotle's *Metaphysics*. Althoff[53] makes similar claims about *Morb.* II.[54]

Whatever the intended audience, though, it is quite likely that most of the writings in the Hippocratic Corpus - as well as other similar ones - were accessible to the interested layman. This was certainly the case in later times, too. Galen (II.282 K) speaks of medical books, if only as a nostalgic reference to a past in which oral learning had been sufficient. It is quite obvious that medical books such as his own were available to the public and that they were read by doctors, those training to become doctors and amateurs alike.[55] Further proof for this is given by Aulus Gellius (XVIII.X.8), who recounts how he started to read medical books

---

[49] Cited by Daremberg (1869), p. 67.
[50] Lloyd (1979). Cf. Langholf (1990).
[51] Ed. Edlow, p. 92. (Edlow [ibid., p. 8] considers the work a training manual for philosophers and physicians.)
[52] τοὺς ἀκηκοότας ἤδη.
[53] (1993), pp. 218ff.
[54] On *Aph.*, see also Althoff (1998).
[55] See Manuli (1985), p. 394, on Galen's intended audience.

in order to become more knowledgeable on medical matters: "I occupied myself also with books on medical learning which I considered appropriate for studying [lit.: for teaching]".[56]

Another way by which the amateur could acquire medical knowledge was through public lectures (ἀκροάσεις) given by professional doctors. Such lectures are mentioned already in the Hippocratic Corpus: the author of *Precepts* (IX.266f. L) warns his audience - which he apparently expects to consist, at least in part, of professional doctors - against citing the poets in their public lectures if they have to give them at all (an endeavour the author obviously wants to discourage). Galen writes about his own public anatomical demonstrations and lectures, which were attended by his professional rivals as well as by interested laymen. (When speaking of medical lectures for a general public, one has to keep in mind that some professionals in the field of medicine may well have been professional lecturers or teachers rather than practitioners.)

The practice of giving lectures appears to have been fairly common and we can see it reflected in a decree of the city of Perge.[57] It expresses the gratitude of the council and the people of Perge towards the physician Asclepiades, thanking him for, among other services, lectures he gave to the general public on topics related to health: (1.5-9).[58] From the phrasing of the inscription it would not seem that the practice of giving lectures itself was unheard of and novel, but rather that Asclepiades is praised for giving them free and of his own accord. A similar inscription from Phocis[59] thanks the doctor Asklepiodoros who had given "lectures ... over several days".[60] The giving of lectures does not appear to have been limited to medicine either, as there is also an inscription from Tanagra in Boeotia[61] thanking two musicians for giving "theoretical as well as practical lectures".[62] It also appears that at a fairly late stage the training for ephebes in Athens comprised some formal education other than weapon training, including lectures.[63]

---

[56] *medicinae quoque disciplinae libros attigi, quos arbitrabar esse idoneos ad docendum.*
[57] Cited in Fraser (1972), vol. IIa, p. 526.
[58] ἀποδείξεις μεγάλας πεποίηται τῆς ἑαυτοῦ ἐνπειρ(ί)ας, διά τε τῶν ἐν τῷ γυμνασίῳ ἀκροάσεων πολλὰ χρή(σι)μα διατεθεῖναι ἐν αὐταῖς πρὸς ὑγείαν τοῖς πολίταις ἀνήκοντα.
[59] *SEG* III (1929), 416.
[60] ἀκροάσεις ... ἐπὶ ἀμέρας πλείονας.
[61] *SEG* II (1925), 184.
[62] ἀκροάσεις λογικάς τε καὶ ὀργανικάς.
[63] Grasberger (1881), vol. III.

The third possible source of information on medical topics was personal contact with men in the medical profession. Thus Aristotle's father was a doctor and no doubt so were some of his father's friends, and it is unlikely that he was brought up without medical knowledge. Plato (or rather Plato's Socrates) had friends such as Eryximachos whom he could consult on anything concerning medicine and who - as we can see in the *Symposium* (185e-188e) - would readily launch into theoretical explanations, even at a banquet. Another example is Plutarch, whose works abound in references to medical topics. There appear to have been some doctors among his close friends[64] and among friends of the family.[65] For all we know, members of his family may have been doctors, too. It may well be that Plutarch acquired his knowledge of medicine from conversations with his friends or relations, perhaps combined with book-learning.

The lower status of the doctor in Roman society made him a less likely candidate for friendship. Galen may have been an exception (and he himself would have been the first to agree that he was), his wealthy family background freeing him from the obligation to work for gain, therefore giving him higher social standing. When Cicero and Seneca speak of their respective doctors in apparently very friendly terms, it is obvious that these doctors are commendable because of their good services, but they are not men of Cicero's or Seneca's own social class and can therefore only be 'friends' in the wider sense of *amicitia* between patron and client. Nevertheless, Cicero[66] writes of his grief at the death of his doctor, the slave Alexius, despite the social gap.

It has to be stressed again for both Greek and Roman antiquity, that however profound the medical knowledge acquired by the layman, its purpose was not professional use in the sense of full-time practice. The amateur aspect was indeed part of the attraction and made medicine as an object of inquiry a worthy pursuit for the free man. The importance of this aspect is made clear in the *Protagoras* (312a), where Plato says, speaking of music and sports, that one would not learn them "for an art, in order to become a craftsman, but for education, as it becomes the layman and the free man".[67] In the opening sentence of *De Partibus Animalium* (639a), Aristotle makes a similar distinction between two states of mind in any kind of speculation or investigation: the

---

[64] Cf. *Table-Talk* VII.1.698 (Nikias of Nikopolis).
[65] His grandfather's friend, Philotas of Amphissa, mentioned in *Ant*. XXVIII.
[66] *Fam*. XVI.1.1; cf. Mudry (1980).
[67] οὐκ ἐπὶ τέχνῃ ἔμαθες, ὡς δημιουργὸς ἐσόμενος, ἀλλ' ἐπὶ παιδείᾳ, ὡς τὸν ἰδιώτην καὶ τὸν ἐλεύθερον πρέπει.

knowledge of the thing[68] and some kind of education or culture (παιδειά τις). In *Polit.* 1282a he distinguishes between three ways of pursuing medicine and of being an *iatros*: the practitioner or craftsman (δημιουργός), the skilled 'master craftsman' (ἀρχιτεκτονικός) and the man who is educated with regards to the art (ὁ πεπαιδευμένος περὶ τὴν τέχνην). The latter would have equal standing with the experts (τοῖς εἰδόσιν) in making judgements regarding medical treatment.

Beginning from the fifth century BC, medicine had become more and more a part of general culture - of the *enkyklios paideia* - and Jaeger[69] calls it a leading cultural power factor (*führende Kulturmacht*) leading to a new concept, the medically educated person (*der medizinisch Gebildete*). The pursuit of medical studies for purposes other than professional practice continued throughout antiquity. It may well have been based, as Marrou[70] hypothesises, on a refusal of technical orientation, the aim of ancient education being not the creation of specialists, but something resembling the German idea of *Allgemeinbildung*.[71] His hypothesis is that the only exception was medicine, which alone had a "proper training" (*formation propre*) - although this point is highly debatable. The feeling of inferiority thus created among professional doctors would be at the bottom of doctors' claims that they were also philosophers. Although Marrou's idea in itself seems too modern, his hypothesis is nonetheless very attractive and may be true in a way for certain groups within the medical profession, who aimed at being integrated into the system, while others went out of their way to stress the difference between their in-group and laymen. (Either position could, of course, have been mere rhetoric.)

The "collective feeling of inferiority" among professional doctors imagined by Marrou would certainly have been more appropriate in Rome. When Cicero[72] distinguishes between disgraceful and honourable pursuits, medicine and architecture are among the latter, but only for "those for whose position they are appropriate".[73] According to Vitruvius, who in *De architectura* (I.10) counts medicine among the *enkyklia mathêmata*, the arts consist of *opus,* which is reserved to the expert, and of *ratiocinatio* or theory, the practical part of which can be understood by all the

---

[68] ἐπιστήμη τοῦ πράγματος.
[69] (1947), vol. III, p. 11.
[70] (1965), pp. 330f.
[71] Cf. Kühnert (1961).
[72] *Off.* I.XLII.150f.
[73] *iis, quorum ordini conveniunt.*

CHAPTER FIVE

educated. One can easily imagine that the theoretical aspect would have been more highly estimated among the upper classes.

Often the gap in knowledge and even experience may not have been so great between a professional and a *philiatros* layman,[74] but it was rather the individual's self-image that decided whether he wanted to call himself a doctor or not. It is therefore less surprising that the awareness of a difference between expert and layman was quite pronounced on both sides - far more pronounced than the difference itself would appear to have been.

Thus, for example, in Plutarch's *Dinner of the Seven Wise Men* (158.A-B), Kleodoros says that Hesiod had been *iatrikos*, because he spoke about topics such as regimen with accuracy. This is a surprising statement to appear in a work by Plutarch, an author whose own medical knowledge appears to be above average. It could be that he considers himself an exception (or that he disagrees with Kleodoros), but it could also be that for some reason he prefers to draw a firm line between the *idiôtês* and the *iatros*.

This difference is also pointed out by Lucian (*Abdic.* 7) when he makes the young physician (disowned by his father for not curing his stepmother's insanity) say that his father could not possibly have known the cause and the intensity of the disease and had therefore ordered his son - "for lack of expertise"[75] - to cure it by the same remedy that had cured him. At 26 he again repeats that this would have appeared very logical, especially "to a layman and one inexperienced in medicine".[76] Plato, too, despite his own familiarity with medical matters, makes a point of stressing the dichotomy between a person who is *iatrikos* and, e.g., one who is "an imitator of ... medical discourse" (*R.* 599c).[77]

If this point is pressed by non-medical authors, it is made even more strongly by the medical ones, in particular by the Hippocratics and by Galen. The author of *VM* expresses it in an entire paragraph (II.13-25/I.572f. L): he declares that one has to talk about things familiar to lay people (... δεῖν ... γνωστὰ λέγειν τοῖσι δημότῃσι), because understanding the cause and course of their disease is no easy matter for them, being laymen (δημότας ἐόντας οὐ ῥηίδιον), and if one misses being understood by them (εἰ δέ τις τῆς τῶν ἰδιωτέων γνώμης ἀποτεύξεται), one misses one's aim.

---

[74] Some of the works in the Hippocratic Corpus may even have been written by non-practitioners.
[75] ὑπὸ ἰδιωτείας.
[76] ἰδιώτῃ καὶ ἀπείρῳ ἰατρικῆς.
[77] μιμητὴς ... ἰατρικῶν λόγων.

The author of *Aff.*, who expects at least some medical knowledge from laymen, nevertheless points out (VI.254 L) that - regarding food and remedies - such things as are discovered by medical understanding (τῇ ἰητρικῇ γνώμῃ) have to be learnt from those who are able to discern the matters of the art. This viewpoint is shared by the author of *Flat.*, who, after the statement that medicine is a burden to those who have mastered it but a benefit to the *idiôtai*, goes on to say that the negative aspects are harder to know and "can be understood only by the doctors and not by the lay people, as this understanding is the work of the intellect rather than of the body" (VI.90 L).[78] Note that this is the contrary of what Vitruvius claims; obviously the drift of the argument depended largely on which side the author was, or pretended to be, on.

Galen often uses the same distinction between expert and layman, for instance in his remark in the commentary on the *Timaeus* that it was not astonishing that Plato, being a philosopher, did not know anatomy.[79] One could also quote his statement (VII.416 K) that even a non-*iatros* could understand his explanation except for the variations of the pulse, or a similar one in *Medical Names* [Med. N.][80] that small changes could only be noticed by a doctor, while considerable changes were obvious to the layman as well (106v). In *Simul.* (XIX.1ff. K) he also distinguishes between the *idiôtai*, who are easily fooled by malingerers, and the *iatroi* who are not. The perceived lack of knowledge of the former is also clearly stated in the expression (XIV.245f. K) "seeing only what has happened in the manner of a lay person".[81]

The same superiority of the expert, who cannot be fooled, over the layman appears in Plutarch's *Dion* (XXXIV.4f.), to my knowledge the only example of forensic medical expertise in classical literature.[82] Several unnamed *iatroi* examine a wound in order to give a verdict on whether it was caused by an attack or self-inflicted, and are able to conclude from certain characteristics of the wound that it was the latter. Here we have a clear case of expertise being used to obtain knowledge which is not accessible

---

[78] τοῖσιν ἰητροῖσι μούνοισι ἐστιν εἰδέναι, καὶ οὐ τοῖς ἰδιώτῃσιν. οὐ γὰρ σώματος, ἀλλὰ γνώμης ἐστὶν ἔργα.

[79] The fragments of the commentary were published by Daremberg (1848).

[80] Surviving only in an Arabic translation, translated into German by Meyerhof (1931).

[81] τὰ γιγνόμενα μόνον βλέπειν ἰδιωτικῶς.

[82] In Demosthenes, 54.10-12, the doctor who sutured the assault victim's wound is merely called as a witness.

to the layman. (Note, however, that again Plutarch appears to know these characteristics as well as the doctors involved.)

It appears from our numerous examples that there was a conscious effort on both sides to stress the difference between expert and layman, the reason varying according to which definition the respective author saw appropriate for himself. The medical experts preferred to stress their expertise in order to give their authority firm grounding, probably both in their dealings with their patients and in their stance against other types of practitioners. Much of this emphasis on expertise may indeed have been rhetoric deployed in order to cover a certain insecurity concerning the doctor's position in society. As for the laymen, it will have been preferable for them to emphasise the amateur character of their involvement as more becoming to themselves as members of a literate élite.

2. *Medical terminology*

The investigation into the general proliferation of medical knowledge leads to the next issue, namely how this knowledge was expressed - in writing, for that is all on which we can give a verdict. In the case of anatomy and surgery in particular the written word was likely to become a restrictive element, given that teaching would have been preponderantly by demonstration. Some passages reflect the author's struggle to represent in writing something that could be understood easily if demonstrated - and that would normally be demonstrated rather than explained. Wilamowitz[83] admires the "intellectual labour and linguistic training" making the description of fractures, dislocations and surgical operations in the Hippocratic Corpus possible, but it is one of these very authors who points out the difficulty of written description (*Art.* XXXIII/IV.148 L): "... for it is not easy to describe the entire surgical treatment in writing",[84] he writes halfway through the instructions for the treatment of a broken jaw, as if suddenly exasperated with his task. The subsequent instructions for bandaging are indeed not obvious at first sight.

One can distinguish between three categories of description which appear to suffer in particular from the limitations of written expression: 1) that of the visual aspect of an object, especially a

---

[83] (1912), p. 99.
[84] ἀλλὰ γὰρ οὐ ῥηίδιον ἐν γραφῇ χειρουργίην πᾶσαν διηγεῖσθαι.

surgical instrument in our case; 2) of the consistency of a substance, e.g. a drug; and 3) of a surgical technique.

In *De Anat. Admin.* (VIII/II.682f. K), Galen describes a type of knife which he himself has made (or probably designed) and which he calls πρόμηκες μαχαίριον, i.e. 'elongated [small] knife'. It is "thicker than the *skolopomachairia*" and "has two sharp sides coming together into one point at the tip".[85] The description appears unequivocal at first reading, but it gives no details on the length or width of the instrument nor on the angle at which the blades meet, and it is doubtful whether the reader would recognise the instrument if he saw one, or distinguish it from similar knives.

The ambiguity of the written word is even more evident in Celsus' description of the 'spoon of Diocles' (VII.5.3B/309.20f.), which has given rise to fanciful reconstructions.[86] Here again the apparent clarity of the sentences is deceptive. Its first part is fairly unambiguous: "An iron, or also bronze, blade has on one end two hooks turned backwards on both sides ...".[87] However, the second half is less so: "At the other end it is turned up on the sides and slightly inclined at the end towards that side which is concave, and furthermore there it is also perforated ..."[88] As mentioned in Ch. 2.3.3, it had appeared that an instrument in the Meyer-Steineg collection was such a 'spoon', and it fits the description very well. While it was considered genuine, it seemed that its shape had always been the obvious answer, but the text on its own is not that unequivocal. Thus *inclinata* could refer to an angle rather than a curve, and neither does *sinuata* tell the reader anything about the depth of the concavity nor does *perforata* inform him about the shape and size of the perforation. Nor does Celsus ever mention the overall size of the instrument. Other examples for the descriptions of instruments in written texts are the 'Hippocratic bench' (*Mochl.* 38/IV.384f. L), the *diôstêr* (Paul VI.88.3/II.131.20) and the 'instrument the shape of the Greek letter' (Celsus VII.5.2B/309.6f.), which could be the shape of any one of several letters.[89]

---

[85] καὶ μέντοι καὶ παχύτερον τῶν σκολοπομαχαιρίων ... δύο πλευρὰς ὀξείας ἔχον ἐπὶ τοῦ πέρατος εἰς μίαν κορυφὴν ἀνηκούσας.

[86] The translator of the Loeb edition, W. G. Spencer, was led to disregard the text in his certainty of what the instrument looked like.

[87] *Lammina vel ferrea vel aenea etiam ab altero capite duo utrimque deorsum converso uncos habet ...*

[88] *ab altero duplicata lateribus, leviterque extrema in eam partem inclinata, qua sinuata est, insuper ibi etiam perforata est..*

[89] See Jackson (1991), who opts for 'Y', identifying the instrument as a bivalve speculum, a suggestion also made by Garnerus (1979)

The consistence of a substance, a drug for example, is another concept which is hard to express unambiguously in writing. Thus Celsus (VI.6.38/274.16f.) writes of a mixture of ground purslane seeds and honey that one should add honey "until the mixture no longer drops from a probe"[90] and Scribonius Largus (CCXL) recommends applying a remedy to ulcers with a probe that is dipped into it and to which "the mixture adheres almost like dust".[91] Similar phrases can also be found in the Hippocratic Corpus, referring to excretions or pathological alterations. The author of *Morb.*, e.g., uses the following comparisons to visualise what he wants to describe: at II.47/VII.72 L he describes pus as being "like gruel" (λεκιθοειδές),[92] at II.49/VII.74 L as being "like a knot or lump" (οἷον χάλαζα)[93] and at III/VII.146 L he compares a "bubble" (i.e. a blister) appearing on the tongue in pleurisy to those created when "dipping a [red-hot] iron into oil".[94] In *Aff. Int.* (I /VII.166 L) the scales torn from the trachea by coughing are compared to those coming from pustules.[95]

When it comes to the description of surgical skills, the handicap caused by having to explain them in writing is particularly obvious. The written instructions would be superfluous to those who have seen a practical demonstration - as Galen says in *De Anat. Admin.* (II.628 K): "For those who have seen me operate [lit.: cut], there will be no need for long discourses, but as for those who did not see it, for those it is necessary to say this."[96] This sentence introduces a detailed description of vivisection involving opening of the thoracic cavity, beginning with instructions on how to deal with the haemorrhage. As soon as you first see the blood spurting from the artery, he says, you must

> having finished the downward incision, turn the scalpel as quickly as possible to the position of the tranverse cut - as has been said - and with the two fingers of the left hand, i.e. the index and the thumb, grasp that part of the sternum where you can see the haemorrhaging artery, so that at the same time one finger becomes a cover for the

---

[90] *eatenus ne id ex specillo destillet.*
[91] *quod ei quasi pulvis adhaeserit.*
[92] This meaning appears to be more plausible than "like egg-yolk" as suggested by Littré.
[93] Again Littré's translation "like hail" seems less convincing.
[94] οἷα σιδηρίου βαφέντος ἐν ἐλαίῳ.
[95] λεπίδας ἀπὸ τῆς ἀρτηρίης ἀποβήσσων ἀποσπᾷ, οἵας περ ἀπὸ φλυκταινιδίων.
[96] τοῖς μὲν ἑωρακόσιν ἐμὲ τέμνοντα οὐ μακρῶν δεήσει λόγων. ὅσοι δ ' οὐκ εἶδον, ἐκείνοις εἰπεῖν ἀναγκαῖον, ...

orifice and both fingers have a sure grip on the entire bone (ib. 628f.).⁹⁷

Here the account is sufficiently visual to be understood without a practical demonstration, but, for example, the author of *Haem.*(VI.440 L) has to resort to a comparison. Discussing the removal of a condyloma, he writes: "for it is no more difficult than to pass [lit.:penetrate] the finger between the skin and the flesh of a sheep which is being skinned".⁹⁸ (This passage also seems to suggest that the author expects his audience to have had the personal experience of skinning a sheep, or at least to have watched the skinning of a sheep.)

The difficulty of writing clear instructions is even more obvious in a lengthy - and rather puzzling - passage, in *Off.* (III.278-82 L). The author depicts the correct way for the doctor to sit and stand while examining or treating his patients - a straightforward topic and an action which could easily be demonstrated, but which can barely be understood through the smoke-screen of writing. Galen's commentaries (XVIII.B.694-700 K) on the passages in question suggest that they were far from clear even for his contemporaries.

One particularly good example of a relatively simple technique requiring extensive explanation - in the absence of diagrams - is Celsus' description of a two-handed suture for abdominal wounds, holding a needle in each hand (VII.16.4f./333.26-334.2):

> Therefore thread is to be passed through two needles and they are to be held in both hands [i.e. one in each hand]; and first the stitches are to be inserted into the inner membrane in such a way that the left hand conveys the needle through the right margin, the right hand through the left margin, beginning from the end of the wound, from the inside towards the outside. ... When each margin has been pierced once, the needles are to be changed between the hands, so that the needle which had been in the left hand is in the right hand and the needle which the right hand had been holding comes into the left hand; ...⁹⁹

---

⁹⁷ τελευτώσης ἤδη τῆς κατάντους τομῆς, ἐπιστρέφειν μὲν ὅτι τάχιστα τὴν σμίλην εἰς ἐγκαρσίου τομῆς σχῆμα, καθ' ὅτι λέλεκται, τῆς δ' ἀριστερᾶς χειρὸς τοῖς δύο δακτύλοις, λιχανῷ τε καὶ μεγάλῳ, περιλαμβάνειν τοῦ στέρνου τὸ μέρος ἐκεῖνο, καθ' ὃ τὴν ἀρτηρίαν αἱμορραγοῦσαν ὁρᾶτε, ἵν' ἅμα μὲν ἐπίθημα στόματος ὁ ἕτερος ᾖ δάκτυλος, ἅμα δ' ἀσφαλὴς ἐξ ἀμφοῖν γίγνηται λαβὴ τοῦ παντὸς ὀστοῦ.

⁹⁸ οὐδὲν γὰρ χαλεπώτερον ἤπερ προβάτου δειρομένου τὸν δάκτυλον μεταξὺ τοῦ δέρματος καὶ τῆς σαρκὸς περαίνειν.

⁹⁹ *Igitur in duas acus fila coicienda, eaque duabus manibus tenendae; et prius interiori membranae sutura inicienda est sic, ut sinistra manus in dexteriore ora, in sinisteriore dextra a principio vulneris orsa ab interiore parte in exteriorem acum mittat. ... semel utraque parte traiecta, permutandae acus inter manus sunt, ut ea sit in dextra, quae fuit in sinistra; ea veniat in sinistram, quam dextra continuit; ...*

More examples can be found both in Greek authors (e.g. Galen's instructions for abdominal sutures, mentioned in Ch. 2.3.4) and in Celsus and it is not surprising that Soranus' *De fasciis* was illustrated, since otherwise it would have been nearly impossible to apply a dressing following his instructions.

Lonie[100] suggests that with the advent of literacy doctors were "among the first to see certain advantages in prose writing and to make systematic use of it in their craft", and that literate form modifies the information it conveys.[101] This can certainly be said for writings concerning medical theory and 'lists', based on a subjective decision on what was relevant and worth recording - the *Epidemics* in particular. In the case of anatomy and surgery, however, a particular set of information had to be conveyed, and the teaching received at the other end of the line of information had to be the same whatever the means of communication.[102] This made those fields not so easily adaptable to diffusion by writing and what Galen says regarding the differences in pulses (VIII.678 K) applies very well to surgical techniques: "If it cannot be said but can be shown, then do not write anything about it, but only show us the thing."[103] As far as the layman was concerned, although surgical treatises were physically available, they would have been less accessible than, e.g., writings on medical theories or on pharmacology, and their teachings could only be applied if they were joined to practical training.[104]

Besides a few glimpses of non-literary transmission of medicine, all our sources are literary and therefore medical writing is what we have to focus on. We tend to expect medical writing to differ in style and terminology from works of 'literature' such as the writings of philosophers, historians and poets, but it has to be examined if this difference can be found in antiquity, too.

When Thucydides (VII.15.1) speaks of Nikias suffering from *nephritis*, Irigoin[105] assumes that it is a term "borrowed from

---

[100] (1983) p. 147.

[101] Ib., p. 154. Pigeaud (1988), p. 324, puts it more strongly: "Coming back to Hippocrates, it is quite correct to say that writing is the founder of medicine."

[102] This is not to say that medical books played an important part in medical training, the bulk of which rested on apprenticeship. On medical education, see Kudlien (1970). Cf. Aristotle (*EN* 1181b2ff.), who writes that one does not become a physician by reading medical writings (συγγράμματα).

[103] εἴπερ ἐστὶν ἄρρητος μὲν, δεικτὸς δὲ, μηδὲν μὲν γράφων ὑπὲρ αὐτοῦ, δεικνὺς δὲ μόνον ἡμῖν τὸ πρᾶγμα.

[104] It would be useful to compare surgical writings with treatises on other non-literary crafts, such as horsemanship or tactics, in order to determine whether the same difficulties are apparent in all of them.

[105] (1988), p. 249.

medical vocabulary", but this presupposes the existence of a 'medical vocabulary' - as opposed to everyday language - as a given fact. The medical terminology of modern (Western) languages consists almost entirely of words derived from Greek or Latin, but the Greeks at least had to use the resources of their own language.[106]

If one looks at the words used, e.g., for anatomical nomenclature or names of diseases, it becomes clear that they are often originally straightforward popular terms used metaphorically.[107] Terms such as πῦρ (pyr), πύρετος (pyretos), θέρμη (thermê) and καῦσος (kausos) for fever only describe the symptoms in everyday language and would initially have been understood by everybody, the same as *nephritis* or *pleuritis* would have been, the suffix *-itis* being used only in the vague sense of 'disease of' or 'trouble with'.

This was evidently a common situation for words used in medical texts, if one is to believe Galen. In *On the [Critical] Times in Diseases /De morborum temporibus [Morb. Temp.]*, VII.417f. K, after a discussion of the terms for different cycles of tertian fevers, he explains how medical terms are formed, namely that there is

> something like a law, common to all Greeks, for those things for which we have names given by the ancients, to use those. For the things for which we do not have them, to transfer [*metapherein*] from something for which we have them, or to make them up by some analogy with things that are named, or to make use of [*katachrêsthai*][108] the names belonging to other things.[109]

This outline of the creation of medical terms - another fruit of Galen's interest in linguistic problems - reflects very well the way the process worked in reality, as far as we can judge from our sources. There are numerous examples in Galen for the authority of the 'ancients'. Thus, to quote but one of them, in *Morb. Temp.* (VII.414 K), Galen speaks of the absence of fever [*apyrexia*], "which shall be called intermission [*dialeimma*] by us, because

---

[106] Of the scholars who have touched upon the subject, Wilamowitz (1912, p. 99), Cadbury (1919, pp. 53f.) and Skoda (1988, preface) agree that there was a medical terminology in Greek, while Nutton (1988a, p. 31) opts for the absence of a specifically medical terminology.
[107] Cf. Lloyd, (1987), p.203
[108] According to *Comp. Med.* III (XIII.573 K), *katachrêsis* in a linguistic context appears to be a specialist term used by grammarians.
[109] καθάπερ τις νόμος ἐστὶ κοινὸς ἅπασι τοῖς Ἕλλησιν, ὧν μὲν ἂν ἔχωμεν ὀνόματα πραγμάτων παρὰ τοῖς πρεσβυτέροις εἰρημένα, χρῆσθαι τούτοις· ὧν δ' οὐκ ἔχομεν, ἤτοι μεταφέρειν ἀπό τινος ὧν ἔχομεν ἢ ποιεῖν αὐτοὺς κατὰ ἀναλογίαν τινὰ τὴν πρὸς τὰ κατωνομασμένα τῶν πραγμάτων, ἢ καὶ καταχρῆσθαι τοῖς ἐφ' ἑτέρων κειμένοις.

Hippocrates named it thus".[110] In a passage in *De Anat. Admin.* (II.682 K), on the other hand, Galen is obviously not basing his nomenclature on earlier authors, when he says of the aforementioned type of scalpel called πρόμηκες μαχαίριον (elongated knife) "thus I call it". As so often, the passage continues with a criticism of the more recent doctors, who disregard linguistic conventions. (His argument that one has to agree with these doctors in order to avoid their garrulity, because they are "aggressive and shameless", remains unconvincing in view of his own behaviour in confrontations with other doctors).

The word generally used for technical terms is *onomata* (ὀνόματα) - names -which is also used in other cases where we would speak of terminology, but one cannot say that the meaning of the term was anything like the modern concept of terminology. It was rather a very vague and general expression, also used for names of objects (and, of course, proper names), which makes one wonder whether there actually was a concept of specialist terminology as opposed to common language. The word *onomata* was almost certainly used in the title of the treatise translated from the Arabic as *Über die medizinischen Namen* [*Med. N.*] by Meyerhof and Schacht, and it also featured in titles of other lost Galenic works. Thus in *Libr. Propr.* (XIX.43 K) we find such titles as παρὰ 'Αριστοφάνει πολιτικῶν ὀνομάτων, τῶν παρὰ Κρατίνῳ πολιτικῶν ὀνομάτων or τῶν ἰδίων κωμικῶν ὀνομάτων παραδείγματα. Rufus also uses the same word in *Onom.* 6 (p.134), where he states that one should begin the study of medicine by learning the 'names', first of all those of the parts of the body - the exact opposite of what Galen says in *Med.N.* *Onomata* is also the word used in the *Index* of Iulius Polydeuces, who has a chapter (IV.171) περὶ ἰατρικῶν ὀνομάτων ('On medical names'), containing such words as κένωσις (emptying), κρίσιμος (the adjective of *krisis*) and ἴσχαιμα (haemostatics), and a separate one περὶ ἰατρικῶν ὀργαλείων ('On medical instruments'). Apparently for him surgical instruments are not part of the 'medical names'. Other authors never explicitly exclude instruments when speaking of words 'used by the doctors', but they never include them either, so it may well be that the term *iatrika onomata* was only used for anatomical details, for names of diseases and perhaps for surgical techniques.

The reality of these terms corresponds largely to the explanation given by Galen (VII.417f. K). Many of the words

---

[110] ἥτις ἡμῖν καλείσθω διάλειμμα, διότι καὶ ὁ 'Ιπποκράτες οὕτως ὠνόμασεν [for Kühn's ὠνόμασιν].

used in medical, especially anatomical, contexts are words that had been in use for some time, although in some cases the references had changed in the course of time. Although Homeric Greek already had a fairly rich - if imprecise - anatomical vocabulary, the existing vocabulary became insufficient with anatomical discoveries, especially in Hellenistic times, and new terms had to be forged.[111]

According to Irigoin,[112] two thirds of the anatomical terms used in *Loc. Hom.* (about one hundred) had been known to Homer already, albeit three of them with a different reference. Half of the remaining third appear in lyrical poetry, especially in Archilochus, and in Herodotus. Not all the remaining words are neologisms, some of them - e.g. νέφροι (kidneys) and πλεύμονες (lungs) - being very ancient words, their age reflecting, among other things, the importance of the viscera in sacrifice and divination. Although these are interesting results, the choice of Hippocratic treatise has certainly influenced the outcome. The ratio would be quite different if one were to chose one of the surgical or gynaecological treatises, where most of the terminology would not appear in non-medical authors writing earlier than the fifth century BC, either because it was unknown or simply because it was not needed for the topic they wanted to treat.

Thus the absence of a word in the extant sources does not prove that it was not yet in use and one should abstain from rash decisions on the age of a particular word or of a meaning for it. An example from Celsus should serve as a warning. At VII.7.10/318.17 he writes that a certain condition of the eyelid is called *ectropion* by the Greeks, but the earliest extant medical author using this word in the same sense is Galen (XIX.439 K).[113] Although this is only one example, it should draw attention to the fragmentary character of our evidence and the conjectural nature of conclusions based on this evidence.

The flexible nature of the language offers many possibilities for the creation of new words or expressions in Greek. Some of the nouns in anatomical terminology are formed by attaching suffixes, such as μυκτήρ (nostril) from the verb μύσσομαι (blowing one's nose), others are descriptive compositions like ἐπιγάστριον (the covering of the abdominal cavity from thorax to pubes, literally 'on the stomach') or ἀντικάρδιον (the hollow

---

[111] Cf. Irigoin (1988), pp. 247ff.; Roura (1972), on the semantic persistence of some terms which become more specific in the Hippocratic Corpus; Leumann (1950) on Homeric words in the Hippocratic Corpus.
[112] Ib., p. 249.
[113] Cf. Spencer's note on this passage in the Loeb edition.

above the clavicle, literally 'against the heart/cardiac orifice'). Adjectives formed by attaching the suffix -*eidês* are frequent: ἀραχνοειδής ('spider/cobweb-like'), κερατοειδής ('horn-like') or βελονοειδής ('needle-like'), to name but a few. Some terms are descriptive expressions such as κοίλη φλέψ ('hollow vein'; the vena cava), but many are metaphorical expressions based on familiar objects; κάλαμος ('reed'; the shin or also a type of splint) or στεφάνη ('crown'; the rim of the cornea) would be examples of this category.

In his book *Ptolemaic Alexandria*,[114] Fraser claims that Herophilus was the pioneer of medical terminology. While this is a rather bold sweeping statement, it is true for some of the anatomical vocabulary. The best-known example may be the duodenum, of which Galen explicitly says in *De Anat. Admin.* (II.780 K): "... the attachment called duodenum by Herophilus. So he calls the beginning of the bowel".[115] At VIII.396 K. he explains the reason for this name: "applying to it the name derived from its length"[116] - another example of one of the ways of creating new names, namely by a descriptive expression. Again according to Galen, Herophilus apparently also named the procedure of removing the upmost layer of tissue in dissection *darsis*.[117] In this case the new word was formed from the well-known verb δέρω ('to skin' or 'flay') and its approximate meaning would have been understood by most Greeks, but it appears to have been used first by Herophilus in this specific sense.

In general anatomical terms have the advantage of being easier to trace back and date than other words used in medical writing, as the great majority of them originated in Hellenistic times. The terminology for the internal anatomy of the human body used by the writers in the Hippocratic Corpus had been more or less restricted to the major organs, e.g. καρδία (heart, but also used for the stomach), ἧπαρ (liver), κύστις (bladder), etc., and therefore, when previously unknown anatomical structures were discovered, a new vocabulary had to be created for them. The means for these new creations were mainly description, such as ὑαλοειδής χιτών ('glass-like membrane'), and metaphor, for example ληνός ('wine-vat', for what is now called the torcular Herophili).

In the case of names of diseases and surgical techniques the development is less easy to follow and there appears to be a

---

[114] (1972), vol. I, p. 354.
[115] τὴν δωδεκαδάκτυλον ὑπὸ Ἡροφίλου καλουμένην ἔκφυσιν. ὀνομάζει δ' οὕτως ἐκεῖνος τὴν ἀρχὴν τοῦ ἐντέρου.
[116] ἀπὸ τοῦ μήκους αὐτῷ τὴν ἐπωνυμίαν θέμενος.
[117] II.349 K: κατὰ δάρσιν, ὡς Ἡρόφιλος ὠνόμαζεν.

gradual increase. It would appear that the new discoveries in anatomy also widened the horizon of surgery and that therefore its vocabulary had to be expanded, but the lack of extant Greek authors writing on surgery between the Hippocratics and Galen makes it difficult to trace the appearance of new terms. Celsus' occasional references to "X as the Greeks call it" shows that by his time a far greater variety of terms was in use than we can see in the extant works of the Hippocratic Corpus. The situation is similar when it comes to surgical instruments: other than the implements and levers used for the reduction of fractures and dislocations, the Hippocratic writings mention little more than scalpels, probes, cauteries, catheters, specula and needles. The range becomes more varied in Celsus, and in Galen there appears to be a fine differentiation between different types of instruments (e.g. II.682.f. K; ib. 686).

Some highly inventive expressions can be found among the qualifiers for different types of pulse movements, ulcers or pain, often with very little actual link between the word and the reference. This group of adjectives in particular gives an idea of the imaginative nature of the associated ideas in the creation of metaphors in Greek. The most striking examples are probably to be found in the range of vocabulary used for different types of pulse movement; some of the most frequently used are παρεμπίπτων ('broken'), δίκροτος ('with a double beat'), μυρμηκίζων ('moving like an ant'), δορκαδίζων ('moving like a deer') and σκωληκίζων ('moving like a worm'). The line of thought leading to the creation of the first and the second term is straightforward and easy to follow, but not so much for the other three. One can imagine (although perhaps the layman was not meant to) the basic difference between a pulse that 'moves like a deer' and one that 'moves like a worm', but it is difficult to see what distinguishes the latter from one that 'moves like an ant', given that the reference always has to be a pulsating sensation. It would probably not have been more difficult to create words with a more obvious meaning and it is unlikely that the aforementioned terms were sufficiently evocative to be understood without practical demonstration and without an underlying pulse law, which had become highly complicated and controversial by Galen's time.

In the case of some terms used for different types of ulcers and of pain it can equally be said that they were not self-explanatory and were most likely a core of expressions used only by the doctors. Thus patients were unlikely to complain about their pain being ἑλκώδης ('like a sore'), ἐνερείδων ('thrusting'), σφακελώδης ('like gangrene') or νυγματώδης ('like pricking'): these are only a few of the adjectives used by Galen (*Loc. Aff.* VIII.92 K). It may well be that these terms were coined with an intentional obscurity built into them in order to create some kind of medical language that would not be understood by everyone. The same could be said about the desire to create separate expressions for every variety of fracture, criticised by Galen (*MM* X.424 K). It is tempting to see a parallel between this growing profusion of terms and the trend towards polypharmacy in late antiquity, perhaps as an attempt to make medicine more prestigious and less accessible.

Along with a particular vocabulary one would also expect a style of writing peculiar to medical writings, but there is little evidence for this on a large scale. The single medical authors differ too much between themselves to allow for an overall similarity in style, although there may have been certain styles for certain types of writing, e.g. the books of the *Epidemics* or the *Aphorisms*.[118] One must also keep in mind that some authors (e.g. Oribasius) quote others verbatim - not always acknowledging it - and are therefore bound to take over the other author's style in that passage.

This assumption is the basis of Wellmann's[119] hypothesis that most of Celsus' work is a translation and that one can distinguish between the translated text and Celsus' interpolation by the difference in style. Senn[120] makes a similar claim concerning some of the Hippocratic texts. According to him the descriptions of experiments can be distinguished from those of experiences made in everyday life by means of their style. His conclusion is that therefore the experiments must have been copied from an earlier treatise. These two hypotheses cannot be proved beyond doubt, and it is also clear that style was more a matter related to the individual or a small group of writers than to a whole literary genre. The main difference between exclusively medical writings and other types of literature remained the content and often the purpose for which they were written and would be read. In Ch. 1 I have quoted Galen's remark (*De Anat. Admin.*/II.393 K) that one should not read his book as one would read Herodotus, for the sake of enjoyment, but rather with the intention of learning its contents. However, Erotian (frgm.18/p.105) appears to have a

---

[118] Cf., for example, Redondo (1992) on rhetorical forms in the Hippocratic Corpus; Nutton (1991) on Galen's *MM* and Langholf (1990) on the *Epidemics*.
[119] (1913), mentioned above.
[120] (1929), p. 221.

different opinion on Herodotus' authority and usefulness, when he quotes both 'Hippocrates' and Herodotus to support his own explanation of the word *sphakelizô* - appearing to attribute to both authors equal value as evidence.

It may be a logical consequence of the apparent freedom in creating new words or expressions[121] that one can observe a high degree of indecision and disagreement concerning medical terminology. Despite assertive statements such as "as we doctors call it", the situation is often close to being chaotic. Not only is there often a shift in denotation over time, but also within the same time period there is little agreement on the use of certain terms and no one was able to impose a standard - or perhaps, to be more accurate, nobody attempted to.

The indecision occurs on different levels. One is that of a general conceptual vagueness, illustrated by the example of *pepsis* (πέψις) by G. E. R. Lloyd:

> As a portmanteau concept, it *both* enables a variety of different processes to be related and brought under the scope of a single theory, *and* it pays a price for this in the indeterminacy of the theory and a corresponding lack, at many points, of predictive or explanatory power.[122]

This is true also for other words used to express medical concepts, the possibility of semantic stretch proving both an advantage and a handicap.

On a different level various types of fluctuation made the meaning of words hard to pin down. One of these was a shift in denotation, as it happened with *neuron* (νεῦρον), *helkos* (ἕλκος) or *phrenes* (φρένες). In these three cases the reference of the term changed over time. In the first case this was once again influenced by new discoveries in the field of anatomy, namely the discovery of the sensory nerves. The use of a single term to cover a range of references with similar characteristics - in this case the elastic, 'stringy', aspect - is a common phenomenon in the language used in medical writing, as for example *chitôn* (χιτών, the common word for 'tunic') used for pleura (e.g. *On the Opinions of Hippocrates and Plato / De placitis Hippocratis et Platonis* [*PHP.*] 8/V.715 K), a membrane covering the eye (*VM* 19/I.616 L) or a membrane containing pus in empyema of the liver (*Aph.* VII.45/IV.590 L), because of a visual association. Even in later

---

[121] E.g. *Oss.*, II.745 K: "In that place there is also the styloid process, which I call needle-like and *graphoeidês* ['stylus-like']." (ἐν τούτῳ καὶ ἡ στυλοειδὴς ἀπόφυσίς ἐστιν, ἥν ἐγὼ βελονοειδῆ καὶ γραφοειδῆ καλῶ.)
[122] (1987), p. 206.

writings, however, *neuron* is not used for 'nerve' exclusively, but occasionally it can still mean 'sinew' or 'tendon'.

Helkos is the word used for a fresh wound in the *Iliad*, e.g. at XI.267, XVI.511, or XXIV.420 (however, Homer never speaks of ulcers,[123] so we cannot tell what word he would have used), along with *ôteilê* (ὠτειλή: e.g. XI.266, IV.140, XVI.862), whereas the word *trauma* (τραῦμα) appears to be unknown before the fifth century. In the Hippocratic writings τραῦμα/τρώμα is beginning to appear for the reference 'wound', as can be seen in the titles of *On Wounds in the Head* (Περὶ τῶν ἐν κεφαλῇ τρωμάτων) and the now lost *On Wounds and Arrows* (Περὶ τραυμάτων καὶ βελῶν). However, the reference of *helkos* is still ambiguous.[124] Thus the treatise *Peri helkôn* (Περὶ ἑλκῶν; *Ulc.*) mainly describes the treatment of wounds and, explaining a passage from this treatise, Erotian writes (frgm.47/p.113) that *helkea* 'now' (i.e. in this passage or in his time?) means fresh wounds, while in Περὶ τραυμάτων καὶ βελῶν it meant chronic wounds or ulcers. *Aph.* appears to use both words to mean wound, for example at V.2/IV.532 L - "A convulsion supervening upon a wound: deadly." (ἐπὶ τρώματι σπασμὸς ἐπιγενόμενος, θανάσιμον) - or in two consecutive aphorisms: V.65/IV.558 L: "those cases in which swellings appear on the wounds do not get strong convulsions" (ὁκόσοισιν οἰδήματα ἐθ' ἕλκεσι φαίνεται, οὐ μάλα σπῶνται ...) and ib. 66 (IV.560 L): "when the wounds are grievous and painful and swellings do not appear [on them]: a great evil." (ἢν τραυμάτων ἰσχυρῶν ἐόντων καὶ πονηρῶν οἰδήματα μὴ φαίνηται, μέγα κακόν. However, at VI.8/IV.564 L, where the author speaks of *helkea* appearing on patients suffering from dropsy, the word clearly means ulcer, as it does in *On the Sacred Disease* [*Morb. Sacr.*: VI.370 L]. Later writers consistently use *trauma* for 'wound'[125] and *helkos* for 'ulcer',[126] so that one can definitely speak of a shift of reference over time.

As for *phrenes*, Onians[127] argues that in Homeric Greek it is a synonym for πλεύμονες (lungs), basing his fairly convincing argument on the aspect of the diaphragm which does not agree with the description, the fact that the term *phrenes* is plural, and on

---

[123] With the possible exception of *Il.* II.723, where he speaks of Philoctetes "suffering with a bad wound/ulcer" (ἕλκει μοχθίζοντα κακῷ).
[124] On its shift in meaning, cf. Wöhrle (1991).
[125] E.g. Soranus, *Gyn.*I.36.6/26.4 or *Fract.*15/157.17; Galen I.239 K, XVIII.B.568 K; Aetius VII.24./II.271.
[126] Sor.*Gyn.* III.36/116.18, ib. II.53/90.17; Galen XIII.668 K, XVIII.B.548 K; Aetius VIII.49/I.476.
[127] (1951). For the full argument, see pp. 23-40.

several passages in which the *phrenes* are wounded. They are "holding the liver" (*Od.* ix.301), the part behind them is between the shoulders (*Il.* V.40f., VIII.258f., XVI.806f., etc.), and when Patroklos pulls his spear out of Sarpedon's chest, the *phrenes* prolapse (*Il.* XVI.504), all of which makes far more sense if we assume that Homer is thinking of the lungs.[128] At the same time the *phrenes* are also the organ of consciousness, the seat of thoughts and emotions, and the two uses of the word obviously continue side by side. One of a great number of examples for this second reference would be the frequently used phrase (e.g. *Il.* XVI.851):"... put that well into your mind" (σὺ δ' ἐνὶ φρεσὶ βάλλεο σῆσιν).

By the time the word is used by the Hippocratic writers, its anatomical object of reference has obviously shifted to the diaphragm, e.g. in *VM* 22 (I.634 L) or in Plato (*Ti.*70a). The latter passage appears to be the oldest one to use the word *diaphragma* (διάφραγμα) in an anatomical context, but it is used as an explanation of *phrenes* rather than as a technical term: "... putting the diaphragm as a subdivision between them".[129] Aristotle (*PA* 672b), who uses the word *diazôma* (διάζωμα), reports that the diaphragm is also called *phrenes* "as having a part in thinking [*phronein*]",[130] whereas, he emphasises, in reality they have no part in the thinking process. In this reasoning he follows the author of *Morb. Sacr.* - although this need not mean that Aristotle had actually read any of the Hippocratic writings - who declares (VI.392 L) that the *phrenes* have obtained their name by coincidence and by custom, but not from reality or nature.

Other factors of indeterminacy are: 1) the use of a variety of terms for one reference, e.g. *phrenes*, *diaphragma*, *diazôma* or *hypozôma* for the diaphragm, the different names for the retina (Rufus, *Anat.* 15), or the variety of terms used for the uterus according to Soranus (I.3.6/6.13: *mêtra*, *hystera*, *delphys*); 2) a variety of references for one word, such as the aforementioned *neuron*, *kardia* or *phleps*, and 3) a combination or overlap of the two. This is the case, for example, again with *neuron*, which can have the references 'nerve', 'sinew' or 'tendon' and which in the latter case is a synonym for *tenôn*. *Phleps* presents the same

---

[128] The last passage on its own would still leave open the question whether the poet knew that the diaphragm was not likely to prolapse, but in combination with the other evidence it corroborates Onian's thesis (in which he follows Justesen [1928]). Cf. also Ireland/Steel (1975), who suggest (p. 194) that the term might refer to a group of organs rather than any one particular organ.

[129] τὰς φρένας διάφραγμα εἰς τὸ μέσον αὐτῶν τιθέντες.

[130] ὡς μετέχουσαί τι τοῦ φρονεῖν.

difficulty, as it can be used to mean any type of vessel in the body, transporting blood, *pneuma,* milk or semen, and it can, in some cases, be substituted by *angeion* or *artêria.*

It can furthermore be observed that in some cases the term was changed following a shift in associated ideas (e.g. *phrenes*), but in other cases the old term was kept although the reasoning upon which it was based was no longer valid. An example of the latter can be seen in the *karôtides* (καρωτίδες). In *PHP* I (V.195 K) Galen explains that the pair of large arteries "... is not correctly called *karôtides,* but the name has already been established because of the great lack of understanding of all philosophers, and even doctors, after Hippocrates".[131] Having promised to explain in the second book that it is wrong to think that *karos* (κάρος), stupefaction, is an affliction of these arteries, he continues: "But in the present discourse I shall not begrudge the arteries the name, but let them still be called *karôtides* even now".[132]

The confusion and uncertainty is by no means a phenomenon that started in post-Alexandrian times. Within about a century of the youngest works in the Hippocratic Corpus the first commentaries on the Corpus began to appear - according to Erotian (31/p. 4) written by both doctors and grammarians (the latter out of linguistic interest, regarding, e.g., 'Hippocrates" use of dialect): "Many famous men, not only doctors but also grammarians, made efforts to explicate the man and to lead his words towards a more common usage."[133] We have to keep in mind that one can assume a variety of motivations for making the works of the Hippocratics an object of research, including the construction of a canon of medical writings, and a strong philological interest among the 'grammarians'. However, even so it is obvious that the writings in the Hippocratic Corpus presented difficulties of comprehension soon after they were written - or perhaps even at the time when they were written.

The difficulties are not limited to a vocabulary which would require specialist knowledge of the field for understanding - names of bones[134] or of categories of fevers, for example - but

---

[131] οὐκ ὀρθῶς μὲν ὀνομάζονται καρωτίδες, ἀλλ' ἤδη κρατεῖ τοὔνομα διὰ τὴν πολλὴν ἄνοιαν ἁπάντων μεθ' 'Ιπποκράτην φιλοσόφων τε καὶ ἰατρῶν.

[132] ἐν δὲ τῷ παρόντι λόγῳ τοῦ γε ὀνόματος οὐ φθονήσω ταῖς ἀρτηρίαις, ἀλλ' ὀνομαζέσθωσαν ἔτι καὶ νῦν καρωτίδες.

[133] πολλοὶ τῶν ἐλλογίμων οὐκ ἰατρῶν μόνον, ἀλλὰ καὶ γραμματικῶν ἐσπούδασαν ἐξηγήσασθαι τὸν ἄνδρα καὶ τὰς λέξεις ἐπὶ κοινότερον τῆς ὁμιλίας ἀγαγεῖν.

[134] On these, see Irmer (1980).

encompass seemingly straightforward terms such as *ôteilê, helkos, armena* (ἄρμενα) or even *thanasimon* (θανάσιμον). In fragment 46 (p. 113) Erotian claims that *ôteilê* usually means *oulê* (οὐλή; scar) and rarely *helkos*, that it is however used with both references in *Fract.*, but with the first only in *Art.*; it would seem that not even within the Hippocratic Corpus there was much unity in expression. Erotian disagrees with an earlier commentator, Baccheius, who had apparently said that *oulê* was a synonym for *helkos* and *trauma*, and who, according to Erotian, was misled by the Homeric use of the term. For *armena* Erotian suggests surgical instruments as a reference, making it a synonym of *ergaleia*, again disagreeing with Baccheius.

The seemingly unambiguous adjective *thanasimon* (fatal) would appear to be an unlikely candidate for semantic confusion, but in his *In Hipp. Aph.* Galen obviously felt the need to consecrate two paragraphs to an explanation of the word (XVII.B.785f. K). In the commentary on *Aph.V.2.*, "A convulsion supervening upon a wound: deadly.",[135] Galen states that here, as in the preceding aphorism, *thanasimon* means "dangerous, and often ending in death ... bringing about death, not necessarily and in every case, but very often".[136] Commenting on V.3., "Convulsion supervening when much blood has flown: bad.",[137] he explains that one should not assume that the *kakon* (bad) means anything different from the *thanasimon* in the preceding aphorism, and that this is how Hippocrates used to call those symptoms upon which death often follows. "If it seems that the words differ from each other by the greater or lesser degree", he writes, "the word *thanasimon* would be likely to show greater danger than *kakon*."[138] This explanation suggests deviation from ordinary word use, where *thanasimon* would simply be 'deadly'.

Di Benedetto[139] approaches the same problem regarding *thanatôdes* (θανατῶδες), which is the corresponding adjective used by the author of *Prognosis/Praenotiones [Prog.]*. Expressions like θανατῶδες σφόδρα ('vehemently fatal'),[140] with

---

[135] ἐπὶ τρώματι σπασμὸς ἐπιγενόμενος, θανάσιμον.
[136] κινδυνώδη τε καὶ τελευτῶντα πολλάκις εἰς θάνατον ... οὐκ ἐξ ἀνάγκης τε καὶ διὰ παντὸς ἐπιφέροντα θάνατον, ἀλλ᾽ ὡς πάνυ πολλάκις.
[137] αἵματος πολλοῦ ῥυέντος σπασμὸς ἐπιγενόμενος κακόν.
[138] εἰ δὲ τῷ μᾶλλον τε καὶ ἧττον ἀλλήλων δόξειεν τὰ ὀνόματα διαφέρειν, μείζονα τὸν κίνδυνον ἐνδείξαιτ᾽ ἂν ἡ θανάσιμον φωνὴ τῆς κακόν.
[139] (1966), pp. 333ff.
[140] The Littré edition, II.118 L, has λίην (excessively). It appears that Di Benedetto used the Loeb edition.

the similar expression ὀλέθριον κάρτα ('very pernicious') at II.122 L, or θανατωδέστερα ('deadlier'; II.138 L) and the statement that sneezing is good in "the other deadly diseases",[141] make it clear that the translation 'lethal' or 'deadly' is inappropriate. Di Benedetto, very much along Galen's line of thought, speaks of a "gradation of deadliness" and an indication of probability rather than certainty. The fact remains that, even with words for which the meaning was confirmed by common usage, the medical authors did not feel compelled to conform to it.

This anarchic state of affairs is not limited to anatomical and pathological vocabulary, but appears also in pharmacology: Dioscorides often lists different names used for the same plant,[142] frequently offering more than one alternative.[143] It would, however, appear that surgical instruments were an exception - and there may be some link between this fact and the aforementioned one that instruments were never mentioned among the *iatrika onomata*. Rare instruments such as the 'spoon of Diocles' were described, but most of the time instruments are only referred to by name (e.g. "using the X") - without providing synonyms or showing confusion about the reference - as would be normal for an object known to the reader. Some examples should illustrate the point: *Mochl.* XXXIII./IV.376 L: "...[for] the reduction, the small levers";[144] *Morb.* II.33/VII.50 L: "placing the forked probe under the uvula";[145] Galen, *De Anat. Admin.* (II.686 K): "...using the doubly convex scalpel, ... place underneath a thin membrane-protector or a broad spatula-probe";[146] Paul VI.88.9/II.134f.: "One must lift these [i.e. the sling bullets] by levering with levers or the spoon of the small wound probe and, if the wound allows for it, even extract them with tooth forceps or root forceps."[147]

One could say that the surgical instruments are a case apart and their peculiar position may be related to the fact that the majority of these words were specially created, often composite terms.

---

[141] τοῖσι ἄλλοισι τοῖσι θανατώδεσι νοσήμασιν [II.146 L; Littré has the superlative θανατωδεστάτοισιν].

[142] E.g. II.165/I.230.11: κυκλάμινος ἑτέρα, ἥν ἔνιοι κισσάνθεμον καλοῦσι.

[143] For example at II.166 [RV]/I.231.15ff.: δρακόντια μεγάλη, οἱ δὲ ἄρον, οἱ δὲ ἴσαρον, οἱ δὲ ἴαρον, οἱ δὲ ἱεράκιος, οἱ δὲ ἄμι ἄγριον, οἱ δὲ κύπερις, ...

[144] ἐμβολὴ δέ, οἱ μοχλίσκοι.

[145] χήλην ὑποθεὶς ὑπὸ τὸν γαργαρεῶνα.

[146] χρώμενος ἀμφικύρτῳ μυρσίνῃ. ..., ὑπόβαλλε μηνιγγοφύλακα λεπτὸν ἢ σπαθομήλην πλατεῖαν.

[147] δεῖ δὲ ταῦτα μοχλεύσαντα δι' ἀναβολέων ἢ κυαθίσκου τραυματικῆς μηλωτίδος ἀναβάλλειν, εἰ δὲ προσδέχοιτο, καὶ δι' ὀδοντάγρας ἢ ῥιζάγρας ἐξέλκειν.

These had not existed before the invention of a particular instrument and therefore had no established reference to compete with. The reason that the instruments are not referred to as *iatrika onomata* may be related to the fact that many of them - e.g. *staphylagra* (σταφυλάγρα; 'uvula-forceps'), *mêningophylax* (μηνιγγοφύλαξ; 'membrane-protector') or *embryoulkos* (ἐμβρυούλκος; 'foetus-extractor') - would indeed not count as an *onoma* according to the Aristotelian definition (*Int.* 16a20f.): "a word ... no part of which has a meaning separately".[148] (However, this would disqualify some of the anatomical vocabulary as well.)

Another puzzling problem related to terminology is the use of the expression 'the [so-]called' - *kaloumenos/-ê/-on* (καλούμενος/-η/-ον). Often in medical writing, in the Hippocratics and Galen in particular, a medical term is preceded or followed by this, for example: *Medic.*11/IX.216 L: "the so-called [ulcers]";[149] *Fract.* 9/III.448 L: "the so-called palm";[150] Sor., *Gyn.* I.18.1/12.19: "it ends in the so-called clitoris'[151] (followed by an explanation why it is called so); Galen, *De Anat. Admin.*VIII /II.682 K: "with the so-called pointed scalpel".[152]

It has been suggested[153] that this usage indicates "technical words belonging to a particular art, here to medicine". Louis[154] follows basically the same reasoning for Aristotle's use of *kaloumenos*, stating that when prefacing anatomical terms it introduces a word taken from 'medical vocabulary'. Lanza's theory,[155] on the other hand, is that *ho kaloumenos* precedes words which have been taken into medical language from current spoken language and which are not yet "convalidated and nobilitated" by literary use. However, as Lloyd[156] points out, expressions of that kind "may indicate merely that the term is not a common one", i.e. for the audience in question, and are used in non-medical literature as well, such as *Il.* V.306 or Plato, *Ti.* 69e. However, when, in *De Anat. Admin.* III [II.345 K], Galen writes about "those who are called gladiators",[157] one can hardly speak of

---

[148] φωνή ... ἧς μηδὲν μέρος ἐστὶ σημαντικὸν κεχωρισμένον. This is Lanza's ([1972], p. 420) argument in explaining why Aristotle refers to the *malakostraka* as *anonyma*, nameless, in *H. A.* (490b13).
[149] τὰ καλεόμενα [sc. ἕλκεα].
[150] τοῦ ταρσοῦ καλεομένου.
[151] εἰς τὴν καλουμένην ἀπολήγει νύμφην.
[152] τῷ καλουμένῳ σκολοπομαχαιρίῳ.
[153] Festugière (1948), pp. 68f.
[154] (1965), p. 145.
[155] (1972), p. 410.
[156] (1983), pp. 154f.
[157] τῶν καλουμένων μονομάχων.

a rare word or a specialist term and it is unlikely that his audience had never heard of gladiators before. Similarly, Paul of Aegina (VI.88.1/II.129.21). refers to a fairly common term for the shaft of an arrow, *atrakton*, by saying τῶν καλουμένων ἀτράκτων.

In *Med. N.* (95) Galen offers a helpful explanation: speaking about a passage in which Hippocrates mentions "the so-called semi-tertian", he points out that Hippocrates uses this expression to emphasise the fact that names and their references are not indissolubly linked and that therefore names can be exchanged. It may well be the case therefore that the expression *kaloumenos* was often used as we would italicise a word or put it in quotation marks, but that at times it was more or less a mere rhetorical figure, at least in Galen.

Galen also shows remarkable inconsistency when it comes to the importance or unimportance of 'names'. In the first chapter of *On the Natural Faculties* (*De naturalibus facultatibus* [*Nat.Fac.*]), II.1f. K, he stresses the overwhelming importance of distinctness for a word: "... but we are convinced that a word's greatest virtue is clarity, and we know that this [virtue] is destroyed by nothing as much as by unusual names, as is the habit of the many".[158] This is similar to Aristotle's *Rh.*1404b: "It is the virtue of a word to be clear ... if a word does not explain, it will not do its job."[159] Galen makes the same demand on words in *Capt.* (p.35) as well. However, in some other passages his approach appears to be different. Thus in his *Commentary on the Timaeus*, 10 (p.8), referring to Plato's use of the words μέρη and μέλη,[160] he discards the question as being a problem of names, not of knowledge (*epistême*), continuing: "but let us rather see what he says on the things themselves".. In *Med. N.* he repeatedly emphasises (e.g. pp. 14, 35) that it is the things themselves which count, the names being of lesser importance. In *Morb. Temp.* IV (VII.418 K) he becomes even more off-handed, when he writes that one has to follow the more recent doctors, "because the sick will take no harm from the transgression of order in names".[161] How this would fit with the demand for clarity is hard to see.

---

[158] ἀλλ' ἡμεῖς γε μεγίστην λέξεως ἀρετὴν σαφήνειαν εἶναι πεπεισμένοι, καὶ ταύτην εἰδότες ὑπ' οὐδενὸς οὕτως ὡς ὑπὸ τῶν ἀήθων ὀνομάτων διαφθειρομένην, ὡς τοῖς πολλοῖς ἔθος.

[159] ὡρίσθω λέξεως ἀρετὴ σαφῆ εἶναι ... ὁ λόγος, ἐὰν μὴ δηλοῖ, οὐ ποιήσει τὸ ἑαυτοῦ ἔργον.

[160] Here Galen points out that Plato imposed a different meaning upon the two words and that it is impossible to be certain about his use of those words - an indication that semantic confusion was not limited to medical texts.

[161] οὐδὲ γὰρ οὐδὲ βλαβήσονταί τι διὰ τὴν ἐν τοῖς ὀνόμασι παρανομίαν οἱ κάμνοντες.

Now that I have discussed the type of vocabulary found in medical writings, there remains the question whether this vocabulary was something that one might call 'medical terminology' and whether its use was restricted to medical authors. Again, the scarcity of literature surviving from the early fifth century and before often makes it extremely difficult to decide whether certain words which seem to appear in the Hippocratic Corpus as new creations or with new references were actually creations within medical language or whether they form part of the larger scenario of the development of the Greek language at the time.

As far as tragedy is concerned (and in some cases comedy[162] as well), there is a considerable overlap with medical writings in vocabulary concerning physiological or pathological concepts, and the problem of terminology there has been explored by several scholars. The disparity of their conclusions shows the complexity of the topic: Miller ([1944], p.157) and Dumortier ([1935], *passim*) see an influence of medical language upon the language of tragedy, while Lanata ([1968], p. 25) and Berrettoni ([1970], p.68f.) suggest that the language of poetry was taken up by the medical writers, Berrettoni offering also the alternative of an autonomous development. According to Psichari ([1908], p.106) the medical vocabulary used by the writers was actually everyday language. Lanza ([1981], p.185) professes the most convincing (if rather easy) theory, namely that the creation of medical terms was part of a larger process, the creation of prose language.

Many terms which are common in medical literature are also frequently used in non-medical prose literature - e.g. words such as *cholê* (χολή; bile), *phlegma* (φλέγμα; phlegm), *phlegmonê* (φλεγμονή; inflammation), *pyretos* (πύρετος; fever) etc., can often be found in philosophical or historical writings. To cite only a few of a large number of examples: Plato's *R.* 564b: "... like phlegm and bile in the body",[163] or *Leg.* 691e: "beholding our government still inflamed";[164] Procopius, *Goth.* VI.II.31.: "when the membranes in that place [i.e. the head] began to be inflamed, he was seized by the disease phrenitis and died not much later;"[165] Plut. *Crass.* XV.5.: "Attempting with force to pull out the

---

[162] See Zimmermann (1992) about medical terms in Aristophanes and Gil/ Alfageme Rodriguez (1972) on doctors in Attic comedy.
[163] οἷον περὶ σῶμα φλέγμα τε καὶ χολή.
[164] κατιδοῦσα ὑμῶν τὴν ἀρχὴν φλεγμαίνουσαν.
[165] ἐπεὶ δέ οἱ φλεγμαίνειν αἱ τῇδε μήνιγγες ἤρξαντο, φρενίτιδι νόσῳ ἁλούς οὐ πολλῷ ὕστερον ἐτελεύτησε.

arrowheads which were barbed and buried among veins and nerves, they lacerated and mangled themselves."[166] However, there remains a core of terms which cannot be seen outside medical literature. Along with surgical instruments - apart from the occasional mention of scalpels in non-medical literature - these include the aforementioned adjectives for types of pulse, ulcers or fractures, as well as many pathological terms, e.g. *empyos* (ἔμπυος: suppurating), *leienteria* (λειεντερία; the passing of undigested food), *kolpos* (κόλπος) in the sense of fistula, etc.. It is arguable whether their absence in non-medical literature alone qualifies them as medical terminology, as there is generally no context for them to be used from the point of view of the contents - in very few cases pathological details would have added to the interest of the story. This core, if anything, though, could be called specialist terminology - although it was a problem of medical knowledge rather than of vocabulary: most Greeks would have understood the words, but might have failed to understand what exactly they referred to.

Despite this rather limited extent of purely medical language, the fact that certain words are used by the doctors is repeatedly stressed by authors in the Hippocratic Corpus as well as by Galen, and this insistence is obviously part of a certain rhetoric. These occurrences of expressions such as "they/we call" or "the doctors call" should be considered separately from the more vague *kaloumenos*, as they narrow down the group of people who call something by a certain name. While the Hippocratic authors generally use "they/we call", Galen tends to say "the doctors/we doctors call" - a difference which may be caused by the fact that Galen is often writing with a lay audience in mind, and perhaps also by his general defensiveness and desire to corroborate his authority beyond the range of attack.

Thus, for example, in *De Anat. Admin.* (II.633 K) Galen obviously classifies *syntrêsis* (σύντρησις) as a term specifically used by doctors, when he says that he suggested performing an excision of the sternum without doing "what is called *syntrêsis* peculiarly by the doctors".[167] His phrasing in *On Antidotes* (*De Antidotis* [*Ant.*]), XIV.1 K, suggests that he also considers the word *antidotos* (ἀντίδοτος) as a 'medical' term: "the doctors call (ὀνομάζουσιν οἱ ἰατροί) internal remedies against poisoning

---

[166] βίᾳ τε πειρωμένους ἐξέλκειν ἠγκιστρομένας ἀκίδας καὶ δεδυκυίας διὰ φλεβῶν καὶ νεύρων προσαναρρηγνύναι καὶ λυμαίνεσθαι σφᾶς αὐτούς.

[167] τὴν καλουμένην ἰδίως ὑπὸ τῶν ἰατρῶν σύντρησιν.

antidotes". In *M.M*, Galen distinguishes between the term for fracture used by laymen and that used by doctors (X.423f. K). He states that a lesion to the bones is called *katagma* (κάταγμα), a name customary to almost all those who speak Greek, but "*apagma* (ἄπαγμα) is a name proper to the doctors, unfamiliar to most people".[168]

Medical authors admit, however, that non-doctors can know some terms: in *Nat. Fac.* (II.31 K) Galen writes of people calling themselves *nephritikous* (νεφριτικούς) and, in *Loc. Aff.* (VIII.414 K), of women referring to themselves as *hysterikai* (ὑστερικαί), having heard this name from the midwives. Likewise, the author of *Acut.* states (II.236f. L) that it is easy for non-doctors to appear as doctors, because they can easily learn the names of remedies, for example "barley juice ... and melicrate".[169] In *Med. N.* (p.17) Galen claims that "ordinary people"[170] know words like 'fever' or 'fracture', while they do not know others, e.g. *sphakelos*. At least for this particular word this is patently untrue, given that Herodotus (VI.136) uses the term *sphakelizô*.

As with the problem of medical knowledge - which overlaps with that of terminology - the consciousness of a difference is stronger than any actual, visible, difference. There is a small number of expressions which may not have been understood by those who were not doctors, but the awareness of a specialist terminology appears to extend to a degree beyond this. However, it can be noticed only in medical writing and the question seems of no interest to laymen. One could say that there is a certain element of defensiveness in the attempts at the creation of a medical terminology and, in particular, in the way such terminology is presented by the authors. At the bottom of it there may be a need, on the doctors' side, for an identity as a professional group, given the lack of unification among doctors in reality - unification being made impossible by the competitiveness of the field. It may also be an artificially created exclusivity of medical language in order to counteract its easy accessibility for laymen.

So far the discussion of medical terminology in this Chapter has been restricted to the Greek language. This is justifiable insofar as any efforts to create a specialist terminology in Latin are very much dependent on Greek. When there is the need for a

---

[168] ἄπαγμα δὲ τῶν ἰατρῶν ἴδιον ὄνομά ἐστι τοῖς πολλοῖς ἀνθρώποις ἀηθες.
[169] πτισάνης τε χυλὸν ... καὶ μελίκρητον.
[170] In the original the word used was presumably *idiôtai*.

specific term in Latin, a Greek word is often used, introduced by expressions such as *Graeci vocant/dicunt* (e.g.: Celsus, VII.18.3/ 335.25, ib. 7/336.17; Scribonius Largus, *Comp.* CCVI). Other ways of creating a terminology were the use of proper names (for remedies, for example), metaphor, semantic extension (such as *ustio*, burning, for cauterisation), descriptive terms and suffixation (e.g. *rubor* or *sanies*).[171]

Despite the fact that Greek medical terminology is richer and often more inventive, it is the language of Latin medical writings (Celsus in particular) that has attracted the atttention of scholars in the recent decades. General studies include the contributions by Boscherini and Mazzini in Sabbah (1991), an entire volume of the *Mémoires du Centre Jean-Palerne* dedicated to 'medical Latin', Baader (1970) and Vazquez Buján (1988). The adaptation of Greek nosological terms in Latin is discussed in Grmek (1991, in the same volume of the *Mémoires*), the use of Greek terms in Latin medical writings in Mazzini (1978) and the use of Graecisms in Celsus by Capitani (1975) and Sconocchia (1994). (Capitani [p. 450] suggests that Celsus used Greek terms not from an inability to find Latin equivalents, but from a sense of continuity *vis-à-vis* the Greek tradition.)

The use of Greek words by Roman authors could be seen to reflect several motivations. It may be a means to make their writings more apparently technical by using a foreign language, or a means to emphasise their authority and give themselves prestige by showing how knowledgeable and well-read they are in the relevant medical literature. It could also be seen as resignation to the fact that Latin is a less expressive and flexible language than Greek, or perhaps rather pride in the simplicity of the authors' own language. (In *Tusc. Disp.* II.XV.35, Cicero comments on the richness of the Greek language compared to Latin: "... these little Greeks whose language is richer than ours..."[172] - only to reveal the comment as a pose by pointing out the deficiency of Greek in distinguishing between *labor* and *dolor*.)[173] However, the use of Greek terminology for medical writings may well have been a way of highlighting the fact that medicine always remained essentially

---

[171] See Langslow (1991) for a more detailed explanation, as well as id. (1994), where he focuses on the language of Celsus.

[172] *Graeculi illi, quorum copiosior est lingua quam nostra ...*

[173] Cf. de Meo (1986), p. 225: "It was the poverty of the Latin language as far as medical terminology was concerned as well as the level reached by the Greeks in that field that induced [the Roman writers] to use Greek widely and open-mindedly."

un-Roman and that there was no desire to integrate it as a part of Roman culture.[174]

---

[174] According to Wilamowitz (1912), Latin did develop a specialised terminology for law - which was always considered an intrinsically Roman activity.

PART TWO

WOUNDING AS A CODE

CHAPTER SIX

THE *ILIAD*

It has already been mentioned that non-medical literature abounds in scenes of wounding and also of wound treatment; the scope of this second part of the book is to explore the motivations and reasons for this 'treatment' of wounds - both in a medical and in a literary sense. At first sight it may seem as if those scenes were there as part of the realistic rendering of a story, simply for the reason that "that was what had happened". However, even when the authors were rendering actual events - as we can sometimes assume for the material regarding Alexander the Great - the writing down of such descriptions was the result of a conscious choice between a large number of actual happenings. There are obviously reasons why certain scenes were chosen to feature in the narrative while others were deliberately left out. The element of conscious choice becomes even more evident with such literary creations as we would call fiction, especially epic poetry, where the account is not, or only loosely, based on any historical event and every component of the story has been put there by the poet for a particular purpose and with a particular intention. I intend to shed some light on those intentions and to show that the inclusion of scenes of wounding in works of essentially non-medical literature was based on the idea that these scenes were a way of representing a heroic ideal. We shall see that scenes of wounding and wound treatment are often used to emphasise the hero's courage and endurance and that they are as essential a part of Greek and Roman literature as passages describing fighting or death in battle.

Because of the close conceptual link between the theme of wounding and the image of the hero it will be necessary, in this part of the book, to digress occasionally from the topic of wounding strictly speaking and to discuss other themes pertaining to heroism, such as death in battle or the virtues of the warrior.

The first literary work to be examined is the *Iliad* - not only because it is chronologically the first major work[1] of Western literature, but also because its ideals and imagery had a lasting influence throughout antiquity and it can be seen as the origin of the permanent core in Graeco-Roman concepts of heroism, as well

---

[1] And, in the words of R. L. Fox ([1980], p.12), "still quite comfortably the best".

as the prime object of emulation and imitation and the main source of literary motifs for generations of authors.

It is well known that the *Iliad* contains a large number of detailed descriptions of fatal wounds and some of non-fatal ones. Given the almost unlimited quantity of works of Homeric[2] scholarship concerning almost any aspect of the epics, it is not surprising that these scenes have found ample treatment in secondary literature. Roughly speaking, one can distinguish between two main types of approach, although they are sometimes combined. One is based on an interest in the *Iliad* as a source of information on medicine in the poet's time, discussing the degree of accuracy and realism to be seen in these descriptions. The main champions of this line of research are Malgaigne (*Etude sur l' anatomie et la physiologie d' Homère*, 1842), Ch.-V. Daremberg (*Etudes d' archéologie médicale sur Homère*, 1865), the Saxon military surgeon H. Frölich (*Die Militärmedicin Homers*, 1879), who even summons the support of statistics, supplying, e.g., percentages of mortality,[3] B. Coglievina (*Die homerische Medizin*, 1922) P.-Th. Justesen (*Les principes psychologiques d' Homère*, 1928), O. Körner (*Die ärztlichen Kenntnisse in Ilias und Odyssee*, 1929), F. Kudlien (*Zum Thema "Homer und die Medizin"*, 1965), A. Throuvalas ('Η ἰατρικὴ ἐν 'Ελλάδι κατὰ τους ὁμηρικοὺς χρόνους, 1970),[4] A. Albarracin Teulón (*La cirugia homerica,*1971], S. Laser (*Medizin und Körperpflege*, 1983) and I.-E. Leschhorn (in her unpublished thesis, 1985).

Another angle on the topic - although, as said before, the two are not always clearly distinguished - consists in examining the formulaic expressions used in depictions of dying and wounding in order to support hypotheses on authorship or earlier and later versions. Some of the scholars taking this approach are W. Schadewaldt (*Iliasstudien*, 1938), W. H. Friedrich (*Verwundung und Tod in der Ilias*, 1956), who also shows an interest in different degrees of realism, B. Fenik (*Typical Battle Scenes in the Iliad*, 1968) and Niers (*Struktur und Dynamik in den Kampfszenen der Ilias*, 1975). The purpose of the scenes of wounding is usually

---

[2] This is not the place for a discussion of questions regarding the creation or 'authorship' of the Iliad and the Odyssey, nor is it my purpose to discuss them. The terms 'Homer' or 'the poet' will be used interchangeably to designate whoever is responsible for the epics as we have them. A useful short overview of Homeric scholarship can be found in Fantuzzi (1980).
[3] Ibid., pp. 58f.
[4] It is to be hoped that his description of the myth of Pelops as an example of plastic surgery in prehistoric Greece is intended as a joke.

viewed as a means to delay or advance the plot.⁵ The situation is similar with the scholiasts. In their comments on scenes of wounding their interest seems to be divided between medical aspects and difficulties of grammar and word use.

In contrast to those views, I believe that there is more to the scenes of wounding than meets the eye - something beyond a mere, clinically more or less accurate, description or a ploy to remove certain warriors from the battle. This possibility is only rarely hinted at in secondary literature and appears to have been not even considered by the majority of authors. Furthermore, most scholars take the presence of these scenes for granted, as something that had to be in the epic because it would happen in a war, disregarding the fact that the poet was under no constraint to have certain scenes feature in his epic, but had instead chosen to do so. And indeed, many events which would occur in a war do not figure in the *Iliad* or are only hinted at, and the scenes in question are not essential for the development of the story.

On those premises one can assume that scenes of wounding and wound treatment feature in the *Iliad* for a particular reason or purpose, and it is my opinion that they are an element in the depiction of the hero. Most scholars would agree that the central theme of the *Iliad* is heroism and the right way for a hero to live and die, and I believe that the scenes of wounding and wound treatment are an integrated part of this theme.

Generally speaking, the passages referring to wounds fall into three groups: fatal wounds, those (inflicted on both humans and gods) cured or alleviated by divine intervention, and the wounds receiving some kind of treatment - however rudimentary - either by others or by the casualty himself. Wounds in the *Iliad* are always either immediately fatal or are cured in a relatively short time and the poet never describes protracted agony before death,⁶ long-term effects of wounds, or crippling. This alone should be sufficient proof that Homer's scenes of wounding are not merely part of the realistic depiction of a war. There is only one reference to warriors suffering from the effects of their wounds long after they were hit, namely in Hector's threat (VIII.513ff.) that, after their flight from Troy, some of the Achaeans, wounded as they leapt aboard their ships, would still labour at home with - literally

---

⁵ This approach is particularly pronounced in Marg (1976) and Lossau (1989).

⁶ With the exception of the few moments given to Sarpedon (XVI. 492-501), Patroklos (XVI.844-54) and Hector (XXII.338-43) for a last speech.

'digest' (πέσσῃ) - a wound made by an arrow or a sharp spear.[7] This short remark shows clearly that the poet was aware of the real consequences of war wounds, and presumably so was his audience, but the theme was not developed in the *Iliad*. It obviously lacked drama or some other quality that made fresh wounds worth describing in epic poetry. Perhaps, as Griffin[8] puts it: "there are to be no mutilated and hideously suffering warriors to blur the overriding contrast between heroic life and heroic death", or, as Redfield[9] suggests, these features "combine to establish an epic distance".

The first group - the fatal wounds - is by far the largest, though not necessarily the one which has received most elaboration in detail by the poet. Frölich[10] tells us that the mortality of those wounded in battle in the entire *Iliad* is of "almost 77,6%". I have not checked this percentage but whether it is correct or not, what counts is the fact that the majority of wounds described result in almost immediate death. In these cases it is not the wounding as such that is of interest for the poet and his audience, but the killing.

The descriptions emphasise the effectiveness of the blow and the competence of the slayer. The anatomical details help to make these facts more visible to an audience who would be able to appreciate such details - or at least that is one of their purposes. In Marg's words,[11] the exact location and the type of wound are important "just as a hunter, an expert - and such is the warrior and soldier - would notice and discuss these things". Thus the audience would understand the reference to the spot where the collar-bones meet the neck, "where a wound is most quickly fatal"[12] (XXII.325) - incidentally the only throw in the *Iliad* specifically aimed at any part of the body in particular, perhaps in order to highlight Achilles' outstanding marksmanship. The audience would also appreciate the famous explanation (XXII.328f.) that Hector was still able to speak after being struck, because Achilles' spear had missed the trachea, or the detail of Meriones' spear hitting Adamas

---

[7] ἀλλ' ὥς τις τούτων γε βέλος καὶ οἴκοθι πέσσῃ, / βλήμενος ἢ ἰῷ ἢ ἔγχεϊ ὀξυόεντι. The sufferings of Philoctetes, referred to at II.721-4, are not the result of a war wound but of a snake-bite.

[8] (1976), p. 48.
[9] (1975), p. 37.
[10] (1879), p. 60.
[11] (1976), pp. 10f.
[12] ἵνα τε ψυχῆς ὤκιστος ὄλεθρος. (Literally "where destruction of the soul is swiftest").

between the genitals and the navel, the most painful spot to be wounded (XIII.568f.).[13]

Nevertheless, there is an insistence on anatomical and medical details in these passages, as if the poet had some interest in those subjects and wanted to communicate his knowledge to his audience. (Passages of this kind led Frölich to the startling conclusion[14] that Homer was an army surgeon.) One gains a similar impression from the explanatory "they call it the socket" [15] (V.306) in designating the spot where the rock thrown by Diomedes strikes Aeneas, i.e. at the hip joint.

Another possible reason for the use of anatomical details is the need for variety in the large number of duels and killings so as to make the narrative more vivid. In particular, descriptions such as that of the spear moved by the dying man's heartbeat (XIII.442ff.) would contribute greatly to the visual impact of the account. Friedrich classes this killing as one of the *Phantasmata*,[16] like the description of Mydon's corpse sticking head down in the sand (V.585ff.). Similarly, the verses describing the bone-marrow spurting from the vertebrae of a severed neck (XX.482f.) certainly make for strong visual effects.

We can also see some distinctions between the deaths of Greeks and those of Trojans. The more gruesome wounds, e.g. severed heads (XX.482f.) or arms (XI.145), even a shoulder (V.147), or prolapsing intestines (XXI.180f.) appear to be reserved for the Trojans, while the Greeks are usually allotted 'cleaner' deaths. It is also more often the Trojans who are hit in the back while trying to escape[17] - perhaps as a parallel to the fact that it is only the Trojans who plead for their lives.

Details of deaths are not normally used as a means to elicit sympathy for those who are slain; this is usually achieved by the 'biographies' preceding or following the fatal blow, i.e. short

---

[13] ἔνθα μάλιστα / γίγνετ ' "Αρης ἀλεγεινὸς ὀιζυροῖσι βροτοῖσιν. ("There Ares is most painful for miserable mortals.")

[14] (1879), p. 64.

[15] κοτύλην δέ τέ μιν καλέουσιν. The expression is reminiscent of the many occurrences of *kaloumenon* and similar terms in medical texts, discussed in Ch. 5.2.

[16] However, Coglievina (1922), p. 40, n. 16, following Körner, considers the description plausible. If one is to believe Paul (VI.88.6/II.133.21), the pulsating movement was one way of recognising an arrow wound to the heart, but it is uncertain whether the heartbeat would move a heavy spear.

[17] To our modern mind, shooting a man in the back, whether he is trying to escape or not, would seem even more cowardly, but this does not appear to be the case in Homer. Presumably a man who had turned his back to run had forfeited his right to honourable treatment and put himself on the same level as women or children, to whom the warriors' code of honour did not apply.

accounts of the warrior's reasons to come to the war, his special skills and his family.

The reason why the topic of fatal wounds has to be treated to some extent here is the prevalent emphasis on death in the *Iliad*, which has often been commented upon by scholars. Thus W. Marg[18] has called the *Iliad* "a poem of dying and death" and this opinion is shared by J. de Romilly[19] who calls it "a poem of battles and death". This may be an extreme view, mitigated by J. Griffin[20] to: "The great theme of the *Iliad* is heroic life and death", but the omnipresence of violent death in the *Iliad* cannot be denied. By an illusion of realism[21] the poet contrives to highlight the gruesomeness of war, but also its fascination as the only acceptable setting for a heroic way of life, as well as for a heroic death. The fact that the Homeric heroes conceive of themselves as made for this particular way of life is obvious in Odysseus' words (XIV.85ff.), when he says that it was given to them by Zeus to spend all their lives fighting: "... we ... to whom Zeus has given it to endure painful wars from youth to old age, until we each perish".[22]

The inescapability of death, combined with the absence of a belief in an afterlife as anything more than a shadow-like existence, imparts paramount importance to the way this death takes place and the *Iliad* is our earliest testimony of the ideology of the 'good death', that is, death in battle. This idea is developed by F. Kudlien:[23] "The wound alone is 'honest', therefore, old people or women who cannot be active on the battlefield, pretend to be killed by an arrow from Artemis."

We can see the contrast between good and bad death in two passages in particular The first is at XIII.663-72: the Corinthian Euchenor knows from his father's prophecy that he will either die of an illness in his own home or be killed by the Trojans (a less glorious version of Achilles' choice). He chooses the latter fate "shunning the troublesome penalty imposed by the Achaeans as well as the hateful sickness" (XIII.669f.).[24] The passage is remarkable not so much for the choice of violent death over death

---

[18] (1976), p. 18.
[19] (1979), p. 3.
[20] (1980), p. 44.
[21] In Redfield's words ([1975], p. 59), "an unreal world which is about the real world".
[22] ἄμμιν ..., οἷσιν ἄρα Ζεὺς / ἐκ νεότητος ἔδωκε καὶ ἐς γῆρας τολυπεύειν / ἀργαλέους πολέμους, ὄφρα φθιόμεσθα ἕκαστος.
[23] (1968), p. 312.
[24] τῷ ῥ ἅμα τ' ἀργαλέην θωὴν ἀλέεινεν Ἀχαιῶν / νοῦσόν τε στυγερήν, ...

from disease, but for the explanation attached to it: "so that he would not suffer grief in his heart" (XIII.670).²⁵ Thus obviously illness involves suffering for the *thymos* which death in battle does not entail (conceivably because it is a swifter death, but this may not be the only reason), since the *thymos* merely leaves the body. It does so here in the following line (XIII.671) and it seems like a deliberate arrangement that the word *thymos* appears in both phrases, to make the contrast more poignant. In the second passage contrasting death in battle with other ways of dying (XXI.273-87), Achilles prays to Zeus to save him from being drowned by the river Scamander, but it is clear that he is not doing so from fear of dying, since he is prepared to suffer any fate later.²⁶ What Achilles complains about so bitterly is that he has been cheated of the death by Apollo's arrows that has been promised to him, and that he is about to die a wretched death,²⁷ "like a swineherd", etc. The last remark may suggest that death by drowning was acceptable for people of lower social standing, but not for a warrior. Thus both passages emphasise the importance of the quality and perhaps the appropriateness of death according to who and what a man is.

It is important to die a hero, not because it gives the dying warrior himself much satisfaction or comfort, but because of what will be said about him after his death - because the *klea andrôn* (κλέα ἀνδρῶν; 'renown of men') is the only thing that survives after a man's death, and being remembered by future generations in tales or songs is the only way to transcend mortality.²⁸

This is the thought that makes Hector stop and face Achilles, although he realises that "the gods have called [him] to his death"²⁹ (XXII.297): he decides not to die without glory, but performing great deeds "and be remembered by future generations" (ib. 305).³⁰ The importance of fame after death finds its most unambiguous expression in Sarpedon's speech to Glaukos (XII.310-29, esp.322-5):

---

²⁵ ἵνα μὴ πάθοι ἄλγεα θυμῷ.
²⁶ XXI.274: ἔπειτα δὲ καί τι πάθοιμι.
²⁷ XXI.281: λευγαλέῳ θανάτῳ.
²⁸ Cf. Jaeger (1965), p. 137: "Poetry is man's immortality".The thought of this kind of immortality was an incentive for the Homeric warrior to choose the death that would guarantee it.
²⁹ ... θεοὶ θάνατόνδε κάλεσσαν.
³⁰ καὶ ἐσσομένοισι πυθέσθαι.

Good man, if we could escape this war and live forever ageless and immortal, I would neither myself fight amongst the foremost nor would I send you [out] into the battle which brings renown to men.[31]

The epithet for battle, *kydianeira*, seems deliberately chosen for this passage, because the sole fact that death is inescapable would not be a sufficient explanation for why men have to fight; the incentive to do so is the *kydos* to be gained in fighting.

Idomeneus' words to Meriones (XIII.275-94) also demonstrate how much the battle is seen as a test of manhood. The *lochos* (here presumably meant as a pars-pro-toto expression for battle) is "where the value of men is most [clearly] discerned" (XIII.277),[32] and where it becomes clear who is a coward and who is brave. These words follow Meriones' claim that he is always fighting among the first - again using the epithet *kydianeira* for battle.

Frequent mention is made not only of the importance of dying as a warrior but also of the youth - and often also the beauty - of the dying warrior. The warriors who die in the *Iliad* are all young, e.g. the two sons of Diokles (V.550f.): "They had, still young, followed the Argives on the black ships to horse-abounding Troy."[33] Often their youth is illustrated by those whom they leave behind: aged parents, newly-wed wives and new-born babies if any children at all, e.g. Sarpedon (V.480): "I left behind a dear wife and an infant son."[34] None of them has sons of fighting age, they all belong to the generation of 'sons'. Obviously the bereaved parents and brides are meant to stimulate our pity for them[35] - all the survivors are potential victims and spoils of war - but also for the warrior himself who is fated to die young, despite the *kydos* in store for him.

At the same time those deaths set an example of how and when a man should die. Priam states this clearly (XXII.65-76) in his comparison between the dead young warrior where "everything is beautiful, though he is dead"[36] and the pitiful spectacle of the old man lying slain - a motif to be expanded later in literature, by Tyrtaeus in particular. The link between manhood and youth is

---

[31] ὦ πέπον, εἰ μὲν γὰρ πόλεμον περὶ τόνδε φυγόντε / αἰεὶ δὴ μέλλοιμεν ἀγήρω τ' ἀθανάτω τε / ἔσσεσθ', οὔτε κεν αὐτὸς ἐνὶ πρώτοισι μαχοίμην / οὔτε κε σὲ στέλλοιμι μάχην ἐς κυδιάνειραν·

[32] XIII.277: ἔνθα μάλιστ' ἀρετὴ διαείδεται ἀνδρῶν.

[33] τὼ μὲν ἄρ' ἡβήσαντε μελαινάων ἐπὶ νηῶν / Ἴλιον εἰς εὔπωλον ἅμ' Ἀργείοισιν ἐπέσθην.

[34] ἄλοχόν τε φίλην ἔλιπον καὶ νήπιον υἱόν.

[35] The excessive old age of fathers whose sons are barely out of adolescence also appears to be intended to highlight the tragedy of their bereavement.

[36] XXII. 73: πάντα δὲ καλὰ θανόντι περ, ὅττι φανήῃ.

also made explicit in the verse describing the souls of respectively Patroklos (XVI.857) and Hector (XXII.363) fluttering away to Hades "bemoaning its fate, leaving behind manliness and youth"[37] - obviously leaving behind what makes life most valuable. *Androtês* - the word *andreia* for manliness or courage does not appear in Homeric Greek - is something that can be noticed by other warriors or communicated to them. Thus, at XXIV.6., Achilles lies sleepless, longing for Patroklos' "manliness and courage",[38] although this may be used in the sense of an adjective, i.e. "longing for manly, brave Patroklos".

To "be men" would appear to be a similar concept, appearing in exhortations to fight. Thus it is used by Agamemnon at V.529: "Friends, be men and take a stout heart",[39] and by Hector at VIII.174. and XI.287: "Be men, friends, and call to mind your impetuous courage".[40] Agamemnon goes into more detail, when he calls upon his men "to show regard for one another [Or is it meant in the sense of 'being ashamed'?] in the fierce battle"[41] (V.530) and points out that there is neither glory nor defence for those who flee (ib.532).[42] In these passages we can see the development of what is later to become the ideal of *andreia*, the warrior's virtue *par excellence* throughout classical antiquity.

Beauty is another attribute used to heighten the tragedy of the warrior's actual or impending death. We can see this, to list but a few examples, in the reference to Hector's good looks, after Achilles has killed him,[43] his formerly comely head lying in the dust,[44] Euphorbos' lovely tresses, decorated with gold and silver, now defiled with blood (XVII.51f.), or Patroklos' beautiful eyes when he appears as a ghost (XXII.66). The tragic quality is most conspicuous in Achilles' rejection of Lykaon's plead for his life: Achilles' reference to his own beauty (XXI.108): "... do you not see how I, too, am beautiful and big ...?"[45] is not a boast, but a dramatic build-up towards the statement that Achilles, too, is doomed to die soon: (XXI.110): "... but after you, there is death and dire destiny for me, too".[46] His beauty, strength and good parentage are the background designed to make the tragedy of his

---

[37] ὃν πότμον γοάουσα, λιποῦσ᾽ ἀνδροτῆτα καὶ ἥβην.
[38] ἀνδροτῆτά τε καὶ μένος ἠύ.
[39] ὦ φίλοι, ἀνέρες ἔστε καὶ ἄλκιμον ἦτορ ἔλεσθε.
[40] ἀνέρες ἔστε, φίλοι, μνήσασθε δὲ θούριδος ἀλκῆς.
[41] ἀλλήλους ... αἰδεῖσθε κατὰ κρατερὰς ὑσμίνας.
[42] φευγόντων δ᾽ οὔτ᾽ ἄρ κλέος ὄρνυται οὔτε τις ἀλκή.
[43] XXII.370: φυὴν καὶ εἶδος ἀγητόν.
[44] Ib. 402f.: κάρη ... πάρος χαρίεν.
[45] οὐχ ὁράᾳς, οἷος καὶ ἐγὼ καλός τε μέγας τὲ ...
[46] ἀλλ᾽ ἔπι τοι καὶ ἐμοὶ θάνατος καὶ μοῖρα κραταιή.

death stand out more powerfully. However, when male[47] beauty is not directly connected with death, reference to it is always used as an insult, to emphasise a man's lack of courage or fighting prowess - e.g. the "most good-looking one"[48] used by Hector against Paris at III.39. and by Glaukos against Hector at XVII.142. Beauty without the heroic touch is appreciated in women and is therefore a negative attribute in a man, something that makes him less of a man.

Despite the poet's pronounced interest in topics related to death and dying, not all of those wounded in the *Iliad* die, and the poem contains many descriptions of woundings leading to non-fatal wounds. In six cases of wounds or injuries the gods intervene (V.416f.; V.121-32; V.445-50; V.899-904; XV.235-70; XVI.527-31) and in two of these cases the casualty is actually one of the Olympians, as the Homeric gods are obviously not invulnerable. Both Aphrodite and Ares are wounded by Diomedes during his *aristeia* in Book V and are healed by other gods. Dione[49] heals Aphrodite's hand by merely wiping off the *ichor* (V.416f.), and Ares is treated by Paean, who - in a curious parallel to human treatment - applies "pain-killing drugs" (V.900).[50] According to Dione's tale about other gods who had in the past been wounded by mortals, he used the same treatment on Hades, wounded by one of Heracles' arrows (V.401).

Four times in the *Iliad* the gods assist wounded or injured mortals, giving varying degrees of assistance (V.121-32; V.445-50; XV.235-70; XVI.527-31). In the case of Diomedes, wounded by Pandaros' arrow, Athena merely boosts his energy, without actually healing his wound - V.122: "she made his knees light, his feet and the hands above"[51] - and when she finds him later, cooling his wound which is still giving him trouble (V.794-8), it seems to be only her taunting words that make Diomedes return to the fight.

Apollo is, at least in part, involved in the three remaining divine interventions. Aeneas is taken away by Apollon to his temple in Pergamon, where his wound is cured by Leto and Artemis in an unspecified way (V.445-8). It is obviously a miraculous cure, which is effected very quickly, because Aeneas is brought back

---

[47] Women are expected to be beautiful as well as skilled in handicrafts in order to be worth having.
[48] εἶδος ἄριστε.
[49] She is the only female involved in wound treatment in the epic, and the reason for her appearance here may well be that the casualty is female as well.
[50] ὀδυνήφατα φάρμακα.
[51] γυῖα δ' ἔθηκεν ἐλαφρά, πόδας καὶ χεῖρας ὕπερθεν.

and joins the battle again in verses 512ff. In Hector's case Apollon, sent by Zeus, breathes *menos* into him (XV.262) after Zeus had already revived him (XV.242).

The healing in which Apollon plays the most active part is that of Glaukos, who, unlike the others, specifically prays to Apollo for help. In Glaukos' case - as with the wounded gods - the healing is instantaneous; the pain and the bleeding stop and Glaukos is filled with new courage (XVI.528f.): "... immediately he stopped the pain, dried the black blood from the painful wound and infused courage into his soul".[52]

Glaukos' case shows most clearly what divine healing stands for: it is the ideal of wound treatment, unobtainable in the human world. The pain and the haemorrhage - the main problems with wounds in real life and often mentioned in connection with wounds in the *Iliad* - are dealt with immediately and for good.

It is interesting to see, however, that the wounds healed by the gods do not appear to be fatal in the first place. The gods never save a dying man, or rather we are never told that the man could or would have died without their help. Only in Hector's case the injury, with its internal damage, could have been beyond the scope of human assistance and Hector himself says to Apollo that he had thought he would die (XV.251f.). However, this is Hector's personal opinion in a moment of weakness and does not imply that he really would have died. Aeneas' wound is not fatal, although it could be disabling, and for Diomedes and Glaukos their wounds are a nuisance and an impediment to fighting, but not a danger to their lives. Even the gods only facilitate the healing process or speed it up, but they do not interfere with fate.

Many warriors in the *Iliad* are wounded and survive without divine help, and the first question to be examined here is who helps them. The image conveyed by the poet corresponds very closely to the actual situation as we know it for later times and presumably also to the situation in his own times: assistance is given either by what we might call experts, or by other warriors, or attempts at treatment are made by the wounded man himself.

Men who were expected to treat the wounded and who had a far more specialist knowledge of wounds than the average warrior are mentioned on several occasions in the *Iliad*. We hear of nameless *iêtroi*, without any mention of their numbers, at XIII.213 and XVI.28. At XIII.210-14 the poet describes Idomeneus as coming from the side of a wounded companion, whom others had carried

---

[52] αὐτίκα παῦσ' ὀδύνας, ἀπὸ δ' ἕλκεος ἀργαλέοιο / αἷμα μέλαν τέρσηνε, μένος δέ οἱ ἔμβαλε θυμῷ.

back; Idomeneus had then "given orders to the physicians".[53] Returning to report the situation to Achilles at the beginning of book XVI, Patroklos tells him that all the best fighters are wounded[54] and that their wounds are being treated (XVI.28f.): "The doctors with many remedies are tending them, healing their wounds."[55] There appears to be a certain number of men whose (sole?) job it is to look after the wounded and the former passage in particular supports Edelstein's claim[56] that "physicians, in the Homeric world, are of inferior standing' : the warriors - at least the leaders - are in a position to give them orders. This also appears to be the message of the passage in the *Odyssey* (xvii.383ff.), where physicians are said to belong to the *dêmioergoi*, together with carpenters, soothsayers and bards.

Other than those anonymous *iêtroi* - and probably not identical with them - two men are referred to by that term, namely Machaon and Podaleirios, the sons of Asclepius. Apparently Asclepius is not yet a god in Homeric times, only a hero or prince, and he is not involved in any of the divine healings. His sons, too, are "leaders of men", who have come from their territory, Trikka, bringing their own ships and men.[57] Edelstein[58] argues convincingly that originally they were merely physicians, craftsmen (and at II.732 they are only called "good doctors"), but "since he [sc. Machaon] must appear on the Homeric stage in the costume of a hero, [he] is dubbed a knight and invested with a train of vassals".

Podaleirios is mentioned only in passing, as being busy fighting, so that Eurypylos, hit by an arrow, cannot ask him to treat his wound (XI.833-36). In the passage in question Eurypylos speaks of the two brothers as the obvious people to turn to for medical help and this appears to be their main function in the Achaean camp. They are always referred to as doctors and the main, perhaps even the only, reason for the other warriors' concern when Machaon himself is wounded seems to be his usefulness as a healer - as expressed in the much-quoted lines (XI.514f.): "For a physician is a man worth many others for cutting out arrows and applying soothing remedies."[59] Although

---

[53] ὅ δ' ἰητροῖς ἐπιτείλας ...
[54] Machaon, after whom he was supposed to inquire in the first place, is never mentioned again.
[55] τοὺς μέν τ' ἰητροὶ πολυφάρμακοι ἀμφιπένονται, ἕλκε' ἀκειόμενοι.
[56] (1945), II, p. 6, n. 17.
[57] Cf. their appearance in the catalogue of ships, II.729-33.
[58] (1945), II, p. 16.
[59] ἰητρὸς γὰρ ἀνὴρ πολλῶν ἀντάξιος ἄλλων / ἰοὺς τ' ἐκτάμνειν ἐπί τ' ἤπια φάρμακα πάσσειν.

Paris' arrow is supposed to have stopped Machaon distinguishing himself in the fight (ἀριστεύοντα; XI.506), we hear no more of his fighting and his equivalent of a hero's *aristeia* is his treatment of Menelaos' wound in book VI, where he is even described as a god-like hero (ἰσόθεος φώς; IV.12). This passage is the only description in the *Iliad* of the treatment given by a 'professional'.

It appears that in the post-Homeric epics Podaleirios and Machaon played a more important role and also that - perhaps with the inclusion of internal disease into the domain of the doctor - they were each allotted a particular skill, namely surgery for Machaon and the treatment of internal illness for his brother. This can be seen, e.g., in Eustathius or the scholia ad XI.515 (BT), quoting Arctinus: "To the one he gave lighter hands for taking and cutting arrows out of the flesh and for healing all wounds, and he put it into the other's heart to know exactly all the invisible things and to cure what cannot be healed."[60] Aristonicus' scholion ad V.193, i.e. the scene in which Agamemnon sends for Machaon to treat his wounded brother, says the same: "He does not summon both, given that the one was [knowledgable] about wounds, the other about the other diseases."[61] This subdivision is essentially un-Homeric and XI.514 tells us exactly what is expected from the *iêtros*, namely surgical and pharmacological treatment of wounds. This seems to be what both sons of Asclepius would do in the *Iliad* and the wounded Eurypylos would have asked either of them for assistance had they been available.

However, there is something curiously impersonal about the figure of Machaon in the *Iliad*. Although he is physically present in five passages - treating Menelaos' wound in book IV, being wounded by Paris, carried off the battlefield on Nestor's chariot, and being entertained by Nestor, in books XI and XIV - we hear no biographical details or characteristics other than his being the son of Asclepius and an excellent physician - and he never speaks a word. The latter is particularly surprising in the Homeric epics, where much time is spent in discourse (even one of Achilles' horses talks). It would seem as though Machaon was seen as 'the healer' and an expert valued for his skills, as a personification of his office rather than as a person.

In the majority of cases of wounding, though, we do not hear of professional help and the wounded man is looked after, more or

---

[60] τῷ μὲν κουφοτέρας χεῖρας πόρεν ἐκ τε βέλεμνα / σαρκὸς ἑλεῖν τμῆξαί τε καὶ ἕλκεα πάντ᾽ ἀκέσασθαι, / τῷ δ᾽ ἄρ᾽ ἀκριβέα πάντα ἐνὶ στήθεσσιν ἔθηκεν / ἄσκοπά τε γνῶναι καὶ ἀναλθέα ἰήσασθαι.
[61] οὐ μεταπέμπεται ἄμφω, ὅτι ὁ μὲν περὶ τὰ τραύματα ἦν, ὁ δὲ περὶ τὰ ἄλλα νοσήματα.

less expertly, by other warriors. Sometimes he is only led or carried to a chariot and then taken back to Troy (e.g. Deiphobos at XIII.533-9) or to the Achaean ships (e.g. Odysseus at XI.487f. or Hypsenor at XIII.421ff.) and we are not told who will treat his wounds there and how. We are told in the case of Hector, who is struck on the chest by a rock thrown by Telamonian Aias and is also carried to his chariot by his companions and driven towards the town (XIV.428-32): they decide to stop by the river Xanthos, where they deposit him on the ground and pour water over him. This only revives him momentarily, he vomits blood and faints again, but, as we have seen, he then recovers with divine help. The more energetic of the heroes do not rely on others to help them leave the battlefield: Agamemnon (XI.273) and Diomedes (XI. 309) leap on to their chariots and return to the ships.

The most active type of assistance given by a wounded warrior's companion is the removal of the spear or arrow. This is done by Sthenelos for Diomedes (V.112), by Pelagon for Sarpedon (V.694f.), by Agenor for Helenos (XIII.598) and by Patroklos for Eurypylos (XI.844-8), although the latter is a case to be considered separately. The treatment of a wound by a battle companion seems to be something like a set theme,[62] as well as the rescuing of a body, dead or alive, and these themes are to survive in later poetry and prose as some of the warrior's virtues. The consideration for fellow warriors is obviously part of being a hero, mainly perhaps because its prerequisites are fighting prowess and courage: only a good fighter will be able to stop for another warrior rather than being entirely occupied with defending himself.

Patroklos differs from the other warriors assisting their comrades in the 'professionalism' of his treatment. In fact, his is the only wound treatment in the *Iliad* corresponding to the description of what makes the *iêtros* 'worth many men", namely the cutting out of arrows - as opposed to the pulling out, which requires only physical strength but no particular skill - and the application of soothing drugs. And indeed, through Achilles, Patroklos' knowledge goes back to the same source as Machaon's: the centaur Cheiron, who taught Achilles the use of *pharmaka* (XI.830ff.), had also transmitted their use to Machaon's father Asclepius (IV.218f.).

In his discussion of Menelaos' wounding, Edelstein[63] makes the enlightened suggestion that Machaon is introduced into the story

---

[62] Cf. Brelich (1958), p. 117.
[63] (1945), II, pp. 15f.

at that point as a substitute for Achilles. While Achilles and Patroklos are the two heroes best versed in wound treatment, he argues, Agamemnon could not possibly ask either of them to help his brother, Achilles having retired from the fighting. However, because of the casualty's status the situation requires an outstanding physician, and thus Machaon takes Achilles' place so that Menelaos' wound can be treated properly.

Following the same lines, I would argue that Patroklos, in his treatment of Eurypylos' wound, stands in fact for Achilles. Patroklos' identity as Achilles' *alter ego* has often been stressed[64] and at that point in the *Iliad* it would be impossible for Eurypylos to ask the as yet unreconciled Achilles for help. It is possible that Achilles' medical knowledge is transferred to Patroklos for this particular scene - with the explanation "they say that you were taught these things first by Achilles"[65] (XI.831) in order to make it plausible. However, it is more likely that in his function as Achilles' *alter ego* Patroklos also has his share in Achilles' healing skills - a trait which fits well with the former's repeatedly emphasised kindness and gentleness. (Here Patroklos may well be meant to represent Achilles' kinder self: this could have been Achilles, were it not for his pride.)

One curious detail regarding Patroklos' medical assistance to Eurypylos is difficult to explain, unless one is prepared to assume a break in the narrative: upon his return from Nestor's hut Patroklos tells Achilles that Diomedes, Odysseus, Agamemnon and Eurypylos are wounded[66] and that they are being looked after by the physicians with many remedies (ἰητροὶ πολυφάρμακοι; XI. 28). Even if this is true for the other warriors and there are *iêtroi* other than Machaon and Podaleirios, it is patently untrue as far as Eurypylos is concerned. It would rather seem that this scene is a deliberate twist in the plot and that Patroklos is meant to conceal the fact of his assistance to one of the Achaeans from Achilles so as not to anger him further.

In two cases the wounded warrior himself removes the missile, namely Diomedes extracts Paris' arrow from his foot (XI.397f.) and Odysseus draws out Sokos' spear, which has pierced his armour and caused a superficial wound to his side (XI.456f.). On the one hand this is a realistic feature, as attempting to remove the spear or arrow would be most men's spontaneous reaction, but on

---

[64] See, e.g., Lowenstam (1981) or MacCary (1982).
[65] τά σε προτὶ φασὶν 'Αχιλλῆος δεδιδάχθαι.
[66] Here the poet uses two verbs for 'wounding', perhaps distinguishing between arrow wounds (βέβληται) and spear wounds (οὔτασται).

the other hand it is also used as an action illustrating heroic behaviour, as we shall see.

In Glaukos' case we do not know how he manages to rid himself of the arrow that has hit him in the arm (XII.388f.), when he prays to Apollo in book XVI, the arrow appears to have been removed and Glaukos only asks for relief from the pain and the haemorrhage of the wound. With Machaon's wound, treatment is not mentioned either: Nestor merely speaks of Hekamede washing off the blood (XIV.6f.), but the bath would appear to be part of the ritual of hospitality rather than therapeutic, and the removal of the arrow does not feature in the poem. It may be that to dwell on the treatment received by a man who was normally expected to administer treatment to others would have been considered improper or an unnecessary irony. It would have been an effective irony, however, and it may well be that Homer chose to hint at it rather than exploit it.

As one can see already from the aforementioned passages, all the wounds that are treated or healed are spear or arrow wounds. Sword wounds are always lethal, and when the first blow in a killing - using a spear or a stone - is not fatal, the sword is often used for the *coup de grâce*.

The question of *how* the wounds are treated is a question which was discussed already by the scholiasts. "He knew three types of the removal of a missile (*beloulkia*)", comments Aristonicus in the scholion ad IV.218 (AT), "extraction, as with Menelaos; excision, as with Eurypylos and *diôsmos*, as with Diomedes."[67] This is more or less the distinction as we know it from Paul of Aegina (VI.88.3/II.130.25f., except that for him excision was a sub-category of extraction), and, as this scholion proves, it dates back to at least Hellenistic times.[68] As said above, the *ektomê* or 'cutting out', as the most strictly expert treatment, appears only once, while most spears or arrows are simply pulled out. This is the obvious thing to do with the spear, or javelin, at XIII.598, but as far as the arrows are concerned, it may be a case of pseudo-realism,[59] if one considers some of the references to them. At IV.151 the barbs of the arrow are mentioned, not as an extraordinary detail, but as something that one is accustomed to see on an arrow, just as the string attaching the metal point to the shaft. At V.393 and XI.507

---

[67] ἐξολκήν, ὡς ἐπὶ Μενελάου· ἐκτομήν, ὡς ἐπ' Εὐρυπύλου· διωσμόν, ὡς ἐπὶ Διομήδους.

[68] It is not unlikely that the scholiasts had read some medical treatises, or had acquired medical knowledge in some other way (cf. Ch. 5.1).

[69] Or, to use a term coined by Friedrich (1956) for similar phenomena, *Scheinrealismus*.

arrows have the epithet τριγλωχίς - three-barbed - again suggesting that we are to imagine most, if not all, arrows used in the fighting as barbed. However, if this is the case, they can only be pulled out by an enormous physical effort and at the cost of extensive damage to the wound, because it is precisely the objective of the barbs to complicate the extraction and aggravate the wound. In the case of Diomedes' second wound it is possible to imagine him breaking off the point before the extraction, given that the arrow has gone right through the foot and is stuck in the ground, but there is nothing in the text to suggest it. Here, as in other scenes of wounding, the poet moves on the thin line between a realistic description which would appeal to his audience and a certain cavalier attitude towards the reality of wounding and wound treatment.

Another example of this pseudo-realism is verse IV.214, the meaning of which already puzzled the scholiasts (A, T): Machaon pulls out the arrow that has wounded Menelaos superficially - the barbs being visible outside the armour - and "when he had pulled [it] out, the sharp barbs broke backwards".[70] Whether πάλιν is meant to go with ἐξελκομένοιο or with ἄγεν, the fact remains that the barbs break and, even more puzzling, they break after the extraction. Given the shallowness of the wound, Machaon is presumably using his bare hands,[71] so he could hardly be meant to bring to the task sufficient violence to break a bronze arrowhead. Even reading πάλιν ἄγεν as "were bent backwards" with the scholiast (Nic., A) does not help, and it would also be a misrepresentation of the meaning of the verb ἄγνυμι. However, the description is couched in realistic terms and gives no cause for suspicion at first sight.

While the cases of *ektomê* and *exolkê* are fairly uncontroversial, the presence of the technique of *diôsmos* in the *Iliad* is less unequivocal. At V.660ff., Tleptolemos' spear strikes Sarpedon in the left thigh, the point penetrating almost to the bone, Sarpedon's companions carry him off the battlefield and his companion Pelagos removes the spear from the wound. The way in which he does this has been a source of controversy in secondary literature. The words appear to be straightforward (V.694): "and he pushed the ashen spear out from his thigh"[72] - but it is hard to imagine him doing this in practice. When later medical writers speak of

---

[70] τοῦ δ' ἐξελκομένοιο πάλιν ἄγεν ὀξέες ὄγκοι.
[71] At least no instruments are mentioned.
[72] ἐκ δ' ἄρα οἱ μηροῦ δόρυ μείλινον ὦσε θύραζε.

diôsmos,⁷³ it is only as a technique used for the extraction of arrows, not for javelins or spears - for obvious reasons, because the latter are too thick to be pulled out through an arm or a leg. Furthermore, it is not to be applied when the arrow has almost reached a bone (which would then get in the way of the *diôsmos*).

For the scholiasts there appears to be no problem, or at least they do not comment on the topic, but more recent scholars have held disparate views on the topic. Frölich⁷⁴ declares himself "not convinced" that the *diôsmos* is used in the *Iliad*, but offers no alternative suggestions as to what actually happens in V.694. Friedrich⁷⁵ develops an elaborate argument in order to explain away the action of 'pushing' the spear, which is quite obviously implied in the text: The use of ὠθεῖν, he argues, is triggered by the word θύραζε, in which the image of pushing an intruder out of the entrance is so strong that the poet could be using ὦσε without actually intending it as the action implied by the verb. This either amounts to a charge of considerable thoughtlessness against the poet or assumes imagery extending to a far more abstract degreee than usual.

Laser, on the other hand, is very taken with the idea of *diôsmos* for the scene in question and sees it described in several other scenes as well. He assumes⁷⁶ that in Sarpedon's case the lance or spear is a barbed javelin and that it is first pushed through to the other side, the point is then detached from the shaft and the shaft pulled out backwards. Although this can be done with an arrow, it is difficult to imagine this kind of procedure with a javelin. Laser also claims⁷⁷ that, when Sthenelos follows Diomedes' appeal to pull Pandaros' arrow from his shoulder,⁷⁸ he pulls it through the shoulder in the direction of the impact "as, because of the barbs, an extraction in the usual sense is not possible without further laceration". This is also the opinion of the scholiast (Nic.) ad V.112(b), according to whom this is "the removal of an arrow by *diôsmos*, so that he be not wounded afresh by the turned-back barbs".⁷⁹ Both the scholiast and Laser forget, however, that,

---

⁷³ Celsus VII.5.2.A-B/309.3-10; Paul VI.38.3/II.131.1-4.
⁷⁴ (1879), p. 61.
⁷⁵ (1956), p. 110, n. 4.
⁷⁶ (1983), pp. 112f., n. 301.
⁷⁷ Ibid., p. 110.
⁷⁸ V.112: "... he pulled the swift arrow out through his shoulder" (βέλος ὠκὺ διαμπερὲς ἐξέρυσ' ὤμου).
⁷⁹ ἡ κατὰ διωσμὸν βελουλκία, ἵνα μὴ πάλιν τιτρώσκοιτο ταῖς ἀκίσιν ὑποστροφούσαις [T]. 112bGe adds the realistic detail that Sthenelos pulls out the arrow forcefully (δυνατῶς), because "to remove it little by little would be more painful".

whichever way the arrow is pulled out, either the point or the flights have to be broken off so as not to tear the wound. Furthermore, since the arrow has already pierced the shoulder (V.100: "it went through utterly"[80]), "he pulled it out through the shoulder" would be correct whether the arrow is pulled forwards or backwards. One could also argue that, given the prevalence of righthandedness, it is more likely for Sthenelos to use his right hand for the extraction. As he would be standing on Diomedes' right side, the right shoulder being wounded, this means that he would rather snap off the point and draw the arrow out backwards. However, I admit that this takes the argument to a point well beyond the possible attention of a listening audience.

Even in the case of Patroklos' treatment of Eurypylos' wound Laser interprets "he cut the sharp arrow from his thigh with a knife"[81] (XI.844f.) in the sense of Celsus VII.5.2/309.6, as Patroklos making a counter-opening with the knife. It would seem, though, that the depth of the wound - while not piercing the leg - and the broken shaft[82] provide sufficient justification for the use of the knife for enlarging the wound, given that all or most arrows in the *Iliad* appear to be barbed.

Finally, when Diomedes, wounded for the second time, pulls out Paris' arrow, which has nailed his right foot to the ground (XI.397f.: "he pulled the swift arrow from his foot"[83]), Laser again envisages him[84] as performing a *diôsmos* - although in this case, too, the limb has already been pierced by the arrow.

The reason why I have gone to some detail concerning discrepancies in interpretation is that they prove one very important point: Homeric descriptions of wound treatment give the impression, at first sight, of great accuracy and realism - which is how they are usually read by scholars - but closer scrutiny reveals that they are by no means step-by-step realistic descriptions, and that much is left out of them. This - presumably deliberate - vagueness admits for a range of differing interpretations and suggests that perhaps the medical details are not the main selling point of these passages. It cannot be denied that the poet shows an interest in those details, but his work is not meant to be a textbook of surgery,[85] and medical details may be

---

[80] ἀντικρὺ δὲ διέσχε.
[81] ἐκ μηροῦ τάμνε μαχαίρῃ ὀξὺ βέλος.
[82] XI.584: ἐκλάσθη δὲ δόναξ.
[83] βέλος ὠκὺ ἐκ ποδὸς ἕλκ'.
[84] (1983), p. 114.
[85] And they can be equally vague; cf. Ch. 5.2.

intended to add the kind of quasi-realism that one tends to find in eye-witness reports.

The treatment following the removal of a missile is only hinted at briefly in two scenes. Machaon, treating Menelaos, sucks out the blood after having pulled out the arrow (IV.218) and Patroklos washes Eurypylos' wound with luke-warm water (XI.845f.) - the correct decision according to the scholiast (ad XI.830.b, T), who comments that "warm water brings about bleeding and cold water causes chills" and (ib. a) that "it [i.e. luke-warm water] soothes the pain".[86] Both Machaon and Patroklos apply "sothing drugs" (ἤπια φάρμακα). In Patroklos' case these are described in more detail and we hear that the *pharmakon* is a bitter root, which he crushes between his hands (XI.845f.) and which has analgesic and haemostatic properties (ib.847f.).

A bandage is mentioned only once: Agenor uses a woollen sling (σφενδόνη), handed to him by his squire, to bandage Helenos' hand after the removal of Menelaos' spear (XIII.599f.). This hardly gives us a clue on the frequency of bandaging for wounds in Homeric times, and the only conclusion we can draw is that in this one passage the poet decided to add this detail while in others he did not.

The only hint that wounds need continued nursing is found in XV.390-94, when Patroklos is still sitting with the wounded Eurypylos, entertaining him with talk, and again applying pain-killing remedies to the wound. Patroklos' *pharmaka* are obviously not meant to be miracle drugs and, unlike the divine healings, the cure is not instantaneous.

One aspect of the scenes in question, which may have been of interest to the audience, lies in the promptness and competence of the treatment, although this is not always proportionate to the wounded man's importance. Menelaos' position as the supreme leader's brother is emphasised by the fact that his wound has to be treated by the best physician available and not by another warrior. The latter is what those of a less elevated status have to make do with, and their companions' attitude towards them is of as much interest as their own. This prompt response to an appeal for help, or even help given without waiting for an appeal, is part of the nature of the epic hero. (It has to be pointed out, though, that help is restricted to the hero's peer group.)

In the case of Eurypylos the position and knowledge of the person treating the wound are disproportionate to the casualty's

---

[86] τὸ γὰρ θερμὸν αἵματος ἀγωγόν, τὸ δὲ ψυχρὸν ἐμποιεῖ φρίκην ... πραΰνει γὰρ τὰς ἀλγεδόνας.

importance and at first sight the assistance of the Achilles-substitute Patroklos seems wasted on a second-class hero. However, if the poet had needed a scene in which to demonstrate Patroklos' particular kindness, at the same time giving him an occasion to hear of the plight of the Achaean army, this is the perfect solution. The heroes of first rank wounded in book XI are Agamemnon - who must still be considered Achilles' enemy - Odysseus, who was a member of the embassy sent to persuade Achilles, and Diomedes, referred to as the "best of the Achaeans" (V.103 and V.414) in Achilles' absence, and thus likely to stir antagonism in Achilles.[87] Therefore Patroklos cannot possibly help any of them. Eurypylos who, though one of the Achaeans, is totally uninvolved in the dissent between Achilles and Agamemnon, serves the purpose very well and it may well be that the way he reacts to his wound (which will be discussed below) is intended to make up for his lack of status as a hero.

The main interest of the scenes discussed here is an aspect which has already been hinted at, namely the wounded man's state of mind, his way of bearing the wound. Along with a fearless attitude in fighting, this is what distinguishes the hero from the ordinary man. For Homer and his audience these were obvious criteria and "they knew what a hero was and what was expected of him".[88] We can also expect them to have known war, fighting and wounds either from their own experience or at least through first-hand information given by others. They would therefore expect a certain degree of realism in order to find scenes of wounding convincing and true to life. Examples of this kind of realism are the natural movements of Diomedes lifting the shield-strap to wipe his wound (V.798) and of Glaukos clutching his wounded arm (XVI.510: "grasping it with his hand, he squeezed his arm"[89]), both strongly visual images. This sense of reality would make the audience appreciate the hero's achievement in dealing with his wound and it is obvious that the poet wants his audience to recognise the heroic dimension of the tale. It is likely that the reason for all the non-fatal wounds being arrow or spear wounds is that this emphasises a particular aspect of the passages in question, i.e. because with the removal of the weapon they make for more spectacular scenes than sword wounds would.

---

[87] It is also Diomedes who, after the failure of the embassy, suggests leaving Achilles alone and continuing the fighting (IX.701f.).
[88] Redfield (1975), p. 78.
[89] χειρὶ δ' ἑλὼν ἐπίεζε βραχίονα.

We shall see that the poet makes use of the difference in the warrior's reaction to stress the distinction between Trojans and Greeks as well as between outstanding heroes and ordinary warriors - and also between mortals and immortals. The example of Thersites shows how a lesser man reacts to the pain of blows - in this case the worst (αἴσχιστος) of all the Greeks. Ugly, deformed,[90] a coward without a sense of honour, Thersites is the perfect antithesis of the Homeric hero and the beating inflicted on him by Odysseus can be seen as the caricature of a hero's wounding.

Although Odysseus' blows leave only a weal, certainly less painful than a wound made by a spear or an arrow, Thersites is bent double - this verb is usual for a dying warrior,[91] e.g. at XIII.618 - sits down in fear (the equivalent of the wounded warrior retreating among his companions?) and sheds tears of pain (II.265-9). While it is not uncommon for a Homeric hero to cry, the reason for these tears is always emotional distress or grief, never physical pain, and Thersites' behaviour makes him an object of ridicule (II.270). One could even see a parallel between "he wiped away a tear" (ἀπομόρξατο δάκρυ) at II.269 and "he [sc. Diomedes] wiped away the blood" (αἷμ' ἀπομόργνυ) at V.798.

While Thersites is a singular and extreme example of what a man should not be like, there appear to be varying degrees of being a hero. To begin with, the poet clearly makes a distinction between Trojans and their allies on the one hand and Greeks on the other. It is mostly the Trojans who are killed while trying to run away (e.g. V.45f.,55f.,65f.; XI.446ff.; XIII.567-70) and the four cases of fainting with non-fatal wounds - Aeneas (V.310), Sarpedon (V.696) and Hector (XI.356, when Diomedes strikes his helmet, but fails to wound him, and XIV.438f.) - all occur on the Trojan side. The woundings of Aeneas and Hector can be compared to that of Teukros, who is also hit by a rock (although his injury may be less dangerous than the two others), collapses and drops his bow (VIII.329), but does not faint. Sarpedon's case could be contrasted with Diomedes having Sthenelos pull the arrow from his shoulder (V.112f.) or later pulling the second arrow out through his foot (XI.397f.): in neither case he faints, although this would not be a surprising reaction.

The same excellence of the Greek warrior can be seen clearly in the difference between Diomedes' and Glaukos' prayers. In these two cases the wounds are very similar: both have been hit by

---

[90] Note again the importance of beauty.
[91] E.g. at XIII.618: "he bent double in falling" (ἰδνώθη δὲ πεσών).

arrows, Diomedes in - or rather through - the shoulder, and Glaukos in the arm. As soon as Sthenelos has pulled out the arrow, Diomedes prays to Athena (V.115-20), but he does not ask the goddess to heal his wound despite the copious bleeding (V.113: "the blood darted up through the pliant tunic"[92]). The wish he expresses in his prayer is only revenge for his wound - to kill the man whose arrow has struck him and who boasts that the wound is fatal.[93] This fact also caught the attention of the scholiast (Did.), who comments: "He does not pray for healing, but for the punishment of the man who shot him."[94] When Athena finds Diomedes later, cooling his wound and still in pain, again he does not mention the wound in his retort (V.815-24) to her taunts about having retired from the battle.

Glaukos' prayer to Apollo (XVI.514-26), on the other hand, is a straightforward appeal for help. It is motivated by the dying words of Sarpedon, who has entreated Glaukos to defend his body, pointing out unambiguously that the failure to do so would be a cause for dejection and shame for the rest of Glaukos' life. Thus it would seem that Glaukos is motivated not so much by a desire for revenge as by concern for his own reputation. (As always in the *Iliad*, only success counts and the good intention alone would not. Hence Glaukos has to succeed in order to win *kydos* for himself.) Glaukos' prayer contains (XVI.517-21) the only complaint about a wound in the entire *Iliad*. "I have this severe wound", he says, "my arm is plagued by sharp pain, the blood will not dry up and my shoulder feels heavy with it. I cannot hold my spear firmly nor can I fight advancing towards my enemies."[95] He asks Apollo explicitly to "heal this grievous wound, lull the pain and give [him] strength" (ib. 523f.).[96] While, ultimately, Glaukos is asking for the strength to defend Sarpedon's body, his main concern is with the pain and bleeding of the wound - which makes the overall impression of his prayer rather less heroic than Diomedes'.

---

[92] αἷμα δ' ἀνηκόντιζε διὰ στρεπτοῖο χιτῶνος. According to the entry for στρεπτός in Liddell and Scott, the 'tunic' is a shirt of chainmail, but it is unlikely that chainmail was worn in such an early period.
[93] V.118f.: δὸς δέ τέ μ' ἄνδρα ἑλεῖν, κτλ.
[94] οὐ περὶ τῆς ἰάσεως, ἀλλὰ τῆς τοῦ βαλόντος εὔχεται τιμωρίας (T).
[95] ἕλκος μὲν γὰρ ἔχω τόδε καρτερόν, ἀμφὶ δέ μοι χεὶρ / ὀξείῃς ὀδύνῃσιν ἐλήλαται, οὐδέ μοι αἷμα / τερσῆναι δύναται, βαρύθει δέ μοι ὦμος ὑπ' αὐτοῦ· / ἔγχος δ' οὐ δύναμαι σχεῖν ἔμπεδον, οὐδὲ μάχεσθαι / ἐλθὼν δυσμενέεσσιν.
[96] τόδε καρτερὸν ἕλκος ἄκεσσαι, / κοίμησον δ' ὀδύνας, δὸς δὲ κράτος ...

A slight pro-Achaean bias can be noticed in the descriptions, but not all the Greeks are great heroes either. First of all there is the distinction between the *plêthys* (πληθύς), i.e. the mass, and the *aristoi* (ἄριστοι), literally 'the best', as it becomes clear in Thoas' advice to send the former back to the ships while the latter stay behind to face the charging Trojans at XV.295ff.: "Let us first command the mass to return to the ships and let ourselves, who boast to be the best in the army, stand our ground."[97] The *aristoi*, those who "fight among the foremost", are the warrior élite, numerically only a fraction of the Achaean forces, but nevertheless the focus of the epic.

Even those true 'heroes', however, are not all on the same level. It goes without saying that Achilles is in a category of his own, above all the others, and everyone respects his right to this status, even the enemy.[98] During his absence from the fighting the 'best' appear to be Diomedes and Aias, followed by Odysseus and perhaps Agamemnon and Menelaos, although with the Atreids it is difficult to distinguish between their social status and their status as warriors.

Menelaos is the first warrior to be wounded in the *Iliad* and - given his position in the army - his wound has the greatest impact on the general events, since the arrow shot at Menelaos constitutes the breaking of the attempted truce and frustrates all hopes for a peaceful settlement.[99] In this case, therefore, the circumstances and consequences of the wounding are matters of great interest for the audience, and so are both Menelaos' and Agamemnon's reaction.

This is the only scene in which the bystander - Agamemnon - reacts in any other way than by giving prompt help and Agamemnon's response to Menelaos' wounding is developed to a considerable extent, completing the picture of Agamemnon's character as we already know it from earlier scenes. When Agamemnon shudders at the sight of the blood flowing from the wound (IV.148f.), we can assume that this is from concern for his brother rather than squeamishness, having misjudged the gravity of the wound. The poet makes it clear in other scenes that Agamemnon loses heart easily, and here again he gets carried

---

[97] πληθὺν μὲν ποτὶ νῆας ἀνώξομεν ἀπονέεσθαι· / αὐτοὶ δ' ὅσσοι ἄριστοι ἐνὶ στρατῷ εὐχόμεθ' εἶναι, / στήομεν. The passage demonstrates that the status of *aristos* has to be maintained by deliberately putting one's life at stake.

[98] Although the exchange of verbal abuse before and during fighting is very common in the *Iliad*, no one insults Achilles For example, at XXI.160 Asteropaios addresses him as "glorious Achilles" (φαίδιμ' Ἀχιλλεῦ).

[99] This is an example of what Lossau (1989) means by 'strategic wounding'.

away with visions of defeat, until the wounded Menelaos himself reassures him (IV.184-7). This is a means for reinforcing the impression, present throughout the poem, that Agamemnon, although a brave man in battle, is easily overwhelmed by emotional pressure.

When Menelaos equally shudders for an instant upon seeing the blood running from his wound (IV.150), again it is not a means to heighten the suspense of the scene, because the audience already know that the wound is not dangerous, from a complex explanation (IV.132-8) of the different layers of equipment pierced by the arrow. The latter is another example of a detailed description that leaves us incompletely informed; we do not know exactly where the arrow has hit Menealos.[100] The detail that Menelaos here and Agamemnon at XI.254 are the only warriors who have a moment of shock and fear when wounded may be intended as a negative trait. Menelaos overcomes his initial terror immediately, but it is worth noting that he only picks up courage on seeing that the barbs and the string attaching the metal point of the shaft are outside the armour - and thus obviously outside the wound. This shows Menelaos' great relief at realising that the wound is not deep and - most importantly - that the arrow will not need cutting out.

We are probably meant to assume that all Homeric heroes have sufficient knowledge of wounds to know how they will be treated, and in later passages both Diomedes and Eurypylos know what has to be done. Considering this, Agamemnon does not have very precise ideas when he says to Menelaos (IV.190f.) that "a doctor will palpate the wound and apply remedies that will still the black pain".[101] It may be that he is not actually thinking of the treatment in practical terms, or that he is being intentionally vague by not mentioning the removal of the arrow. If the latter is the case, it can be meant to reflect upon Agamemnon himself as well as on Menelaos and in either case it may convey a negative image. In his initial shock Agamemnon has obviously not had a close look at the wound - or he would know that it is shallow and that the arrow will be easy to remove - but he does not speak of the fact that it has to be extracted. (This could have been done easily by Agamemnon or even by Menelaos himself.)

---

[100] Presumably somewhere between the waist and the lower abdomen, depending on where the *zôstêr*, *zôma* and *mitrê* were worn.

[101] ἕλκος δ' ἰητὴρ ἐπιμάσσεται ἠδ' ἐπιθήσει / φάρμαχ', ἅ κεν παύσῃσι μελαινάων ὀδυνάων.

The possible reasons for this omission, other than mere lack of precision in speech, are either that Agamemnon, from concern for his brother, refuses to think of the extraction, or that he uses 'palpate' as a euphemism for 'pulling/cutting out' so as not to distress Menealos. The latter would make this the only scene in the *Iliad* in which someone minimises the gravity of a wound in order to comfort the wounded man, and would present a very uncharacteristic attitude. Either hypothesis would cast a suspicion of weakness on Agamemnon or Menelaos, for neither of whom it would be surprising. Agamemnon's weakness in the face of emotional pressure has already been mentioned and Menelaos, although one of the leaders, is not a warrior comparable to Achilles, Diomedes or Ajax. Thus Apollo (who, admittedly, is Menelaos' enemy), speaking to Hector, refers to Menelaos as a "soft fighter".[102] The scene of Menelaos' wounding emphasises his status within the army and his importance for the expedition, but it does not show either of the Atreids in a purely positive light, in conformity with their ambivalent image throughout the epic.

We have already seen how Diomedes differs from Glaukos in his behaviour when wounded, but he also stands out among the Achaean heroes. He is the only warrior to be wounded - non-fatally - twice. It appears that the first wound does not stop him from fighting and soon after the second wound we find him competing in the funeral games for Patroklos. He commands - rather than asks - Sthenelos to pull out Pandaros' arrow and when Paris' arrow has pierced his foot, he does not ask for help, but pulls out the arrow by himself. In the first case the poet speaks of the haemorrhage (V.113, cited above) and in the second case of the pain accompanying the extraction (XI.398: "grievous pain shot through his body"[103]), but in neither case does Diomedes show any signs of suffering. After the second wound he mounts his chariot and orders the charioteer to take him back to the ships; "for his heart was vexed" (XI.400).[104] This is the only reference to the effect that this wound has on Diomedes - he needs no help to reach his chariot, nor do his horses carry him away "groaning heavily" like other, lesser, warriors.

The latter is the case, on the Achaean side, with Deiphobos (XIII.538f.), wounded in the arm by Meriones' spear, whom his brother has to lead to his chariot with his arms around him. It is also true of Teukros, struck on the collar-bone with a jagged stone

---

[102] μαλθακὸς αἰχμητής (XVII.588).
[103] ὀδύνη δὲ διὰ χροὸς ἦλθ' ἀλεγεινή.
[104] ἤχθετο γὰρ κῆρ.

which severs the sinew. Two companions support him and take him to the ships while he "groans heavily" (VIII.332f.). (The same is also said of Hector, whom his companions have to carry to his chariot at XIV.428-32.) The need for help to reach their chariots and the groaning appear to be details accompanying the wounding of heroes who are not considered of first rank. In the same way as tears, groans are only acceptable for expressing emotions such as grief or anguish - and the phrase in the nominative, βαρὺ στενάχων, is only used for such occasions (e.g. I.364, IX.16, XVI.20). For obvious reasons crying out with physical pain is even more unheard of, although it is perfectly acceptable in grief or distress.[105] Therefore it is seen only in the dying, e.g. V.68: "he sank to his knees groaning and death enveloped him",[106] or the groaning of the dying on the battlefield described at IV.450f. and VIII.64f.

Odysseus and Agamemnon, who are both wounded in the great battle in book XI, are clearly meant to stand above the two aforementioned warriors. The scene in which Agamemnon is wounded by a spear-thrust piercing his arm (XI.252-72) contains a feature which appears in none of the other similar scenes: Agamemnon does not stop when wounded - as would be the usual procedure - but he continues to fight after an initial moment of horror (XI.254: ῥίγησεν) until the bleeding stops, the wound dries, and the ensuing pain makes him abandon the battle (XI.267f.). This is the only time in the *Iliad* that a warrior continues fighting until the pain of his wound forces him to stop - and the only case in which the pain itself is dwelt upon at length (XI.268-72) - and it is also the only explicit expression of the notion that wounds are more painful after the bleeding has stopped. (In the simile of the wounded deer [XI.474-81], fleeing while the blood is warm, it is not so clear whether "the swift arrow overpowers him"[107] refers to loss of blood, pain or just exhaustion.[108]) However, Agamemnon never groans nor complains and has the strength to shout encouragement at the Achaeans from his chariot before leaving the battlefield. The description of his retreat (XI.273f.) is word for word the same as Diomedes', including the final "his heart was vexed". In Agamemnon's case this is followed by another reference to

---

[105] These distinctions contradict simplistic views of Homer's integration of mind and body often professed by scholar.
[106] γνὺξ δ' ἔριπ' οἰμώξας, θάνατος δέ μιν ἀμφεκάλυψεν.
[107] τόν γε δαμάσσεται ὠκὺς ὀιστός (ib. 478).
[108] This fact has also been noticed by Fenik (1968), p. 89.

Agamemnon's suffering (XI.284): "carrying the suffering king away from the battle".[109]

The poet has obviously taken great care to bring home the fact that Agamemnon is in pain, but it is not quite clear why he should have wanted to do so in this particular case. What is particularly unusual is the simile used to describe the pain of the wound, namely the comparison with the pains of labour. It is difficult to imagine why the supreme commander of the army, having sustained a battle wound, should be compared to a woman in childbirth rather than, e.g., a wounded lion. The parallels and symbolic associations between war and childbirth in Greek thought are discussed in detail by N. Loraux in her article *Le lit, la guerre*,[110] but it is dubious whether they apply for the epic as well as they do for, e.g., tragedy. The main point concerning the Agamemnon passage seems to be[111] the shift from "the beauty of war towards war that hurts", i.e. the emphasis of the suffering involved.

Comparing another man to a woman (e.g. II.235/VII.96: "Achaean women, not Achaeans";[112] VII.163: "you are made like a woman"[113]) is a popular insult,[114] but in Agamemnon's case the comparison can hardly be meant to diminish him as a warrior. The important point here seems to be that it is not Agamemnon himself who is compared with a woman, but only the pain of his wound being compared with the - presumably - most generally familiar example of pain, an example that would convey an impression of intensity to most people. The overall intention, therefore, may well be to show that Agamemnon cannot be blamed for leaving the battlefield, given the particularly painful nature of his injury.

It is, however, interesting to see that in the simile the woman's suffering is referred to as an arrow or missile (βέλος) and the adjective used for her labour pains is 'pointed/sharp' (πικρός), an epithet for arrows (e.g. IV.217: πικρὸς ὀιστός).It would seem that the comparison works both ways: childbirth is as painful as an arrow wound and vice versa, and both are apparently seen as the most representative examples of sharp pain. According to a

---

[109] τειρόμενον βασιλῆα μάχης ἀπάνευθε φέροντες.
[110] (1981).
[111] Ibid., p. 49.
[112] Ἀχαιίδες, οὐκέτ' Ἀχαιοί.
[113] γυναικὸς ἄρ' ἀντὶ τέτυξο.
[114] However, Achilles likening Patroklos to a little girl waiting for her mother to pick her up (XVI.7-10) must be seen as an exception. It is quite clear from the context that Achilles does not intend to insult Patroklos, but that the simile is rather to be understood as terms of endearment expressing his affection.

person's gender, either the one or the other type of 'wound' would be seen as typical or appropriate.

Shortly after Agamemnon and Diomedes, Odysseus, too, is wounded, by Sokos' spear which pierces his shield and breastplate, separating all the skin from his side (XI.435ff.). As usual, we are informed immediately that this is not a dangerous wound: obviously the interest of scenes of wounding is not dependent on suspense. The difference here is that Odysseus himself realises - as soon as the spear hits him - that the wound is not dangerous (XI.439): "Odysseus knew that fatal doom had not come to him."[115] This detail may be meant to show Odysseus' *sang froid*, as it is also pointed out by the scholiast (Did. b.): "The calm of Odysseus is to be admired."[116] With the spear still fixed in his shield and armour - presumably we are supposed to imagine it in his left side - Odysseus kills Sokos and then pulls out the spear without help, causing a fresh haemorrhage (XI.458: " when he had pulled it out, the blood gushed forth.")[117] In this passage physical pain is not mentioned, only a feeling of worry and discouragement, expressed by (ibid.) "his heart was vexed".[118]

Odysseus' subsequent cry for help can hardly be seen as diminishing his prowess as a hero, as he finds himself wounded and alone, surrounded by Trojans, in a position in which normally another warrior should be coming to help him. Furthermore, he is in this position for having protected the wounded Diomedes (XI. 396f.) and following his decision (XI.404-10) that, although he is left facing the Trojans on his own, it would be cowardly to retreat, he is thus in danger because of the kind of behaviour that is expected from him as one of the *aristoi*, a victim of the "heroic code", as Fenik[119] calls it.

When Ajax and Menelaos come to Odysseus' aid, they find him still fighting off the Trojans. His situation is described by the aforementioned simile of the deer, wounded by an arrow and beset by jackals which are wating for it to drop exhausted. While Ajax covers Odysseus with his shield - the familiar gesture for protecting a wounded companion[120] - Menelaos leads him to his chariot, taking him by the hand. Taking another warrior's hand (χειρὸς ἔχων) is usually a gesture of comfort (e.g. IV.154) and

---

[115] γνῶ δ' 'Οδυσεὺς ὅ οἱ οὔ τι τέλος κατακαίριον ἦλθεν.
[116] ἔστι δὲ θαυμάσαι τὸ ἀτάραχον 'Οδυσσέως.
[117] αἷμα δέ οἱ σπασθέντος ἀνέσσυτο.
[118] κῆδε δὲ θυμόν.
[119] (1968), pp. 30f. and *passim*.
[120] See Fig. 3 for a particularly beautiful representation of that gesture, which appears frequently both in literature and in art.

is not likely to be meant as Menelaos supporting Odysseus. Odysseus' departure from the battlefield is not described, but altogether the scene seems to be constructed to give an impression of Odysseus' valour.

Eurypylos' wounding and his treament by Patroklos constitute a special case, since Eurypylos shows perfect heroic behaviour, although he never appears as one of the great heroes in any other scenes. Wounded by Paris' arrow (XI.583f.) when coming to the aid of Telamonian Ajax who is hard pressed by the Trojans - one of the standard heroic behaviour patterns - Eurypylos retreats among his companions and calls upon them to protect Ajax. He then leaves the battlefield unaided and on foot. This happens nowhere else in the *Iliad*, as all other casualties either mount their own chariot or are taken away by their comrades. This is both a show of fortitude and geared to rouse Patroklos' compassion.

Thus when Patroklos encounters him near Odysseus' ships, Eurypylos is described as limping with the arrow fixed in his thigh, sweat running from his head and shoulders, and blood gushing from his wound (XI.810-13), however (ib. 813) "his mind was steadfast".[121] "So that he can speak to Patroklos steadily", comments the scholiast (T), but this is unlikely to be the only reason for describing Eurypylos' state of mind. It should rather be seen as a signal of his heroic qualities that despite the pain and the exertion "his wits are steadfast", since he continues to display an attitude worthy of a great warrior.

Unlike Agamemnon, Eurypylos is very specific as to the treatment of the wound and appears to know exactly what Patroklos has to do. Since Patroklos knows it as well and does not need telling, the fact that Eurypylos does so appears to be a means of showing how little he is daunted by his wound. The request for soothing remedies (ἤπια φάρμακα; XI.830) is the only hint at the pain of the wound[122] and Eurypylos neither complains nor shows any signs of suffering or apprehension at the prospect of having the arrow cut out. As has been suggested earlier, Eurypylos, who is not one of the famous warriors, has been equipped with all the heroic virtues in order to make him significant enough for his role and for being treated by one of the protagonists of the tale.

Among the scholars writing about battle scenes in the *Iliad*, Friedrich has been the only one to pay any attention to this differentiation in the heroes' reaction to wounds as reflecting their

---

[121] νόος γε μὲν ἔμπεδος ἦεν.
[122] As the scholiast remarks (830.c/T), "being in pain, he wants gentle remedies" (ὡς ἀλγῶν πραέα φάρμακα βούλεται).

heroic status. "Apparently", he writes,[123] "the style in Λ distinguishes the great heroes from the lesser ones." Regarding Diomedes' and Odysseus' wounds he says[124] that the poet is not interested in their treatment, only its prerequesite, the removal of the weapon, mainly "because of the self-control maintained by the heroes despite pain and disability." However, he does not develop the theory in much detail and seems to stand alone with this insight and, to the best of my knowledge, no other scholars have taken this approach.

Two motifs related to wounds, which remain valid throughout antiquity, appear in the *Iliad*, but in a way which makes it appear as if they were already commonly accepted: the low status of the archer and the concept of 'honourable' wounds in front. The word 'archer' (τοξότα) is part of the abuse which Diomedes hurls at Paris when the latter triumphs at having wounded him (XI.385) and he goes on to say that it is as if a woman or a child had hit him, "because the weapon of a cowardly, worthless man is blunt" (XI.390).[125] The bow, by killing from a distance instead of in close combat, is despised as a coward's weapon, and this would explain why Teukros, the only archer among the named warriors in the Greek camp, does not use the bow exclusively, but alternates it (successfully) with the spear. However, the presence of archers adds variety to the fighting and, furthermore, outstanding heroes such as Achilles or Diomedes can only be killed or wounded by a treacherous weapon such as the arrow, since no one can defeat them in hand-to-hand fighting.

The theme of wounds in front resists logical explanation and is clearly of merely symbolical value. While the original reasoning is straightforward - a man who is hit in the back must have been running away and is therefore a coward - it is equally clear that in a pitched battle this is not a realistic assumption, since a warrior can easily be surrounded by enemies. The idea that those who turn to run are struck in the back is expressed at XII.42:

> Many were struck in their bodies by the pitiless bronze;
> when having bared their backs by turning round
> in the fight, and many through their very shields.[126]

---

[123] (1956), p. 33.
[124] Ibid., p. 93.
[125] κωφὸν γὰρ βέλος ἀνδρὸς ἀνάλκιδος οὐτιδανοῖο.
[126] πολλοὶ δ' οὐτάζοντο κατὰ χρόα νηλέι χαλκῷ · / ἠμὲν ὅτῳ στρεφθέντι μετάφρενα γυμνωθείη / μαρναμένων, πολλοὶ δὲ διαμπερὲς ἀσπίδος αὐτῆς.

Twice in the *Iliad* it is made explicit how important it is not to be hit in the back. At VIII.94f. Diomedes calls out to Odysseus: "Where are you escaping to, turning your back like a worthless man in the crowd; [beware] lest someone plant a spear in your back as you flee."[127] and Idomeneus, encouraging Meriones, says (XIII. 288ff.):

> If you are wounded or hit whilst toiling [in the fight],
> let the missile not fall onto the neck behind or in the back,
> but let it strike in the chest or the stomach,
> as you go forward in the company of those who fight in front.[128]

As if to prove the absurdity of this notion, Patroklos - who is certainly meant to be one of the most prominent heroes - is treacherously struck in the back by Euphorbos (XVI.806f.), after being equally struck on the back and stunned by Apollo (XVI.791). It is quite obvious that this wounding is not the result of an attempt to flee. As the death of Patroklos is one of the three most important death scenes in the *Iliad*, this can hardly be an oversight and we have to wonder why the poet has chosen to make it happen the way it does. Also, the fact that Patroklos is struck in the back is not commented upon by any of the other warriors and no one seems scandalised by it. The purpose is presumably to make the death of gentle Patroklos - who is already an object of considerable pity and mourning within the epic - even more tragic and pitiful. Perhaps another objective was to make Hector's victory over Patroklos less of an achievement, since, as the dying man points out to him (XVI.850) he was only the third to strike him, after Patroklos had already been wounded.

There is one further point which makes scenes of wounding a vehicle for the image of heroic virtues: when Aphrodite and Ares are wounded, we can see the difference between the way in which they bear their wounds and the way humans do. It is not so surprising that Aphrodite cries out when wounded by Diomedes (V.343), but even the god of war himself screams when hit (V.859: "and bronze Ares roared"[129]) and behaves in a way which would have been considered undignified in a mortal. As Wilson[130] points out: "Nowhere is the difference between man's and god's experience and viewpoint more strikingly presented", and similar

---

[127] πῇ φεύγεις μετὰ νῶτα βαλὼν κακὸς ὣς ἐν ὁμίλῳ, / μή τίς τοι φεύγοντι μεταφρένῳ ἐν δόρυ πήξῃ.
[128] εἴ περ γάρ κε βλῇο πονεύμενος ἠὲ τυπείης, / οὐκ ἂν ἐν αὐχέν᾽ ὄπισθε πέσοι βέλος οὐδ᾽ ἐνὶ νώτῳ, / ἀλλά κεν ἢ στέρνων ἢ νηδύος ἀντιάσειεν, / πρόσσω ἱεμένοιο μετὰ προμάχων ὀαριστύν.
[129] ὁ δ᾽ ἔβραχε χάλκεος Ἄρης.
[130] (1952), p. 272.

behaviour would be unacceptable in a human warrior in the epic. Wilson goes on to say that "very seldom in the poem does a wounded soldier groan or cry out in pain", but, as I have said above, only the dying cry out, never those with non-fatal wounds. Thus war wounds are the domain where mortals can outshine the gods by showing more courage and dignity - since, as we have seen, mortality is a prerequisite for heroism.

To sum up the argument, one can say that for the Homeric warrior death in battle, fighting among the *promachoi*, is the ultimate proof of heroism and the sublimation of the heroic life. This is his only chance for survival in the memory of future generations. However, a man need not die to become a hero. Prowess in fighting and courage in bearing wounds are qualities which are rated highly by other warriors, the latter being as important as the former. Hence fortitude when wounded in battle is one way of asserting heroic status while still alive and able to enjoy it.

CHAPTER SEVEN

BEAUTIFUL DEATH; THE ADJUSTMENT OF AN IDEAL

In the previous chapter I have pointed out - looking at the *Iliad* - that there is a further dimension to scenes of wounding, beyond the mere description of events which are common in a war. As we have seen, the warrior's attitude in meeting the challenge of fear and pain, when facing either fatal or non-fatal wounds, is an essential element in the image of the hero in literature - and presumably this was also the case in popular imagination.

In the extant literature of the centuries which follow the creation of the *Iliad* as we have it, one can notice a decrease in scenes of wounding and wound treatment, almost to the point of disappearance, before a sudden dramatic increase in the material regarding Alexander the Great, preceded by some references to Philip's wounds. Usually classical scholars either tend to regard scenes of wounding (whether leading to death or not) in literature as an obvious facet of what they consider realistic narrative, or they dismiss them as mere literary topoi without much value for the story. It seems to me that both opinions represent unsatisfactory explanations (if, indeed, they explain anything), and that the reasons underlying the authors' decision to include scenes of death and wounding deserve closer attention. It cannot be pure coincidence that the concentration of scenes of wounding is greatest in those works of literature which are particularly concerned with presenting the image of a hero and with showing what makes a man a hero.[1] It would rather seem that such scenes - along with those depicting heroic death - are a deliberate means to that end and that they are closely related to the concept of individual heroism. (It has to be pointed out that, as with any material concerning classical Greece, our sources are geographically very limited. In great majority they are either of Athenian origin or have come down to us in a selection made by Athenian writers.)

This fact is crucial in explaining the silence regarding the individual's wounds between the late seventh and the early fourth centuries BC. During the same period we can also observe a change in the style of warfare, namely the introduction of the

---

[1] And, in Jaeger's words ([1936], I, p. 133), 'for Greek culture and for the whole of antiquity the hero is the higher form of man in its essence".

hoplite in the later sense of the word and, especially, of the phalanx.[2] This change in warfare is itself based on the political and economical changes involved in the transition from what one could call (anachronistically) a feudal society, in which war was the business of an aristocratic warrior class, to the *polis*, in which every citizen became a warrior in case of war. It is obvious that any change on such a scale would necessarily bring about ideological changes, and for our topic it is the ideology regarding the warrior and his behaviour in battle that matters.

The most visible change reflected in the literature describing wars and battles during this period is the waning interest in the individual warrior. He is no longer of interest as an individual hero, but *qua* citizen who will die or has died for his city. It is not surprising therefore that one can also detect less interest in individual biographical detail such as wounds, since it is the fact of the citizen warrior's death that counts, and not the detailed circumstances of that death.

Although my topic is wounding and wound treatment, the literary 'treatment' of the subject is intrinsically linked with a framework of ideas about heroism, encompassing aspects other than wounding as well. Therefore it would make for an incomplete argument to isolate only passages concerning wounds strictly speaking without discussing other, related topics. In other words, since I argue that wounding in literature is an essential part of the literary depiction of the hero, it would not make sense to ignore the other components of the concept of heroism altogether. In this chapter I am therefore digressing slightly from the topic of wounding in a narrow sense in order to present an approximate outline of the background against which the subject of wounds is usually set.

As one would expect, the most frequently described aspect of heroism is the right way to act in battle, that is, the right way to fight and the right way to die. It is the concept of the right way for a man to fight that undergoes the most conspicuous change because of the new techniques of warfare. In a formation of hoplites in a phalanx each man depended on his right-hand neighbour's shield to protect his right side, as much as the man on his left depended on him, and the phalanx lost its efficacy if the

---

[2] Opinions differ as to which are the earliest literary descriptions that can be taken to represent unambiguously the employment of the phalanx in battle, but the Chigi Vase, dated to about 650 BC, beyond any doubt shows two phalanxes facing each other (Snodgrass [1964], pl. 36).

line was broken.³ The foremost duty of every single member of the line was therefore to stay in his place whatever the situation. I do not wish to discuss the tactical limitations of a hoplite phalanx, such as the choice of terrain, in this context, because I do not believe that practical limitations are reflected to any relevant extent in ideology and ideals. (As I pointed out earlier, the concept of wounds in the back being dishonourable did not appear to be influenced by the practicalities of warfare.)

The Homeric hero's characteristic style of fighting had consisted in either rushing forward to challenge an enemy and engage him in a duel or following another's challenge, but in the new style of fighting such behaviour would not only be uncalled for, but it would be unacceptable and would jeopardise the success of an attack. Thus the desire for individual heroics has to be subordinated to the common purpose and to the commands of the community.⁴ What is expected from the citizen warrior is no longer readiness to die for personal glory, but self-sacrifice for the benefit of the city.

The new technique places strong emphasis on order and discipline, especially self-discipline, rather than on feats of daring. M. Detienne,⁵ speaking of the radical change in expected behaviour, characterises the two attitudes by the words *lyssa*, for the Homeric warrior's way of fighting, and *sôphrosyne* for the hoplite in a phalanx. The order imposed by the city is different from the assistance and protection given by Homeric heroes to fellow warriors by free choice, and this absence of choice as well as the necessity to conform to the system are well expressed in the ephebes' oath: "I shall not disgrace the sacred weapons and I shall not abandon my neighbour [in the battle-line; literally "the one standing next to me"] wherever I stand."⁶ What is required, therefore, is staying-power and not personal initiative or feats of derring-do.

---

³ A story in Plutarch's *Sayings of the Spartans* (220A) spells this out: "When someone asked why among them [i.e. the Spartans] they disdain those who throw away their shields but not those who throw away their helmets and armour, he said: 'Because they put on the latter for their own sake, but the shields they wear for the sake of the common battle-line'." (ἐρωτήσαντος δέ τινος διὰ τι τοὺς μὲν τὰς ἀσπίδας παρ' αὑτοῖς ἀποβάλοντας ἀτιμοῦσι, τοὺς θώρακας οὐκέτι, «ὅτι», ἔφη, «ταῦτα μὲν ἑαυτῶν χάριν περιτίθενται· τὴν δ' ἀσπίδα τῆς κοινῆς τάξεως ἔνεκα».)

⁴ Cf. Tyrtaeus, fr. 9, 15: "this is a common good for the city and the entire people" (ξυνὸν δ' ἐσθλὸν τοῦτο πόληι τε παντί τε δήμῳ).

⁵ Cited in Vernant (1968), p. 123.

⁶ οὐκ αἰσχυνῶ τὰ ἱερὰ ὅπλα οὐδὲ λείψω τὸν παραστάτην ὅπου ἂν στοιχήσω. Quoted in Robert (1938), p. 302.

Despite this change in the practical requirements for a good warrior, it has to be stressed that on the level of ideals the essential values of honour and courage remain those of the epic throughout antiquity (as has been pointed out by Jaeger, Croiset, Detienne, etc.), and equally the concept of war as a testing-ground for manliness remains firmly in place. This fact in itself is a source of complications, since the ethics of an aristocratic warrior élite have to be adjusted to fit the purposes of a citizen army. The gradual adjustment of the aristocratic ideal in general to changing circumstances - over the period between the eighth and the fourth centuries - is described in detail by A. W. H. Adkins as well as by W. Donlan,[7] but here I am only interested in the military aspects. Both authors agree on the survival and adaptation of Homeric values, and according to Donlan,

> The cultural standards and attitudes found in the *Iliad* and *Odyssey*, that make up what is called the 'Heroic Ideal', had a profound effect on the conceptual universe of all subsequent generations of Greeks from the late eighth century on. Historically 'real' or not, the epic system of values was very real to the Greeks of the Archaic and Classical periods (and beyond), who had no doubts about the literal existence of the events, characters and behavioral standard depicted in the epics.[8]

And, for the post-Homeric Greeks, especially for those of higher status, the norms of individual behavior contained in the Homeric warrior-ideal constituted a paradigm which they assumptively accepted as right and proper. The evolution of the Greek aristocratic ideal, formed on the model of the ideals embodied in the 'Homeric' epics, is the story of how the upperclass Greeks conformed to, deviated from, or altered this fundamental set of normative values in response to changing social realities.[9]

Our earliest post-Homeric source speaking of the correct way to behave in battle is the seventh-century Spartan poet Tyrtaeus, whose poems[10] consist largely in exhortations to stand one's ground firmly in the battle-line and to fight bravely, e.g. 7.1-4:

> Young men, fight staying next to each other,
> begin neither disgraceful flight nor fear,
> but make your heart great and strong in your breast,
> and do not be faint-hearted when fighting against men.[11]

---

[7] Adkins (1972); Donlan (1980).
[8] (1980), p. 1.
[9] Ibid., p. 2. Cf. also Adkins (1972), pp. 1, 10, etc.
[10] Or, to put it more precisely, the extant fragments of his poems.
[11] ὦ νέοι, ἀλλὰ μάχεσθε παρ' ἀλλήλοισι μένοντες / μηδὲ φυγῆς αἰσχρῆς ἄρχετε μηδὲ φόβου, / ἀλλὰ μέγαν ποιεῖσθε καὶ ἄλκιμον ἐν φρεσὶ θύμον, / μηδὲ φιλοψυχεῖτ' ἀνδράσι μαρνάμενοι·

Tyrtaeus appears to be referring to a phalanx (hence the 'staying together'), and, judging from their equipment, we can assume that the panoploi (πάνοπλοι; 8.38) are hoplites, although F. Lammert[12] refuses to see them as such. While the vocabulary and diction are closely akin to epic language, shifts in reference have already occurred. Thus the *promachoi* (e.g. 6.1) are no longer Homeric warriors but hoplites fighting in the front ranks. The word also appears - presumably with the same reference - on sixth-century funeral inscriptions, e.g. "he fell among the foremost fighters"[13] or "he perished among the foremost fighters".[14] We find the same style of fighting, and the same ideology, in the poems of the Ephesian Callinus, roughly Tyrtaeus' contemporary, who equally calls the young men (νέοι) to battle, e.g. 1.9-11:

> ... but go straight ahead, holding up your spear, with a firm heart under your shield, when battle is first joined.[15]

The motions of battle themselves have changed as well: it is no longer the dynamic charge, but the power to stay in place and withstand an attack - the emphasis is on the action of 'staying' (μένειν), e.g. in the Tyrtaeus passage quoted above (7.1) and 7.31f. (=8.21f.): "... but stay, standing with feet well apart, firmly set with both feet on the earth, biting your lip with your teeth.".[16] (This idea of courage as a form of endurance (καρτερία) will be developed by Plato, e.g. *Laches* 192b-c.)

Another thing that has clearly changed is the motivation for fighting. We find this in both Tyrtaeus: "fighting for his home-country" (6.2) or "fighting ... for the land and the children (9.33f.),[17] and Callinus (1.7): "for [your] land and children and wedded wife".[18] The object of the warrior's protection - the fixed, immovable 'homeland' (πατρίς, for which there is no good English translation) or 'earth/land' (γῆ) - again stresses the image of resistance against the onslaught of external enemies rather than a war of conquest. It can of course be said that the Trojans in the *Iliad* are protecting their city, and the same may be true for some of the Achaeans in earlier wars (e.g. Nestor in his youth), but the

---

[12] 'Phalanx', *RE* XIX.2.1625-46.
[13] ἐν προμάχοισι πέσεν (Peek [1960], p.62).
[14] ἐνὶ προμάχοις ὤλεσε (ib. p.64).
[15] ... ἀλλά τις ἰθὺς ἴτω, / ἔγχος ἀνασχόμενος καὶ ὑπ' ἀσπίδος ἄλκιμον ἦτορ / ἔλσας, τὸ πρῶτον μειγνυμένου πολέμου.
[16] ἀλλά τις εὖ διαβὰς μενέτο ποσὶν ἀμφοτέροισι / στηριχθεὶς ἐπὶ γῆς, χεῖλος ὀδοῦσι δακών.
[17] περὶ ᾗ πατρίδι μαρνάμενον; μαρνάμενον ... γῆς πέρι καὶ παίδων.
[18] γῆς πέρι καὶ παίδων κουριδίης τ' ἀλόχου.

true heroes immortalised in the *Iliad* are the Achaean aggressors. For Tyrtaeus and Callinus the purpose of war is quite clearly the defence of one's country or city as a whole and not merely one's own family, although they are included in the picture. As Jaeger phrased it: "The Homeric ideal of heroic arete is recast into the heroism of patriotism".[19]

Personal glory is still the most desireable aim for the warrior, but it is not pursued to the same extent as it was by the Homeric heroes, since its pursuit has to be co-ordinated with the rest of the army, and the changed fighting style imposes physical limitations. The glory that will be the prize of the warrior - whether returning victorious or dead - is not the universal (one could almost call it international) one expected by Homeric heroes. It is, another new feature, strictly limited to one's own country or city. "The entire *laos* will yearn for the brave man when he is dead, alive he will be worthy of the half-gods",[20] writes Callinus (1.18f.), and similar promises can be found in Tyrtaeus, e.g. 9.27-42, culminating in the phrase (ib. 32) "although he is beneath the earth,[21] he becomes immortal".[22] The mourning by the community is stressed repeatedly, e.g. Tyrtaeus 9.27f.: "both the young men and the old men bemourn him, and the entire city is beset with grievous yearning."[23] The city becomes the mourner, since it is what the warrior dies for, in the same way as in the epic the warrior defending a city (as the Trojans do) would be fighting for, and mourned by, his own kin. Now the warrior obtains immortality in the memory of a specific community.

As Jaeger justly remarked,[24] it appears that the ideology and values advocated by Callinus and Tyrtaeus are not yet generally accepted and established. Both poets are obviously trying to establish and impose a new code (one that was perhaps not likely to be embraced wholeheartedly by their audiences) and to make their presentation of this code as persuasive as possible - possibly not on their own account, but in the name of their patrons. They therefore take great pains to describe not only the rewards awaiting those who fight and die the way a man should, but also the dire consequences of failing to do so. Callinus (I.12f.) uses the

---

[19] (1936), I, p.129.
[20] λαῷ γὰρ σύμπαντι πόθος κρατερόφρονος ἀνδρός / θνήσκοντος, ζώων δ' ἄξιος ἡμιθέων·
[21] The earth which he died defending.
[22] ἀλλ' ὑπὸ γῆς περ ἐὼν γίγνεται ἀθάνατος.
[23] τὸν δ' ὀλοφύρονται μὲν ὁμῶς νέοι ἠδὲ γέροντες, / ἀργαλέῳ δὲ πόθῳ πᾶσα κέκηδε πόλις.
[24] (1934), I, p. 123.

same argument that Sarpedon employs in the *Iliad*, namely that no man can escape death, and develops the theme by adding (ib. 14f.) that many have escaped death in battle only to meet their death upon their return. Unlike those who die for their city, they are not worthy of mourning. Tyrtaeus depicts the fate of the deserter who spends the remainder of his life as a fugitive and a beggar with his family, in poverty and shame (6.3-10), stressing the loss of *arete* for the coward (8.14): 'all the virtue of men who have run perishes".[25]

Both poets also hold up positive incentive for those who fight bravely. They will be mourned by everyone, writes Callinus in the passage cited above (1.17f.), alive they will be as half-gods (ib. 19), and one of them is worth many others (ib. 21), a rephrasing of the famous line describing the healer at *Il.* XVI.514. Tyrtaeus echoes these promises of fame for the dead (9.27-32) and honour for those who survive (ib. 35-42) and, as a further incentive, even claims that those who stay in their rank and fight are less liable to be killed (8.13) - although again the advantages for the army as a whole are stressed (ib.): "they save the people behind them".[26] One could be forgiven for thinking that Tyrtaeus does not quite mean what he says, calling the warriors to "consider life hateful, and the black *kêres* of death as dear as the light of the sun"[27] (8.5f.) - and on the other hand claiming that those who fight courageously have a better risk of survival. It seems almost as if he himself had found it hard to believe that the ideology expressed in his poems would be accepted.

The theory that not all subscribed to the official heroic ideal is corroborated by a famous poem by Archilochus,[28] roughly a contemporary of Tyrtaeus and Callinus, who appears to have been a soldier (according to some a mercenary) most of his life. Although a warrior, he describes how he abandoned his shield and thus saved himself, i.e. he ran away. Since the shield in particular becomes a burden when running, the loss of a hoplite's shield is always associated with ignominious flight and the man who throws away his shield (the ῥιψασπίς) is naturally seen as a coward. Nevertheless, Archilochus unabashedly admits that he preferred losing the symbol of his honour as a warrior to losing his life, and no doubt many who heard his poem agreed with him in private.

---

[25] τρεσσάντων δ' ἀνδρῶν πᾶσ' ἀπόλωλ' ἀρετή.
[26] σαοῦσι δὲ λαὸν ὀπίσσω. (*Opissô* could also be meant in a temporal sense, 'thereafter'.)
[27] ἐχθρὴν μὲν ψυχὴν θέμενος, θανάτου δὲ μελαίνας / κῆρας ὁμῶς αὐγαῖς ἠελίοιο φίλα.
[28] Fr. 5.

However, for obvious reasons this attitude never became part of the 'official version' promoted by those in power, who needed an ideology that called for the individual's sacrifice for the common cause.[29]

Another theme to be found in Callinus and Tyrtaeus - and, as we shall see, in later authors - is one which is already familiar from Homer: the youth and beauty of the warrior, particularly visible in death. Callinus addresses himself to the "young men/youths" (νέοι) and Tyrtaeus emphasises the warriors' youth (e.g. at 9.14) and in fr.7 he gives a graphic description of the horrid sight of an old man, fallen in the front line because the young men have fled. Tyrtaeus uses *aischron* (αἰσχρόν; 'ugly/shameful') and *kalon* (καλόν; 'beautiful') in a moral as well as in an aesthetic sense, e.g. at 7.26: "ugly to the eyes".[30] In contrast to this sight (27-30), "everything is becoming in the young";[31] "while he has the shining flower of desirable youth; he is admirable to look at for the men, desirable for the women while alive, and beautiful when he falls among the foremost".[32]

This is a variation on the Homeric theme insofar as for the Homeric hero youth and beauty are only mentioned in close relation with death and defilement - with the exception of the passages in which Paris' beauty is commented on in a derogatory way. A further variation is that in the *Iliad* all warriors - Nestor and Idomeneus being special exceptions - are very young men, while for Tyrtaeus, and presumably in Callinus as well, the young men are only one part of the fighting force. Old men "with white hair" (Tyrt. 7.23) are also among the fighters, since it is no more an army of 'professionals' of warfare, but one of citizens, and therefore representing the city in its variety of age groups.[33] However, these old men are no longer expected to fight in the front rank, and according to our poets the brunt of the fighting should be borne by the young warriors.

Tyrtaeus is still close to Homer inasfar as he places strong emphasis on the warrior's physical beauty, but in his famous

---

[29] Müller (1989), p. 332, explains fr. 5 as an attack on the hoplite ideal, but not on Homeric or old aristocratic ideals.
[30] αἰσχρὰ τά γ' ὀφθαλμοῖς.
[31] νέοισι δὲ παντ' ἐπέοικεν. This is an almost verbatim quotation of Priam's words in the *Iliad* (XXII.71).
[32] ὄφρ' ἐρατῆς ἥβης ἀγλαὸν ἄνθος ἔχῃ, / ἀνδράσι μὲν θηητὸς ἰδεῖν, ἐρατὸς δὲ γυναιξί / ζωὸς ἐών, καλὸς δ' ἐν προμάχοισι πεσών.
[33] This is part of the phenomenon which Garlan ([1972], p. 85), following C. Nicolet, calls focalisation, by which an army represents an image, albeit distorted, of the social environment from which it has sprung.

opening line (6.1) "to die is beautiful",[34] the beauty referred to is moral beauty, the ethical beauty of heroic deeds. Beginning from the use of the word in Homer, however, there is no clear distinction between the aesthetic and the ethical sense of *kalon*, which always spans both. Even in its most straightforward use for physical beauty in Homer, *kalon* may contain a note of moral praiseworthiness, but despite this ambivalence and tension one can detect a transition in emphasis from the beautiful body of the slain warrior to the beautiful acts performed by the hoplites dying for their community - in N. Loraux's words[35] from the "beautiful dead" to "beautiful death".

Another important theme, equally familiar from Homer, appears in Tyrtaeus: it is the idea of wounds in front being honourable. Thus at 8.19f. he states that a corpse lying in the dust with a wound in the back is *aischros* - although it not quite clear whether this is meant in an aesthetic or in a moral sense, or whether the two overlap. With the changes in warfare, paradoxically reality caught up with ideology: a hoplite is presumably more likely to be hit from the front if he stays in his place. Nevertheless, I do not think that a decrease or increase in likelihood for things to happen would actually have much influence on people's way of thinking or on popular ideology. The idea of the dishonourable wound in the back was associated with an image of the cowardly, runaway warrior, whether this corresponded to a particular reality or not.

Although the sixth-century Megarian poet Theognis[36] mentions war only rarely and speaks mainly about internal strife, some passages are of tangential relevance for our topic. Theognis claims to dislike war (I.885f.) and rates wealth as the foremost *aretê* (I.699f.) - unlike Tyrtaeus' praise of courage (ἀλκή) in 9, in which he places it above all other qualities (in an escalating comparison very much like the praise of *agapê* above all other virtues in St Paul's second letter to the Corinthians). After the first statement Theognis nevertheless goes on to say that it would be (morally) *aischron* not to look tearful war in the face (I.889f.) and in I.209f. he speaks of the stigma attached to the fugitive (from war, one assumes): "if you flee, you have no friend or trustworthy companion; that is grievous about flight".[37] He also advocates

---

[34] τεθνάμεναι γὰρ καλόν ...
[35] (1982), p.34.
[36] Which parts (if any) of the *Theognidea* are actually by Theognis is impossible to determine.
[37] οὐδείς τοι φεύγοντι φίλος καὶ πιστὸς ἑταῖρος· / τῆς δὲ φυγῆς ἐστιν τοῦτ' ἀνιηρότερον.

courage in adverse situations: "the man who is in grievous pains must dare" (I.555).³⁸ ἄλγος could be grief as well as physical pain, and in this case it may well be deliberately chosen to evoke both. Thus, although Theognis appears to glorify a softer life, the values of courage and steadfastness are present as essential for a man's character, relevantly so, since Theognis' poems are educational and his intention is to impart to the youth Kyrnos everything an *agathos* needs to know.

Simonides of Ceos, composing approximately half a century after Theognis, is a rich source of information on the heroic image of death in battle in his age. By the very nature of the material, examples can be found among the dirges (bk. VI), the elegiacs (XIII) and, most of all, the epitaphs (XIV). In Simonides' poems there are no traces of references to the physical beauty of the heroic warriors, but while they themselves are not 'beautiful', their death is, and in 127 (*Anth. Pal.* VII.253) it is suggested that to die well is an important part of virtue: "If to die beautifully is the greatest part of virtue, chance has portioned this out to us of all things."³⁹ The youth of the fallen warriors, however, is still mentioned, e.g. the "Athenian youths" (κοῦροι 'Αθαναίων) in 135 (*Anth. Pal.* VII.254). It is unlikely that all or even many of the Athenian dead (presumably those who fell at Tanagra in 457) were young enough to be called *kouroi,* and the use of this archaic term itself shows its symbolic use. The image of the slain warrior's youth heightens the tragedy of his death and makes his self-sacrifice even more valuable because of the intense quality of the life he has lost.

The motif of the glorious dead becoming immortal is present in Simonides as well, but he does not speak of immortality in song or in their fellow citizens' memory. It is their *aretê* that makes them live on, leading them up from Hades, almost in a physical immortality, comparable to those of the heroes of mythology (126; *Anth. Pal.* VII.251): "They are not dead [despite] having died, because their *aretê* glorifies them, having the upper hand, and leads them up from the house of Hades."⁴⁰ The contrast of "dead, yet living" is also present in 133 (*Anth. Pal.* VII.443), where Simonides speaks of the "animated memorials of the

---

³⁸ χρὴ τολμᾶν χαλεποῖσιν ἐν ἄλγεσι κείμενον ἄνδρα.
³⁹ εἰ τὸ καλῶς θνῄσκειν ἀρετῆς μέρος ἐστὶ μέγιστον, / ἡμῖν ἐκ πάντων τοῦτ᾽ ἀπένειμε τύχη. It is an interesting detail that this is, so to speak, presented as the opinion of the dead.
⁴⁰ οὐδὲ τεθνᾶσι θάνοντες, ἐπεί σφ᾽ ἀρετὴ καθύπερθε / κυδαίνουσ᾽ ἀνάγει δώματος ἐξ᾽ Αΐδεω.

inanimate dead".⁴¹ This play with words and contrasts is reminiscent of the famous saying, supposedly by Heraclitus (47D), about the immortal mortals and mortal immortals, 'living the others' death and dying the others' life".⁴² It may well be that this was a popular way of speaking of the dead at the time, or that both Simonides and Heraclitus were using a common source. Beliefs regarding death in battle would also be influenced by a person's beliefs regarding the afterlife. There was, of course, no one theory for it, but beliefs in different kinds of survival co-existed (e.g. an existence as a shade in Hades, metempsychosis, etc.) and it is practically impossible to know how widespread any particular belief was among the population.

One more aspect of Simonides' epitaphs is worth noting, that is, that in many of them the geographically very limited 'city' for which the warrior dies has been replaced by 'Greece', e.g. 121 (Strabo 9.425): "died ... for Greece"⁴³ or 124 (Plu., *Hdt. Mal.* 39): "we lie [dead], having delivered ... all of Greece".⁴⁴ It is not surprising that this shift in focus occurs at this point in history (although G. Nagy [1979] claims evidence of Pan-Hellenism in the *Iliad*), since it is the first time within historical times that all Greeks are under threat from a foreign invader. The replacement is by no means complete and the city is still mentioned, often along with Greece, e.g. 130 (*Anth. Pal.* VII.442), which speaks of Megara and Greece, or on its own, as is Sparta in what is presumably the best-known epitaph in Western literature, the distych for the Spartan dead at Thermopylae.⁴⁵

The claim (with some variations) that death in battle is somehow nobler and better than death by other causes can be found in literature throughout antiquity, but - as far as one can tell from our extant sources - Heraclitus appears to have been the first to think that an explanation is needed. Having said that both gods and men honour those who die in battle (fr. 24D; Clem., *Strom.* III.16), he also explains that the souls of those who have died fighting are purer than the souls of those who have died from illness (fr. 136D; *schol. Epictet. Bodl.*, p. LXXI). This appears to be the passage which is explained by Clement of Alexandria (*Strom.* IV.14.4), who, although he is writing several centuries

---

⁴¹ μνημήϊα νεκρῶν ἔμψυχ' ἀψύχων.
⁴² ζῶντες τὸν ἐκείνων θάνατον, τὸν δὲ ἐκείνων βίον τεθνεῶτες.
⁴³ φθιμένους ... ὑπὲρ Ἑλλάδος.
⁴⁴ Ἑλλάδα πᾶσαν ... κείμεθα ῥυσάμενοι.
⁴⁵ Fr. 92/Diehl (Hdt. VII.228): "Stranger, report to the Spartans that we lie here, obeying their words (Ὦ ξεῖν' ἀγγέλλειν Λακεδαιμονίοις ὅτι τῇδε / κείμεθα τοῖς κείνων ῥήμασι πειθόμενοι.)."

later, seems to be using earlier material. He explains that the end of those who die in a war is praised, not because of the violence of the death, but

> because he who dies in war dies without fear of dying, cut off from the body, without being weary in his soul before that or [without] becoming soft, as it happens to men in diseases. For these die having become womanish and full of desire for life. Therefore they do not release their souls pure.[46]

It is therefore a kind of corruption before death that makes death from illness less pure and the needed pureness is due to the suddenness of the warrior's death, presumably before he can conceive a desire to live. It is unlikely that this aetiology was very wide-spread, but it is interesting to see that attempts were made to provide an explanation for such a popular belief rather than merely accepting it.

With Herodotus and the beginning of what we are in the habit of calling historiography we are faced with an entirely new type of material - our first example of continuous prose on topics other than philosophy and religion. Since much of Greek historiography consists in descriptions of battles and wars, beginning with Herodotus' account of the Persian Wars, one would expect mentions of individuals being wounded, but in fact these are very rare. The reason for this appears to be the aforementioned one, namely the absence of interest in individual heroism, or, to use A. Momigliano's words: "The Spartans and the Athenians, not Leonidas and Themistocles, are Herodotus' protagonists of the Persian Wars. There is no indispensable Achilles or Hector in them ..."[47]

However, Herodotus does show an interest - or perhaps expected it from his audience - in the concept of heroic death as such, and to my knowledge he is the first to use an expression familiar from later Athenian funeral orations: "having become a good man." (VI.114).[48] This is to become the standard phrase for those who have died in battle, but on one occasion (VII.181.1) Herodotus uses "having become a most excellent man"[49] of a soldier who is merely wounded. This is the only passage in which

---

[46] ὅτι ὁ κατὰ πόλεμον τελευτῶν ἀδεὴς τοῦ θανεῖν ἀπήλλακται, ἀποτμηθεὶς τοῦ σώματος, καὶ οὐ προκαμὼν τῇ ψυχῇ οὐδὲ καταμαλακισθείς, οἷα περὶ τὰς νόσους πάσχουσιν οἱ ἄνθρωποι. ἀπαλλάττονται γὰρ θηλυκευόμενοι καὶ ἱμειρόμενοι τοῦ ζῆν. διὰ ταῦτα οὐδὲ καθαρὰν ἀπολύουσιν τὴν ψυχήν, ... (Quoted in Kirk [1949], p. 385).
[47] (1966), p.40.
[48] ἀνὴρ γενόμενος ἀγαθός.
[49] ἀνδρὸς ἀρίστου γενομένου.

Herodotus ever mentions the treatment of a wound: the Persians who decide to save a wounded Greek fighter, impressed by his courage (δι' ἀρετὴν ἐκείνου), treat his wounds with myrrh and bandage them. Although treatment is mentioned (and both myrrh and linen bandages are familiar from medical writings), it is not the main point of interest. What Herodotus presents is a story of Greek *aretê* recognised even by the foreign enemy[50] and the way in which it is told evokes similar stories of heroic death: The "having become a most excellent man that day"[51] is a phrase usually reserved for the fallen and it would fit the description of death in battle far better than that of wounding. Could this be Herodotus' way of upgrading the story, because to die for one's country was better than being merely wounded?

Three other passages also show that Herodotus was concerned with the right way to fight and to die: When the Spartan Demaratos, in the pay of the Persians, tells Xerxes what kind of men the Lacedaemonians are (VII.104.4f.), he describes them as being ruled by their *nomos* (law/custom). They have to do whatsoever their *nomos* commands, which is always the same: not to retire from the battle whatever the number of enemies, "but to stay in line and be victorious or perish".[52] Nobody in the audience would have objected that it was impossible to know what Demaratos had said, because the essential is that this is what he should have said if this situation had arisen. The story is another opportunity for showing Greek *aretê* at its best in contrast with the morally inferior Persians.

In his account of the battle of Plataea, Herodotus names those who had particularly distinguished themselves:[53] among the Lacedaemonians these are one Aristodemos, the only survivor of Thermopylae (where illness had prevented him from fighting), and one Poseidonios. In the ensuing discussion (IX.71) on who had been the bravest (ἄριστος) it is decided that it must be Poseidonios, because Aristodemos had "clearly wished to die' - to escape the opprobrium of not having died at Thermopylae - whereas Poseidonios, "not wishing to die, had shown himself worthy".[54] This presents a new aspect of death in battle: apparently

---

[50] The topos reappears in later stories about wounded Crusaders treated by Saracens.
[51] ἀνδρὸς ἀρίστου γενομένου ταύτην τὴν ἡμέρην.
[52] ἀλλὰ μένοντας ἐν τῇ τάξει ἐπικρατέειν ἢ ἀπόλλυσθαι. On the *nomos* as a motivation for fighting, see Redfield (1985), pp. 115f.
[53] It should be pointed out that these men have all died in the battle. Those who survive appear to be excluded in the first place.
[54] οὐ βουλόμενον ἀποθνήσκειν ἄνδρα γενέσθαι ἀγαθόν.

the sacrifice is not meant to be easy, and therefore a death-wish makes it less valuable. In order to become an *anêr agathos* a man has to offer up a life which is worth living.

It is not only Aristodemos' desire to end his life which makes him less eligible for the title of a 'good man', but also his way of fighting: " ... he had accomplished great deeds, in a frenzy (λυσσῶντα) and leaving his place in the battle-line (ἐκλείποντα τὴν τάξιν)". This *lyssa* is again the savage courage of the Homeric warrior, undesirable in a hoplite, and to leave one's post is the worst offence. It would seem that by the time of the Persian Wars it is no longer sufficient, in order to be praised, to die fighting bravely, but the warrior ideal has been tamed to fit new criteria.

The passage following the above (IX.72) equally demonstrates the idea of the 'good death', and this time even the theme of physical beauty reappears, obviously to heighten the tragicality of the scene. The Spartan Kallikrates, the "most handsome of all the Greeks", is hit by an arrow while attending the sacrifice offered by the king before the beginning of the battle of Plataea.[55] He is carried from the field and dies, not an easy death. (The meaning of ἐδυσθανάτεε is not quite clear; it could refer to the pain from the fatal wound as well as to the dying man's emotional state.) It does not grieve him, he explains to another soldier, to die for Greece, but to die without fighting or accomplishing great deeds. The tragedy here is not the Spartan's death, but the fact that he dies outside the battle (ἔξω τῆς μάχης ἀπέθανε), he is deprived of his chance to prove himself an *anêr agathos*, and in addition he is killed with an arrow, the coward's weapon *par excellence*.

We can find the lowly reputation of the archer also in Euripides' *Hercules*. There Lykos calls it "the most inferior weapon" (161: κάκιστον ὅπλον), praising the advantages of shield and spear, the only right weapons for a man. Here, however, this view is not unchallenged and Amphitryon retorts that the hoplite is the slave of his weapons, relying only on his one spear. He also adds the suggestion -subversive as far as official values are concerned - that a hoplite runs the risk of dying through the cowardice of those around him if they are not *agathoi* (ib. 191f.).

The contempt for missiles compared to hand-held weapons also seems to be expressed in a stele mentioned by Strabo (X.1.12).[56]

---

[55] From the description it appears that the troops were sitting on the ground in battle order for this occasion.

[56] Although this source is much later than the period treated here, it refers to a situation in that era.

Apparently it ruled out the use of long-range weapons (τηλέβολα) in the ongoing dispute between Chalcis and Eretria over the Lelantine Plain. Presumably practices like this were not common usage - one need only consider the numerous mentions of archers or arrow wounds and the many finds of arrowheads - but it proves that there continued to exist a bias against archers and, presumably, slingers and javelin-throwers, and even in Strabo's time he obviously saw no need to explain the exclusion of those weapons.

The tragedies are rich in hints at the values which were current in their time, and they demonstrate the continuity of certain beliefs and notions. Thus the speech of the herald in Aeschylus' *Seven Against Thebes* (1005-25) spells out why Eteokles deserves burial while his brother does not (1009ff.):

> For he took his death in the city fending off the enemies, from the ancestral temples, being pure without blame, he died for the very thing for which it is beautiful for the young men to die.[57]

So there are further restrictions: dying in battle is not enough and only the warrior who has been fighting for the cause sanctioned by the city will be honoured after his death. For this cause it is worth dying and "beautiful to die".

Another common theme is the contrast between 'manly' self-control in pain or grief on the one hand and of 'womanish' laments and tears on the other. Already in Archilochus (fr.13; Stob. 4.56.30) we find the praise of endurance (τλημοσύνη) as the remedy for irremediable ills. As a metaphor for the unbearable political situation he speaks (ib. 8) of "groaning over a bleeding wound",[58] and his advice is to "bear [it], refraining from womanish grief" (ib. 10).[59]

It is in the same vein that, in Sophocles' *Trachinians*, Heracles, racked with the suffering caused by the poisoned garnment, asks his son to pity him (1070-75) - not so much because of the physical pain, but because its violence is making him behave like a woman, "crying like a girl". He stresses that never before had anyone seen him behave like this and that he had always borne everything "without a groan" (ἀστένακτος). He is therefore particularly aggrieved that the present torment is, so to speak, turning him into a woman (1075):"Wretched me, I find myself

---

[57] στέγων γὰρ ἐχθροὺς θάνατον εἵλετ᾽ ἐν πόλει, / ἱερῶν πατρῴων δ᾽ ὅσιος ὢν πομπῆς ἄτερ / τέθνηκεν οὗπερ τοῖς νέοις θνήσκειν καλόν.
[58] αἱματόεν δ᾽ ἕλκος ἀναστένομεν.
[59] τλῆτε, γυναικεῖον πένθος ἀπωσάμενοι.

[turned into] a woman."⁶⁰ The same high rating of self-control appears again in Heracles' final words in the play (1259-63), which are an appeal to himself not to cry out: "Now, ... stubborn soul, provide a bridle-bit of steel set with stones and put an end to the screams."⁶¹ Although the situation here is a very specific one, we can assume that the same values would apply when a man was wounded.

In Aristophanes' *Acharnians* we can clearly see the caricature of the wounded warrior when Lamachos is carried back, only slightly injured, but lamenting loudly, (1190f.) "Ah, ah, these chilling and abominable sufferings; wretched me",⁶² or (ib. 1205) "Oh, oh, the painful wounds".⁶³ This reads very much like a deliberate parody of scenes in which the hero is assailed by sufferings too great for even his self-control, such as those in the *Trachinians*, Sophocles' *Philoctetes* or Euripides' *Hippolytus*, and it shows a warrior behaving in an unmanly, and therefore ridiculous, fashion (which is highlighted by Dikaiopolis' unsympathetic reaction). The scene obviously features in the play because Aristophanes expected his audience to find it funny: if behaviour like Lamachos' was considered acceptable, it would not offer material for comedy.⁶⁴

The ideals of heroic behaviour, already implicit in the *Iliad*, are with time becoming more explicit and visible and their reasons are explained: tears and cries are a woman's reaction to pain, and a man must at least try not to groan or cry out. This may be a highly theoretical ideal which rarely worked out in practice, but one must not underrate the power of cultural assumptions. In his article on pain perception, already mentioned in the discussion of analgesics in Ch. 3, Melzack points out that "even the significance pain has in the culture in which we have been brought up plays an essential role in how we feel and respond to it".⁶⁵ Thus, what is expected from a man by the other men in his culture may influence his reaction to pain (if not his perception of it), in particular in an agonistic culture such as that of classical Greece. In any case, it is not my purpose to determine how the Greeks

---

⁶⁰ θῆλυς ηὕρημαι τάλας.
⁶¹ ἄγε νυν ... ὦ ψυχὴ σκληρά, χάλυβος λιθοκόλλητον στόμιον παρέχουσ', ἀνάπαυε βοήν.
⁶² ἀτταταῖ ἀτταταῖ, στυγερὰ τάδε γε κρυερὰ πάθεα· τάλας ἐγώ.
⁶³ ἰὼ ἰὼ τραυμάτων ἐπωδύνων.
⁶⁴ Scenes of wounding may have been more common in tragedies than one would assume from the extant examples, if one considers a sentence in Aristotle's *Poetics* (1452b) stating that "death, pain, woundings and similar things" (θάνατοι καὶ περιωδυνίαι καὶ τρώσεις καὶ ὅσα τοιαῦτα) could be seen on stage.
⁶⁵ (1961), p.41.

actually behaved when wounded, but to investigate what they considered to be the right behaviour for a man.

Coming back to Sophocles' Heracles once more, we can see that his suffering is aggravated by the fact that the cause of his death is a woman, which makes it an unworthy death for a great hero like himself. Although his death is Deianeira's crime, Heracles suffers not only physically, but also in a moral sense through being killed by a mere woman,[66] because he is not dying a 'good death'. Speaking of a similar situation, Adkins[67] suggests that it was more *aischron* for Agamemnon to die the way he did than for Clytaemnestra to kill him. In the same way the stigma of having his life taken by a woman makes Heracles' death *aischron*. These examples underline the fact that the right way to die depends on who one is and especially whether one is male or female. This question is explored by N. Loraux (1985), in particular in connection with suicide, where the sword is considered the right means for a man to die while hanging is the appropriate death for a woman.

The right way for a man to die finds it most powerful expression in Athenian funeral oration.[68] The topics of the funeral oration and of the death of the warrior have been discussed in some depth by Loraux in several articles.[69] In her words:

> we can say that, from the world of Achilles to fifth- and fourth-century Athenian democracy, the death of the warrior is a model combining in itself the representations and values which - in the Achaean camp as well as in the classical city - serve as norms.[70]

The official funeral for those who have fallen for the city is an opportunity to state once again the values and expectations of a particular society - and in particular an opportunity to give the living an example of how a good citizen should die. This death itself, or the battle in which it occurred, is never described: the oration commemorates the choice to fight for their city made by the citizens, but not the physiological act of dying. And, as Loraux points out,[71] the city only celebrates the dead citizens; unlike the epic, the orations never mention the wounded, although they had shown equal willingness to give their lives (and some

---

[66] γυνὴ δέ, θῆλυς οὖσα κοὐκ ἀνδρὸς φύσις (1062).
[67] (1960), p.162.
[68] Again, the surviving examples are limited to Athens, but one can expect similar attitudes in other city-states. A useful discussion of the institution of the funeral oration can be found in Argoud (1978).
[69] E.g. (1973), (1974), (1975), (1982).
[70] (1982), p.27.
[71] (1982), p.34.

may be left disabled), and although some of those still alive at the time of the funeral may die soon after it (which would, of course make them part of the praiseworthy dead). Together with the description of death in battle its aesthetic value seems to have disappeared as well. Heroic death is beautiful in a moral sense only, and in Loraux's words,[72] a shift from the 'beautiful dead' to 'beautiful death' has occurred.

Loraux claims[73] that in Athens 'beautiful death' is an abstract model, being a theme of Spartan origin adapted to the needs of the democratic city,[74] whereas in Sparta it is more than an ideological theme. It is, she claims, a categorical imperative, quoting Demaratos' explanation of the Spartan way of fighting (Her. VII.104). I do not think, however, that the sources we have allow us to draw these fine distinctions. The Athenian funeral orations tell us about the self-image the Athenians had, and through which they wanted to be seen by the rest of Greece, but we do not have the Spartan equivalent and we do not know what kind of speech - if any - the Spartans would have heard on a similar occasion. What accounts we have about the Spartans are given by non-Spartans with the purpose of showing either the superiority (Xenophon, Plutarch) or the inferiority (Pericles' funeral oration in Thucydides) of Sparta. Using those available sources, we cannot claim with any degree of certainty that the idea of beautiful death was any more or less abstract in Athens than it was in Sparta or in any other city.

The fact that self-sacrifice for the city was very much an imperative in Athens is visible in 'Pericles'' funeral oration in Thucydides, in which he stresses the example set by the dead: Just as those who died did so in order to preserve their city, those who survive must be prepared to suffer for her (II.415). Thus the funeral oration serves as a moral tale for the survivors, inviting imitation. In his praise of Athens, Pericles depicts the life which her citizens are expected to throw away willingly in order to preserve it for the community. In exchange the city officially bestows on all who die for her the title of *andres agathoi* without restricting it to an élite minority. Adkins claims[75] that in the oration it had to be reiterated that the *aretê* of the deceased was indubitable, because in the case of death in battle "one's *aretê* is not placed beyond doubt by one's own success". However, the

---

[72] Ibid.
[73] (1977), p.105.
[74] Cf. Detienne ([1967], p. 99), who speaks of the 'democratization' of the role of the warrior in the phalanx.
[75] (1960), p. 170, n. 3.

truth that some of the fallen may have had less *aretê* than the others is not forgotten: at II.42.3. Pericles actually draws attention to this fact and makes a point of saying that their shortcomings are more than outweighed by their *andragathia*, "the good outshining the bad".[76] In my opinion we do not see much of the attempt, postulated by Adkins, to justify every dead citizen's *aretê*, since it was justified beyond doubt by his death. It is more to the point to speak, with Loraux, of a displacement within the funeral oration, "which gives *thanatos* the name of *aretê*"[77].

A substantial part of the Hippocratic writings belong to roughly the same time period as these sources and although most of the relevant passages have been discussed elsewhere, it has to be pointed out once more that purely medical writings are not in some mysterious way independent of popular beliefs - since medical historians have tended to present them as if that were the case. Thus we can find the belief in a difference between wounds in front and wounds in the back in two passages. Both *Epid.* II.3/ V.20 L and *Aph.*V.65/IV.558 L claim differing consequences according to where the wound is situated. According to the first passage, if the swelling on a wound disappears suddenly, wounds in the back result in "convulsions (σπασμοί) with pain", while those in front are complicated by delirium, sharp pain in the sides and dysentery. *Aph.*V.65. claims the same, with the addition of suppuration for the wounds in front, and convulsions and 'tetanus' (σπασμοί and τέτανοι) for those in the back. Neither passage offers an explanation why there should be a difference and this divergence in complications is presented as though it were an empirical fact. The authors do not appear to mean wounds to particular organs, where a differentiation would be understandable, but wounds in front or in the back in general, regardless of their depth or position.

Indeed, the case of the casualty described in *Epid.* V.47/V.234 L seems to support the theory about convulsions supervening upon wounds in the back: a man is wounded just below the back of the neck, a wound of little account by the sight of it, since it is not deep. Shortly after the extraction of the arrow, however, he is seized by backwards convulsions like those suffering from *opisthotonos*[78] and dies on the second day. The phrasing 'like those suffering from *opisthotonos*" comes across as rather unusual and makes one wonder why the author chose this expression over

---

[76] ἀγαθῷ γὰρ κακὸν ἀφανίσαντες.
[77] (1974), p.190.
[78] ἐτιταίνετο ἐς τοὔπισθεν ἐρυσθεὶς ὡς οἱ ὀπισθοτονικοί.

saying simply that the man was seized by *opisthotonos*. It may be that the author thought that the convulsions were of a different nature, perhaps the spasms to be expected because the wound was in the back.

There are several descriptions of war wounds in *Epidemics* V (some overlapping with those in VII), and whoever compiled those descriptions obviously practiced in a war zone for some time. Therefore, it is more than likely that what we have is the result of a deliberate choice to record only the most interesting cases, either because they were unusual or because they supported a theory to which the author adhered. In the case in question the latter may well be true, hence the emphasis that the wound was in the back.

Chronologically the next literary works dealing with wars and battles are Xenophon's writings, composed mainly in the early fourth century BC. There are only few references to wounds, and no passages describing their treatment, although what we have includes first-hand accounts by a man who was a commanding officer - or perhaps *because* he was an officer and was therefore more interested in other aspects of the story such as tactics and logistics. The appointing of eight *iatroi*[79] to care for the many wounded is a matter of interest for the author as being one of the problems regarding military administration and organisation. He was after all one of the men responsible for it. An episode about a soldier with an abdominal wound holding his intestines in his hands (*An*. II.V.33) presumably features because of its striking, sensational, quality rather than for any other reasons.

However, it is possible to detect a slightly greater interest in individuals than in earlier authors,[80] and Xenophon mentions the wounds sustained by Cyrus (i.e. his death-wound) and Artaxerxes at the battle of Kunaxa (*An*. I.VIII.26). It appears that these were described in more detail by the latter's physician, Ktesias, whose work was available at the time when Xenophon was writing. Ktesias obviously had a personal interest in the story, because he treated the king's wound. Xenophon also describes (*Hell*. IV.III.20) the Spartan king Agesilaos' magnanimous behaviour against enemies who had taken refuge in a sanctuary: "although he had suffered many wounds, he did not forget the divinity [i.e. respect for the gods]."[81] This is obviously not a mere episode, but a scene meant to demonstrate the Spartan king's self-control

---

[79] *An*. III.IV.30, already discussed in Ch. 4.1.
[80] Cf. Argoud (1978), who detects a move towards a more individualised approach in Hyperides' oration for Leosthenes (fourth century BC) compared to earlier orations (although this source is later than those examined here).
[81] καίπερ πολλὰ τραύματα ἔχων, ὅμως οὐκ ἐπελάθετο τοῦ θείου.

(*enkrateia*; ἐγκράτεια):[82] he is too badly wounded to walk, has to be carried, and is presumably in considerable pain, but nevertheless he does not vent his anger on the suppliants. This sudden interest by a historian in individuals is less surprising if one considers that Xenophon was in the extraordinary position of knowing personally many of the people who feature in his writings, in particular Agesilaos. Xenophon appears to have particularly admired the latter and he wrote his *Agesilaos* [83] in praise of the Spartan king. It is clear from the tenor of the book that he considered Agesilaos a brave man and it is therefore likely that he would incorporate scenes which showed the king's courage and endurance.

We encounter a different, more theoretical, approach to the problem of courage in Xenophon's *Memorabilia*, namely one of the early examples of the definition of *andreia*, courage or manliness. This is not the earliest attempt to define the concept, however, since a short definition of what it means to be valorous is given by Pericles (Thuc. II.40.3), who says that it consists in having firm knowledge of what is frightening and what is pleasant, and nevertheless not shrinking from dangers. The more detailed discussions of the nature of courage are, of course, to be found in Plato's *Laches* and *Protagoras*, with some important remarks in the *Republic* and *Laws*, as well as, at a later date, in Aristotle's *Nicomachean Ethics* and *Eudemian Ethics*, and the quest for the nature of *andreia* is obviously related to similar philosophical investigations into the nature of, e.g., justice or wisdom. However, not all abstract concepts are subject to scrutiny and there are reasons for chosing courage as the object of enquiry other than merely a philosophical fashion of asking for 'the nature of X'. For one thing, it would appear that there was a theoretical interest in war and fighting,[84] and in particular in the right way to do so. As its name shows, *andreia* (from *anêr*, man) was the very essence of ideal male characteristics and war was the male preserve *par excellence*.[85] It is therefore logical that there should be an interest in the nature of courage and (as we shall see) in the question whether it was part of a man's innate character or whether it could be taught.

---

[82] According to J. de Romilly ([1984], pp. 132f.), Xenophon and Plato are the first to use this noun in its abstract and moral sense.
[83] The same story appears there, too (II.13).
[84] In Hanson's words ([1989], p. 220), "battle became an obsessive image'.
[85] The suggestion of military service for women in Plato's *Republic* must have been unacceptable to most of his contemporaries.

It is, however, intriguing that there should be a sudden surge in the concern about a concept which so far had been considered unequivocal. This suggests that by the turn of the fifth and the fourth centuries the ideal of courage was being questioned in a way in which it had not been questioned before. There are two conceivable reasons for this. One is that this interest was triggered by the influence of sophist philosophy - although this implies taking for granted the rise of sophism for no particular reasons. The other possibility is that it was caused by external events. Since, for this area, too, all our sources are Athenian, it may not be without importance that Athens had suffered a humiliating defeat in the Peloponnesian War in the last decade of the fifth century, and it may well be that this blow and the ensuing political unrest had led to a pessimistic attitude towards traditional values[86] - after all, these values had not helped Athens defeat Sparta.

Whatever the reason, in the early fourth century the concept of *andreia* had become an object of philosophical speculation, and we can find this reflected in Plato, Xenophon and, later, in Aristotle. Although Plato's and Aristotle's theories regarding *andreia* are of great interest and would make a rewarding topic of research on their own, I am presenting only a brief synopsis of them here, because their acceptance was limited to a very small intellectual élite. This is particularly true for Plato, whose views were radically different from those of his contemporaries. He attacked the wide-spread ideal of courage, which for large parts of society was still very close to the Homeric concept of *aretê* and which to Plato seemed contrary to being a good citizen. Unlike the popular concept of *andreia*, which is oriented entirely towards war, Plato's own concept was intended to operate in peace as well.

Xenophon's account in the *Memorabilia* is a simplified and condensed version of the discussion of *andreia* in Plato's *Laches* and *Protagoras*. At III.9. Socrates answers the question whether courage can be taught or whether it is an element of a man's character by nature - whether it is teachable (διδακτόν) or natural (φυσικόν). He does so by saying that souls (by nature) differ from each other in their strength in resisting what is frightening, just as some men's bodies are stronger than others'. However, every natural disposition can be improved as far as courage is concerned by learning (μαθήσει) and by care (μελέτη). Similarly, in Plato's *Protagoras* (351b) *andreia* is seen as a combination of nature (φύσις) and nurture (εὐτροφία).

---

[86] Whether purely Homeric or adapted to hoplite warfare.

In *Mem.* IV.6. Xenophon quotes Socrates' definition of *andreia* as knowing how to make good use (καλῶς χρῆσθαι) of what is frightening or dangerous, in a line of argument similar to the one in the *Protagoras*, where *andreia* is defined as (360d) "wisdom of what is frightening and what is not frightening".[87] However, while Plato redefines what is fearful (which is the reason why knowledge of it has to be acquired), Xenophon retains the conventional categories.

Andreia is the central theme of the *Laches*, but the dialogue comes to no final conclusion on its nature. It is, however, stated (197b) that fearlessness is not the same as courage, since madmen and children can be fearless out of ignorance. Hence, here again it is made obvious that courage consists in some kind of knowledge. The *Laches* is of interest for our topic, because in this dialogue one can see what is presumably the popular definition of *andreia*, given by the eponymous Laches (190e): "if a man will stay in his place and ward off the enemies, and does not flee, you may know well that he is brave".[88] This is already the idea of *andreia* adapted to the requirements of fighting in a phalanx. (Socrates does not refuse this definition altogether, but he accepts it only as part of the concept.) No doubt this was likely to be the answer of the men who fought as hoplites, far more so than Plato's elaborate explanation of the term.

Laches makes another remark which may throw some light on the concept of courage. When Socrates names the Scythians as an example of men not standing their ground but fighting while apparently fleeing, Laches retorts (191b) that this is the cavalry way of fighting, "but the hoplite way of the Greeks [is] as I say".[89] This suggests that different fighting techniques and strategies could be reflected in different ideas on courage and the correct behaviour in battle, i.e. what counts as the right way to fight in a cavalry battle may not count as such in a hoplite battle.

Alcibiades' account, in the *Symposium* (219d-221c), of Socrates' courageous behaviour in war also presents a more popular and conventional view of *andreia*, especially in the Homeric motif of Socrates saving his wounded friend Alcibiades as well as his weapons (220e).[90] The remark (221b-c) that those who behave courageously run less risks of being attacked shows a

---

[87] σοφία τῶν δεινῶν καὶ μὴ δεινῶν.
[88] εἰ γὰρ τις ἐθέλοι ἐν τῇ τάξει μένων ἀμύνεσθαι τοὺς πολεμίους καὶ μὴ φεύγοι, εὖ ἴσθι ὅτι ἀνδρεῖος ἂν εἴη.
[89] τὸ δὲ ὁπλιτικὸν τό γε Ἑλλήνων, ὡς ἐγὼ λέγω.
[90] καὶ τὰ ὅπλα καὶ αὐτὸν ἐμέ.

utilitarian view of courage similar to the one voiced by Tyrtaeus at 8.13.

The only mention of wounds in the Platonic discussion of courage can be found in the *Republic*, in connection with the practical concern of educating the young so that they will be brave: according to 399a, one has to make use of the kind of music apt for inducing courage in those who have to "go and face wounds or death".[91] Since the discussions in the *Republic* and in *Laws* are more of the nature of projects than of philosophical theories it is not surprising to see a more realistic approach, including the possibility of wounds. Consequently, in those two works one can also find ideas closer to those which are familiar from other authors: the idea of beautiful and fortunate death[92] in *Laws* 943c, the idea of training one's resistance to pain (the Spartan Megillos, ib. 633b), or the comment that a coward without military skills is not a leader for men, but for women (ib. 639b). At 944d the Athenian regrets that it is impossible to change into a woman any warrior who abandons his weapons, since that would be a just punishment for this offence - this is still the same insistence on 'manliness' we have seen elsewhere, and some of the figures in Plato's dialogues still act as a mouthpiece for conventional views on *andreia*.

I do not intend to give a detailed description of Aristotle's concept of courage here, because again it is limited to a small number of followers, and, most of all, because the time by which it may have come to have any influence lies beyond the time period treated in this chapter. The important point, however, is that Aristotle's views on courage are closer than Plato's to what one can assume to be conservative, commonly accepted views in his insistence on the importance of courage in war. Aristotle, too, insists that one can learn courage - by being brave - (*E.N.* 1103b) and like Plato he states that fearlessness is not courage (ib. 1104a), but he goes beyond Plato's criteria in saying that *andreia* is more than mere appearance; he who is not happy to face the danger is a coward (ib. 1104b).[93] However, an excess, even of courage, is bad (ib. 1116a) - a concept unthinkable in earlier literature; an excess of courage would be impossible in the *Iliad*.[94]

In the *Eudemian Ethics* (1216b), Aristotle criticises Plato for treating the *aretai* like *epistêmai* by claiming that the goal is the

---

[91] ἢ εἰς τραύματα ἢ εἰς θανάτους ἰόντες.
[92] καλὸν καὶ εὐδαίμονα θάνατον.
[93] ὁ δὲ λυπούμενος δειλός.
[94] Although other warriors reproach Achilles for being harsh or cruel, it is never for an excess of *menos* or *androtês*.

knowledge of an *aretê*. According to Aristotle, this is true of theoretical knowledge such as geometry, but not of practical knowledge such as medicine or of *aretê* "For we do not want to know what courage is", he continues (ibid.), "but we want to be brave ...".[95] Thus the emphasis is on the practical applicability rather than on an analysis of the concept

We have seen in the material examined in this chapter that certain standard ideals of courage and heroism continue to be valid over the centuries, although they undergo adaptations to fit new social or political conditions. In the period under discussion here the ideology of the 'beautiful death' is adapted to a new style of warfare, but some basic concepts remain the same throughout antiquity. Although the core of the heroic warrior ideal is still the Homeric hero, his more savage aspects have disappeared and he has become almost unrecognisable in the guise of the citizen hoplite.

---

[95] οὐ γὰρ εἰδέναι βουλόμεθα τί ἐστιν ἀνδρεία, ἀλλ' εἶναι ἀνδρεῖοι.

CHAPTER EIGHT

ALEXANDER THE GREAT

The importance of scenes of wounding in the elaboration of the the hero-image is nowhere as clear as in the figure of Alexander the Great. He is - one can safely say - the greatest heroic figure represented in Greek and Roman literature outside the epics, and at the same time there is no other man in Greek or Roman history about whose wounds we hear as much as about Alexander's. One could of course accept the evidence as signifying that Alexander was wounded more often than any other military commander, but this explanation is unsatisfactory. We know that Alexander's father, Philip of Macedon, for one, was probably equal to Alexander in this aspect, so the number of wounds alone would hardly be a sufficient reason for the amount of accounts we have of Alexander's wounds. There must have been numerous cases of other military leaders being wounded of which we have no records or only a brief mention,[1] at the same time it is obvious that many events in Alexander's life did not survive in written records. Therefore the question that needs to be asked is: Why Alexander and why his wounds?

When speaking about 'Alexander', one has to be aware that this 'Alexander' is the literary creation of numerous ancient (mainly Greek) authors rather than a historical personality. Not only had some of the sources used by our extant authors been 'official versions' of the events, but Alexander became the protagonist of legend immediately after his death, or perhaps even during his lifetime.

One, and perhaps the most important, element in the myths surrounding Alexander is the wealth of Homeric allusions in the extant accounts of Alexander's life. His reported enthusiasm for the *Iliad* and, in particular, his choice of Achilles as his role-model (or rival, whom he strove to surpass) are stressed repeatedly. Thus, e.g., Plutarch narrates (*Alex.* VIII.2) how Alexander always used to keep the *Iliad* under his pillow at night, together with his dagger, considering it the "viaticum of the virtue of war",[2] and

---

[1] E.g. the multiple wounds sustained by Epaminondas in defending the equally wounded Pelopidas (Plu., *Pelop.* IV.5-6).
[2] τῆς πολεμικῆς ἀρετῆς ἐφόδιον.

Arrian (VII.14.4) explicitly states that Alexander had had a rivalry with Achilles since his childhood.

These Homeric connotations were bound to influence the way in which the authors presented events in Alexander's life. They were reinforced by the already existing links (Alexander's alleged descendance from Achilles through his mother's side) and parallels (Alexander's short and glorious life, the obvious pleasure he took in fighting and his rash temper) and vice versa. A discussion of all the Homeric allusions and cross-references in histories of Alexander would fill a book, but here I wish to draw attention to just a few of them. Alexander's adulation and emulation is highlighted most clearly by the accounts of his visit to Achilles's tomb at Troy.[3] This is also an occasion for presenting Alexander's closest friend, and perhaps lover, Hephaistion, as Patroklos to Alexander/Achilles when they each crown the tomb of the respective hero. Arrian stresses this parallel when he says[4] that Alexander would have preferred to die before Hephaistion just as Achilles would rather have died before Patroklos. Likewise, the descriptions of Alexander's frenzied mourning at Hephaistion's death and his subsequent massacre of the Cossaeans as a funeral offering for Hephaistion[5] show strong Homeric influences.

In the same way Alexander's choice of Roxane for his first wife despite the negligeable political importance of her father has strong connotations of Achilles and Briseis. Alexander had defeated Roxane's father and, although he elevated her to the status of a legitimate wife, the image of the beautiful 'captive of the spear' is very strong in this story.[6]

These are only a few of many examples, but they make it clear that it is an impossible task to attempt to reconstruct the 'real' Alexander and his life from our sources. Consequently, I do not pretend to be able to elaborate what happened on the occasion of every wound, and to deduce some information about Alexander, but to examine why and how the scenes of wounding are used and what our authors make of them for their purposes.

In the previous chapters I have drawn attention to the way in which descriptions of wounding or wound treatment are used as a means to enhance aspects of heroism, and this is particularly visible in the material concerning Alexander. The scenes in

---

[3] E.g. Plu., *Alex.* XV.8; D.S. XVII.17.3; Arr. I.XII.1.
[4] VII.16.8.
[5] Plu., *Alex.* LXXII.4.
[6] E.g. Arr. IV.19.5f.

question are a substantial part of the image of 'Alexander the Hero' in literature. I have claimed earlier that wounding - and courage when wounded - are seen in literature as something of a lesser version of heroic death in battle. It may well be worthwile, in this context, to keep in mind that Alexander did not die in battle, and this fact may well be a reason for the emphasis which the authors place on stories concerning his wounds. To spell this out, Alexander is represented as a hero in almost Homeric terms, but he did not die the way a hero should, i.e. fighting. This may be on Plutarch's mind when he writes[7] about stories concerning Alexander's death that some had thought fit to write them "so as to invent a tragic and heart-rending finale for a great drama".[8] The idea expressed by Plutarch seems to be that the more dramatic versions of Alexander's death, especially rumours about poisoning, had been invented by people to whom death from a fever appeared unworthy of a hero like Alexander. Since Alexander did not die fighting, his heroism had to be proved by other means. As we have seen in earlier examples, descriptions of the courage displayed by a man when wounded - the absence of fear when faced with possible or almost certain death, as well as his resistance to pain - are literary means intended to show him as a 'real man', as *agathos* or *andreios*, and to give him special status within the narrative.

Although this courage may not be seen as quite as glorious as a 'beautiful death', it is certainly a way for attaining special renown while still alive. So, one may say, is fighting courageously, and indeed the two are closely linked in practice. Often the wounds sustained in battle are considered the only valid proof for valiant fighting, since no one would have much time to witness another man's behaviour during a battle. Thus, for example, in Diodorus Siculus one of two Messenian warriors competing for the meed of valour claims that his wounds are proof of his superiority, because "it is obvious that a man who endured such great laceration of his body, was offering himself up for his country without fear".[9]

In a similar vein, Arrian's Alexander uses his wounds as evidence for his good leadership and his concern for his men: "Who of you has toiled more for me than I have for him?", he calls out to the soldiers who refuse to follow him any further. "Let any of you who have wounds strip and show them, and I, too, will

---

[7] *Alex.* LXXV.5.
[8] ὥσπερ δράματος μεγάλου τραγικὸν ἐξόδιον καὶ περιπαθὲς πλάσαντες.
[9] πρόδηλος γὰρ ὁ ὑπομείνας τοσαύτας διαιρέσεις τοῦ σώματος ὡς ἀφειδῶς ἑαυτὸν ἐπέδωκεν ὑπὲρ τῆς πατρίδος (VIII.12.8).

show mine in turn. For, indeed, there is no part of my body - in front, that is[10] - which has remained unwounded and there is no weapon, whether hand-held or long-range, of which I do not carry the mark on my body."[11] (This is followed by a list of the different weapons by which he had been wounded.)

A long list of wounds sustained in his campaigns is also one of Alexander's main arguments in attributing his achievements to *aretê*, not *tychê*, in Plutarch's *De Fortuna aut Virtute Alexandri*.[12] The value of scars as the warrior's status symbol is explicit in Plutarch's words expressing Alexander's pride in his wounds, which he calls "images of [his] virtue and manly courage, graven into [his] body".[13] Q. Curtius uses almost exactly the same words - *indicia virtutis* - when he mentions the wounds received by Hephaistion and other officers at Gaugamela.[14] Thus battle wounds, or the scars left by them, are commonly accepted as the visible signs of valour - provided they are in the right places. The obvious fallacy, that is to say that cowards have as much chance of getting wounded as brave men, is never acknowledged by Greek or Roman authors. It is never refuted either, and this would suggest that this fact was never brought up as an argument against the theory that wounds prove a man's courage.

In comparison with the Homeric hero and in particular with later, e.g. medieval, material it is interesting to see that in most of the extant classical, Hellenistic and even Roman material there is great emphasis on the hero's death and on the wounds he suffers rather than those he inflicts. It may be the case that because of the visible and permanent marks which these wounds left upon the hero's body they featured prominently in the authors' and their audiences' ideas of heroism.

Before I begin to discuss Alexander's wounds one by one in their reflection in different authors, some explanation regarding our sources is needed. Although they consist of works of both

---

[10] Note this important restriction. A man would not want to display scars on his back, nor would they be acceptable as proof of martial prowess.

[11] ... καὶ τίς ὑμῶν ἢ πονήσας οἶδεν ἐμοῦ μᾶλλον ... ἢ ἐγὼ ὑπὲρ ἐκείνου; ἄγε δὴ καὶ ὅτῳ τραύματα ὑμῶν ἐστι γυμνώσας αὐτὰ ἐπιδειξάτω καὶ ἐγὼ τὰ ἐμὰ ἐπιδείξω ἐν μέρει ὡς ἔμοιγε οὐκ ἔστιν ὅτι τοῦ σώματος τῶν γε δὴ ἔμπροσθεν μερῶν ἄτρωτον ὑπολέλειπται, οὐδὲ ὅπλον τι ἔστιν ἢ ἐκ χειρὸς ἢ τῶν ἀφιεμένων οὗ γε οὐκ ἴχνη ἐν ἐμαυτῷ φέρω. (VII.10.1-2). Stripping to show one's scars often features in ancient literature as a popular way of asserting one's claim to courage and *aretê*; e.g. Plu., *Cor.* XIV.1.f.; id., *Sert.* IV.2; id., *Mor.* 187C, ib. 241E-F; Val. Max. II.II.24; Livy II.23.
[12] *Mor.* 327A-B.
[13] εἰκόνας ἐγκεχαραγμένας ἀρετῆς καὶ ἀνδραγαθίας (ib. 331C).
[14] IV.XVI.31f.

Greek and Roman authors, written between the first century BC and the second century AD, I treat them all in one and the same chapter (regardless of the chronological order of their compilation), since they can be considered as one group because of their subject matter - the life of Alexander the Great. Whether they take a positive or a negative view of Alexander, they all represent him as an extraordinary figure and therefore have a mutually comparable approach to the description of events which they considered worth recording.

The main works describing the life and exploits of Alexander are: parts of book XVI and most of book XVII of Diodorus Siculus' *Library of History* (first century BC), Quintus Curtius Rufus' *Historia Alexandri* (first century AD), Plutarch's *Alexander* (in the *Lives*) and *De Fortuna aut Virtute Alexandri, Mor.*327-45, (first/second century AD), Arrian's *Anabasis Alexandri* (second century AD), Justin's *Epitoma Historiarum Philippicarum Pompei Trogi* (second century AD) and the *Historia Alexandri Magni* usually referred to as Pseudo-Callisthenes, the earlier versions of which probably date from the first or second century AD.[15] The latter has to be mentioned for the sake of completeness, but - within the sources available to us - his work marks the beginning of the Alexander romance.[16] His main interest lies in tales of miracles and strange, exotic tribes, as well as in fictitious letters written by and to Alexander.

As we can see, all authors are several centuries removed from Alexander's lifetime and from whatever first-hand information there was. This information will have been contained in the official journal, the *ephêmerides*,[17] as well as in the accounts written by Ptolemy and Aristobulos, who had both been on campaign with Alexander. It would certainly be naïve to assume that any of these were mere factual accounts and this is even more true for the extant authors who may still have had access to the earlier sources but were making their choice of material for their own purposes from those sources as well as from intermediate sources based more or less loosely on these. (To give an example of the wealth of material available in antiquity, in his life of Alexander Plutarch quotes no fewer than twenty-four different authors by name). It goes without saying that any attempt at an exact reconstruction of the events is doomed from the start, but

---

[15] The text has come down to us in several different *recensiones* which show considerable textual variants.
[16] Although there is no sharp line between the histories and the legends.
[17] I follow N. G. L. Hammond (e.g. [1983], pp. 5-10), who postulates the genuineness of the *ephêmerides*.

here I am only examining the way in which the extant sources choose to represent Alexander's personality and character.

When it comes to secondary sources the situation is not very encouraging: many of the innumerable books and articles written about Alexander the Great mention his wounds, but only as part of his biography and as just a part of the many events in his life, and two articles and one entire book are concerned with Alexander's wounds from a medico-historical point of view. The articles are J. Rollet's 'Des Caractères particuliers et du traitement de la blessure d' Alexandre le Grand' (1877) and F. Lammert's 'Alexanders Verwundung in der Stadt der Maller und die damalige Heilkunde'[18] (1960) - both discussing Alexander's last and most dangerous wound in particular - and the book is M. Bertolotti's *La critica medica nella storia. Alessandro Magno* (1933), which also includes a discussion of illnesses suffered by Alexander.

The objective of Rollet, Lammert and Bertolotti is merely to determine where and how badly Alexander was wounded, thus treating the literary descriptions as some kind of medical report, as if they were case histories in the style of the *Epidemics* (and even those cannot be taken at face value). Bertolotti's book in particular shows the naïve approach often characteristic of medico-historical research undertaken by retired doctors with no classical or historical training: the author goes as far as illustrating his analysis of Alexander's wounds with anatomical diagrams and even an X-ray photograph to demonstrate the exact site of Alexander's chest wound. Even a brief examination of the primary sources makes it obvious that the information we can gain from them is anything but clear or precise, and therefore any pretence at exact knowledge about Alexander's wounds can only be based on the author's arbitrary judgement.

To my knowledge there is no treatment of the topic in secondary literature taking any different approach. The angle taken by classical scholars is usually a search for earlier sources, but although this is doubtless an important field of scholarship, it still leaves some questions unanswered, since it only delegates the responsibility for a story to a lost author, but does not question the reason for its survival.

However, there is no place in this Chapter for a lengthy discussion of sources - whether primary or secondary - and I shall therefore return to the discussion of the core topic. If we are to

---

[18] The second part of the title makes it clear that the author is mainly interested in the event as an example of how wounds were treated.

believe the testimony of the ancient authors writing about Alexander's life - and there is no good reason for refusing this evidence - Alexander sustained at least seven wounds on his campaigns. While I am convinced that the authors modify the accounts of Alexander's wounds and their treatment and heighten the narrative tension by fictitious additions as well as by the omission of details which they consider unimportant for the purpose of heroisation, I am nevertheless certain that these accounts are based on a framework of some kind of historical reality. It appears legitimate therefore to discuss the events in the chronological order in which they are supposed to have taken place, since the sources agree largely on this order. The wounds as described by our authors fall in the years between 333 and 326. It is possible - and even likely - that Alexander had been wounded in earlier fighting as well, but the only mention of earlier wounds is in Plutarch's *Fort. Al.*,[19] where Alexander speaks of two injuries suffered in combats against the Illyrians.[20] One can imagine different explanations for this absence of information other than just the fact that Alexander was never wounded before Issus. For one thing, as far as we know, no contemporary wrote a systematic history of the earlier years of Alexander's life - only famous anecdotes, such as the taming of Bukephalos, have come down to us. But also, even if Alexander was ever wounded in fights before 333, presumably this would have been of less interest for writers of histories, unless a spectacular story was attached to the incident. The reason for this lack of interest is that at that point the implications of a wound - even a potentially fatal one - would be far less dramatic than at a later stage when Alexander was already the great conqueror at the head of a large army far away from Greece, where his death would have left his men without a leader.

For this same reason I believe that the account of the illness contracted by Alexander in Cilicia should be included here. Although it is by definition not a battle wound, the points that are emphasised are the same. The story is reported, in more or less detail, by all our authors, so they must have considered it particularly worth telling.

The outline of the story is well known. Although there is some disagreement on the cause - fatigue or bathing in the river Cydnus - all authors agree that Alexander is taken severely ill on his passage through Cilicia, shortly before the battle of Issus, and that he is saved by a remedy administered by his doctor Philippos. All

---

[19] 327A.
[20] A stone-throw to the head and a cudgel-blow to the neck.

except Diodorus add the detail that Alexander receives a letter from his general Parmenion warning him that Philippos has been bribed by the Persians to kill him, but Alexander ignores the warning and hands the letter to Philippos while drinking the potion, thus proving his trust in him. (Most authors tell the story with great relish in its theatrical aspects.)[21]

The attraction of this story is self-evident and it has many of the aspects stressed in accounts of wounding: there is danger to Alexander's life (e.g. Arrian II.4.8: "it was not believed that he would live"[22] - he repeats almost the same phrase for a wound at VII.11.1), this by consequence puts the whole army in peril (e.g. Curtius III.V.6-8; Pseudo-Callisthenes, rec.vet., II.8), the story demonstrates Alexander's courage (and, in this case, his trust in his friends) and it emphasises Alexander's importance by spelling out the feelings of others towards him, namely the soldiers' fear for his life, Parmenion's concern (albeit misguided) and Philippos' faithfulness and affection.

Another important aspect of this incident is one which is to appear again in accounts of wounding: despite the gravity of his illness, Alexander is not a passive victim; his choice of the potentially dangerous remedy offered by Philippos is a conscious decision. We shall find the same depiction of Alexander taking control of the situation in Q. Curtius' description of the Gaza wound,[23] Arrian's account of one of the versions of the Mallian incident,[24] the invective of Plutarch's Alexander against his friends' hesitation to saw off the shaft of the arrow that has struck him,[25] and in Alexander's encouraging words to the surgeon, again on the occasion of the wound suffered in the Mallian stronghold, in Curtius.[26]

The style and language in which this episode is told further illustrates that it is constructed on heroic models: Q. Curtius stresses how Alexander does not fear for his life, but only for the outcome of the battle, requiring "not so much a remedy against death as one for war".[27] Similarly, one of the considerations which lead to Alexander's decision to take the draught is that, even if it is poisoned, it will be better to die through another's crime

---

[21] Plutarch, whose Philippos displays rather flamboyant behaviour in his outrage over the accusation, even uses the expression 'a dramatic sight' (θεατρικὴ ὄψις).
[22] οὐκ οἴεσθαι εἶναι βιώσιμον.
[23] IV.VI.18f.
[24] VI.XI.1.
[25] *Fort. Al.* 345A-B.
[26] IX.V.25-27.
[27] *non tam mortis quam belli remedium* (III.V.10).

than through his own fear.[28] Plutarch's choice of words, too, shows his intention to emphasise the aspect of Alexander's courage, when Philippos asks him to "endure and drink".[29] The expression does not fit very well with the context, but it may well be chosen because *hypomenô*[30] is often used for holding one's ground in a fight and therefore has hidden connotations of heroic combat. Finally, Arrian makes it explicit what the story demonstrates as far as he is concerned: it shows not only Alexander's faith in his friends, but also his fearlessness in the face of death.[31]

The story also contains a motif which one can find in scenes of wounding and which may well have been popular in antiquity. By analogy with fighting one could call it the doctor's *aristeia* - i.e. out of several doctors only one, mentioned by name, dares to try his hand at a treatment and saves the patient. The detail that only Philippos ventures to suggest a remedy appears in all authors except in Pseudo-Callisthenes, who, however, also puts Philippos in a special position by mentioning him by name[32] and adding that he was "dearest to Alexander".[33] In Curtius,[34] Alexanders friends and physicians, who entreat him not to take risks, doubt that anyone would dare suggest a new remedy, since it would rouse suspicion, but Philippos alone does so because of his affection for the king.[35] Diodorus[36] again sets off Philippos, who offers to use a hazardous drug, against 'the others', who are disinclined to undertake any kind of treatment, and even Justin, in his relatively short account, states that Philippos was the only one to promise a cure.[37] Plutarch as well[38] makes the already familiar distinction between 'the others' and Philippos.

In all these versions of the story Philippos shows a courage and readiness to take risks which the other doctors do not possess, and by his initiative saves the day - very much in the style of a warrior's *aristeia*. Arrian, Curtius, Diodorus and Plutarch all report that Philippos is from Acarnania, on the west coast of the Greek

---

[28] *at satius est alieno me mori scelere quam metu nostro* (ib.III.VI.4).
[29] ὑπομεῖναι καὶ πιεῖν (XIX.4).
[30] Along with plain *menô*.
[31] πρὸς τὸ ἀποθανεῖν ἐρρωμένος (II.4.11).
[32] In most accounts of medical or surgical treatment the doctors are only nameless *iatroi*.
[33] φίλτατος Ἀλεξάνδρῳ (II.8).
[34] III.V.16-VI.2.
[35] According to Curtius, he had been guardian to Alexander's health since the latter's childhood.
[36] XVII.31.5f.
[37] *unus erat ex medicis, nomine Philippus, qui solus remedium pollicetur* (XI.VIII.5).
[38] *Alex.* XIX.3f.

mainland, and this detail may be an additional point of interest for them. Since Acarnania is neither one of the cultural centres of fourth-century Greece nor famous for its doctors (as Cos would be), the additional motif may be the one of success won by an outsider.

In the same passage Arrian adds the enigmatic comment that Philippos is not only most trusted in things concerning medicine, but also "otherwise not without renown in the army".[39] The editor of the Loeb edition translates this as "moreover, a brave man in the field", but this interpretation seems unlikely and presumably the phrase only refers to Philippos' reputation in general. However, if Arrian had meant to hint at Philippos' qualities as a warrior, it is definitely another Homeric reference in an attempt to equate him[40] with Machaon.

Shortly after his illness - according to all authors except Pseudo-Callisthenes, who leaves it out - Alexander sustains his first battle wound at the battle of Issus, in November 333. The only suggestion that he may have been wounded at the Granicus is in Plutarch's *Fortuna Alexandri* (327A), where he claims that Alexander received a sword-cut to the head,[41] but this would appear to be one of the many fanciful additions to be found in the *Fortuna Alexandri* compared to the *Life* - where Plutarch himself agrees[42] with the other authors[43] in saying that the blow only cracked Alexander's helmet.

The reason why the Issus wound features in practically all accounts may well be the very fact that it is Alexander's first 'real' wound, although it is only a slight wound and there is neither danger nor drama attached to it. The wound itself is a shallow sword-cut to the thigh - a common type of wound for a cavalryman - and treatment is never mentioned. It is worth noting, however, that this is Alexander's only sword wound, while all the other wounds are made by missiles, and this fact may be a point of interest for our authors. Since being wounded with a sword obviously involves hand-to-hand combat, it is a story which is very appropriate for the account of a hero's life, and despite the slightness of the wound the authors make the most of it. Thus Diodorus stresses the fact that Alexander is in the thick of the fight by saying that he is surrounded by enemies[44] and Plutarch

---

[39] καὶ τὰ ἄλλα οὐκ ἀδόκιμον ἐν τῷ στρατῷ ὄντα.
[40] Although presumably no longer a young man.
[41] τὴν κεφαλὴν διεκόπην.
[42] XVI.10.
[43] Arrian, I.15.7; Diodorus, XVII.20.
[44] περιχυθέντων αὐτῷ τῶν πολεμίων (XVII.34.5f.).

explains that Alexander is fighting among the foremost.[45] On the other hand, numerous arrow wounds reinforce the image (present already in the *Iliad* and becoming a topos in later literature) of the hero whom the enemies do not dare approach.

Arrian and Curtius prefer to emphasise the aspect that Alexander does not allow his wound to hamper him: although himself wounded, he visits the wounded on the following day and provides a funeral for the dead[46] and a ceremony to honour those who have distinguished themselves. According to Q. Curtius, Alexander's wound does not stop him from either the pursuit of Darius or from attending the banquet given for his friends.[47] The latter seems incongruous, as lying on a couch at a banquet would hardly be as strenuous for a leg wound as pursuing an enemy on horse-back. It may well be, though, that here Curtius is using his own knowledge that one should not drink wine when wounded.[48]

In the brief remarks regarding Alexander's first battle wound we can already see hints at themes which are to be developed further by our authors at the occasion of later, more serious, wounds. In particular, these themes are Alexander's eagerness to fight and rashness at exposing himself to risk, his concern for his men, and his toughness in bearing wounds and their consequences.

The various authors often voice criticisms regarding Alexander's rashness and lack of regard for his safety, presenting them either as their own opinion or as that of one of the figures in their account, usually Alexander's friends.[49] However, unlike the truly negative comments about Alexander (regarding, for example, his adoption of Persian habits or his heavy drinking), those about his rashness appear to contain a certain ambivalence and a fascination with this aspect of his personality. Given that impetuous daring was very much a Homeric, or more specifically Achillean, trait, it suited the image of Alexander as a second Achilles and the comments can therefore be seen as disguised praise, with rashness perceived as yet another aspect of Alexander's courage.

---

[45] ἐν πρώτοις (*Al.* XX.8f.).
[46] (Arr. II.XII.1). As mentioned in Ch. 4, these two activities - looking after the wounded and burying the dead - traditionally feature together in literature when describing the day after a battle.
[47] III.XII.1-3. The pursuit is mentioned also by Diodorus (XVII.37.2) and Arrian (II.11.6).
[48] Cf., e.g., Celsus V.26.25./223.10-16.
[49] E.g. Arr. VI.13.4.

CHAPTER EIGHT 195

We can see some of the themes mentioned above emerge again in the account of Alexander's next wound, that is, the one sustained in the siege of Gaza in 331. This is mentioned by Arrian, Curtius and Plutarch, the three authors who report all of Alexander's wounds (or at least all the ones we know of), usually with much agreement on the main outlines of events. In this case, too, they agree on the nature of the wound: it is a missile wound - Alexander is hit καταπέλτῃ/*sagitta*/βέλει in Arrian, Curtius and Plutarch respectively - in the shoulder, the arrow (or catapult bolt) having pierced the breastplate.[50]

An additional interest of this story is the aspect of a prophecy come true,[51] when the soothsayer Aristander warns the king that, although he will take the city, there is danger to his life.[52] Thus again Alexander's life is in danger, and this factor serves to highlight his readiness to take risks - or even his pleasure in doing so. Arrian and Curtius in particular spin out the tale how Alexander disregards Aristander's warning when he sees that his men are being pushed back by the defenders: he leads the hypaspists to where the Macedonians are hardest pressed,[53] fighting in the front line himself.[54] This is another depiction of an Alexander valuing the success of a military operation above his life, and at the same time never abandoning his soldiers in difficulties, and it reinforces the image of Alexander as a leader as we find it throughout the sources.

As for the wound itself, it is Alexander's first arrow wound[55] and the way in which he reacts to this wound - considerably more painful than the first - would form an important aspect of the story. As is often the case, Curtius[56] goes into the greatest detail about the treatment and aftermath of the wound and Alexander's behaviour: Philippos pulls out the arrow, apparently without removing the corselet first, and the extraction causes a fresh haemorrhage. This causes much concern among 'all' (this could mean friends, or doctors, or both), as the corselet makes it impossible to judge how deep the wound is, but Alexander himself, "not even changing colour",[57] gives orders to staunch the bleeding and bandage the wound. He then returns to his place in

---

[50] According to Arrian, it has first pierced the shield.
[51] As Curtius puts it (IV.VI.17), "fate is unavoidable" (*inevitabile est fatum*).
[52] Arr. II.XXVI; Curtius IV.VI.11-13; Plu., *Alex.* XXV.4.
[53] ἵνα μάλιστα ἐπιέζοντο οἱ Μακεδόνες (Arr. II.XXVII.1f.).
[54] *dum inter primores promptius dimicat* (Curtius IV.VI.17).
[55] For the purpose of the story it makes no difference whether the weapon was an arrow or a catapult bolt.
[56] IV.VI.17-20.
[57] Ibid. 18: ... *ne oris quidem colore mutato* ...

the front, "having either dissembled or overcome the pain".[58] However, the haemorrhage starts afresh, the bandage having slipped, the wound grows cold, swells and therefore becomes more painful, and finally Alexander faints and is carried back to the camp.

At first sight Curtius' account reads like good dramatic narrative and, at the same time, a fairly realistic account, but on second reading it seems much less of the latter. One can envisage a surgeon pulling out a missile through the breastplate - rather than sawing off the the shaft and removing the breastplate before the extraction, as we shall see at the occasion of Alexander's last wound - and in particular with a tapered catapult bolt this would seem reasonable. However, he is unlikely to do so without first probing the wound[59] and this would give him an idea about the depth of the wound as well. Certainly once the arrow has been pulled out there would be no doubt as to the depth of the wound, which could easily be seen from the blood on the arrow. Hence the detail that because of the corselet no one knows how deep the wound is, is unrealistic. So is the fact that all are alarmed by the haemorrhage following the extraction of the arrow, since this was the natural consequence and would only cause alarm if it was excessive and could not be stopped easily (as, again, it will be the case with Alexander's most dangerous wound). The detail that Alexander returns to the fight immediately after experiencing the treatment of a missile wound for the first time - whether the wound was in the right shoulder or the left - is equally fantastic.

The reason why it is so important to point out the fictitious character of this episode is that it shows the author's intentions. Elements which do not conform with what one would expect in reality have obviously been added by somebody (either by the respective author or by his sources) in order to achieve a particular effect, and in this case the intended effect is quite evident. What all the aforementioned details have in common is that they stress the gravity of the wound and, implicitly or explicitly, Alexander's strength, courage and endurance.

Thus, although everyone else is in panic about the haemorrhage and the potential depth of the wound, Alexander, who has not even turned pale,[60] commands his doctor to staunch the bleeding and bind up the wound. This shows us an Alexander unperturbed

---

[58] *vel dissimulato vel victo dolore.*
[59] Cf. Ch 2.3.3: judging from the descriptions in medical literature, it seems unlikely that extractions of arrows were ever attempted without preliminary probing.
[60] A detail which contradicts the story of the strong bleeding.

by fear or pain, and again in control of the situation. One has to keep in mind that what Alexander orders Philippos to do is precisely what any doctor would do without being told, thus the only point of this command is to demonstrate that Alexander is sufficiently *compos mentis* to take active control of the situation, and that the pain caused by the extraction does not leave him helpless.

Likewise, Alexander's impatience to return to the fight despite his wound is well in keeping with the image projected in other scenes, and the fact that he faints after a renewed haemorrhage only emphasises the gravity of the wound, and therefore the odds against which he is fighting.[61] Curtius stresses this point repeatedly. After being carried back to the camp unconscious, Alexander returns to the siege soon, "the wound not having healed yet",[62] and is wounded on the leg by a stone-throw while leading the vanguard and advancing incautiously. Nevertheless, even after this second wound, he still continues to fight among the foremost, leaning on a spear, "the first wound not having healed over yet".[63] Curtius is hammering in the fact that nothing can stop Alexander, least of all physical pain.

Arrian, who does not revel in drama to the same extent, does not give a detailed account, but we can find similar motifs. Alexander rejoices (ἐχάρη) when he is wounded,[64] since he is now certain that the second part of Aristander's prophecy, the capture of the city, will also come true. Thus, for the sake of a military success Alexander will welcome even the pain and discomfort of a wound.

According to Arrian as well, the wound is not a slight one and Alexander "is treated for his wound with difficulty".[65] Arrian uses a similar expression for Perdikkas, wounded at the siege of Thebes,[66] but it is impossible to reconstruct what exactly he wants to express by it, perhaps summarising material available to him. The expression could refer to difficulties in the extraction or perhaps a protracted or painful recovery. It is unlikely, however, that the phrase was much less ambiguous to Arrian's contemporary audience than it is to us (unless they knew his sources), and his intention may well have been to give a general

---

[61] Even the usually gullible Bertolotti ([1933], p. 187) refutes Curtius' version as "fairy-tales for children".
[62] *nondum percurato vulnere* (IV.VI.21).
[63] *nondum prioris vulneris obducta cicatrice* (ib. 24).
[64] II.XXVII.2.
[65] τὸ τραῦμα ἐθεραπεύετο χαλεπῶς (ib. 3).
[66] "He recovered with difficulty" (χαλεπῶς διεσώθη ; I.8.3).

idea of complications. Despite whatever circumstances complicate his recovery, Arrian's Alexander, too, soon returns to lead the attack in person, again presenting us with the image of an intrepid, even rash Alexander, undaunted by adversity of any kind.

Along with Alexander's many wounds we occasionally hear about those of his officers (as with Perdikkas at Thebes). Thus, in the account of the battle of Gaugamela, Arrian,[67] Curtius[68] and Diodorus[69] mention Hephaistion, Koinos and Menidas, Curtius and Diodorus Perdikkas as well. Alexander is not wounded at Gaugamela, and this may be the reason why the authors take the time to mention others, or else it may be a pretence to completeness of information. Both Curtius and Diodorus report that Hephaistion is wounded in the arm and this piece of information may well have been handed down for its own particular reason. Taking into account the representation of Achilles treating Patroklos' arm wound on the well-known Attic cup by the Sosias painter,[70] it is possible that there was a tradition in the Cyclic Epics (literary evidence of which does not survive) of Patroklos being wounded in the arm. Since, as I explained above, the role of Hephaistion as Patroklos to Alexander's Achilles was stressed in ancient literature, it may well be that the detail of his arm wound was a clear reference to the epic for an ancient audience. This may seem very conjectural, but, considering the amount of Homeric reference contained in the material regarding Alexander, it is not to be rejected out of hand.

While the authors' motives for recording the wounds of some of the officers are difficult to reconstruct, they are much more obvious for Alexander's wounds, and the aforementioned elements emerge in almost every account. The frequency of recorded cases of Alexander being wounded increases during the later years of his expedition and - according to Arrian, Curtius and Plutarch - he is wounded four times in the years between 329 and 327.

The first of these, Alexander's third wound, sustained by the Jaxartes, or perhaps at the siege of Marakanda (today's Samarkand), is another arrow wound. According to Arrian and Plutarch, Alexander is shot in the leg with damage to the bone: "He was shot in the shin, right through, and a piece of his fibula was broken off by the arrow."[71] Plutarch, who does not specify

---

[67] III.15.2.
[68] IV.XVI.31ff.
[69] XVII.61.3.
[70] See Fig. 1.
[71] ἐς τὴν κνήμην τοξεύεται διαμπὰξ καὶ τῆς περόνης τι ἀποθραύεται αὐτῷ ἐκ τοῦ τοξεύματος (Arr.III. 30.11).

the geographical location, writes: "He took an arrow in the shin, through which the bone of the tibia broke off and fell out."[72] Although there is no immediate danger to Alexander's life, the fact that this is the only wound involving the bone - an excruciating and potentially crippling injury - may well be an added point of interest. Along with this, the usual points are stressed: Alexander leads from the front again.[73] and when the Sogdians send their envoys the following day, he conceals the gravity of his wound.[74] Despite his wound, Alexander captures the stronghold,[75] and his wound does not stop him from continuing to expose himself to danger.[76] Curtius[77] also describes the dispute between the infantry and the cavalry vying for the honour of carrying Alexander's litter, Alexander being unable to ride because of his wound. Thus once again we find an emphasis on the motifs of physical courage and rashness in fighting, endurance, and the soldiers' affection for Alexander.

Some or all of these also appear in the following three wounds. In Arrian[78] we read that in the fighting in Hyrcania (329/8), where Krateros and "many others of the officers" are wounded, Alexander himself is hit by a violent stone-throw to the head and the neck, but (again) nevertheless the attack is successful.[79] Arrian does not mention any details regarding treatment or recovery and Alexander does not appear to interrupt his command of the attack, but Plutarch speaks of a temporary reduction of eyesight following the wounding[80] and of the threat of blindness.[81]

It is not quite clear whether the *oculis caligine offusa* in Curtius[82] - who as usual provides the most detailed account - refers to a loss of sight or merely to the loss of consciousness.[83] The latter must be what the author means by "... so that he

---

[72] τόξευμα μὲν εἰς τὴν κνήμην λαβών, ὑφ' οὗ τὸ τῆς κερκίδος ὀστέον ἀποθραυσθὲν ἐξέπεσε (*Al.* XLV.5). In *Fort. Al.* 327A and 341B Plutarch situates the the story in Marakanda.

[73] *inter promptissimos dimicans* (Curtius VII.VI.3).

[74] Ibid.: *magnitudinem vulneris dissimulans*.

[75] καὶ ὧς ἔλαβέ τε τὸ χωρίον (Arr. III.30.11).

[76] ὅμως οὐκ ἐπαύετο χρώμενος ἑαυτῷ πρὸς τοὺς κινδύνους ἀφειδῶς (Plu., *Alex.* XLV.6).

[77] VII.VI.8f.

[78] IV.III.3.

[79] "..., but even so they expelled the barbarians from the market-square." (ἀλλὰ καὶ ὧς ἐξέωσαν ἐκ τῆς ἀγορᾶς τοὺς βαρβάρους).

[80] ταῖς ὄψεσιν ἀχλὺν ὑποδραμεῖν (*Al.* XLV.5).

[81] "For many days he was in fear of becoming blind." (ἡμέρας πολλὰς ἐν φόβῳ πηρήσεως ἐγένετο; *Fort. Al.* 341B).

[82] VII.VI.22.

[83] Although he does not usually express the latter in this way.

collapsed, not even conscious".[84] Curtius repeatedly mentions Alexander's slow recovery and prolonged pain from the wound, e.g. VII.VII.5: "... still suffering from the wound, and suddenly without voice, which the scant food[85] and the pain in his neck weakened", and ib. 6: "He was unable to stand on the ground, ride a horse, instruct or encourage his men."[86] However, as in many other passages, these difficulties do not stop Alexander, who continues the assault before the wound has healed[87] and refuses to capitulate to his poor state of health, claiming to have enough strength to continue: "But if you want to follow me, friends, I am well. I have enough strength to endure this."[88] Or, he continues, if not, what better way to die? Along with the danger - this time of permanent disablement - Alexander's fearlessness and endurance, and his rashness,[89] the motif of the soldiers' concern and affection for Alexander is also present, both in their laments when he is wounded (ib. 22) and their joy at seeing him apparently recovered.[90]

Surprisingly the authors do not make much of the arrow wound suffered by Alexander in the country of the Aspasians in 328/7. Although this time as well, according to Arrian,[91] the arrow has pierced the breastplate, the wound causes no complications.[92] Arrian explains that this is the case because the breastplate has stopped the arrow from going straight through the shoulder. Thus, although this wound is very much like the one sustained by Alexander at Gaza, this one is dealt with rather dismissively. Here, too, it may be the case that our authors had more detailed accounts about the respectively greater or lesser gravity of the two wounds at their disposal and that they are merely summarising their sources. However, it may well be that the resemblance between the two wounds explains the lack of interest in the second, which is after all Alexander's fifth wound and would not rouse the same interest as his first arrow wound.

---

[84] *ut ... collabetur, ne mentis quidem compos.*

[85] The reduced diet is presumably to be seen as part of the treatment.

[86] *adhuc aeger ex vulnere, praecipue voce deficiens, quam et modicus cibus et cervicis extenuabat dolor; ipse non insistere in terra, non equo vehi, non docere, non hortari suos poterat, ...*

[87] *nondum percurato vulnere acrius obsidioni institit* (VII.VI.23).

[88] *Sed si me sequi vultis, valeo, amici. Satis virum est ad toleranda ista* (VII.VII.19).

[89] "Anger stirring up his natural swiftness, ..." (*naturalem celeritatem ira concitante*; VII.VI.23).

[90] VII.VIII.4f.

[91] IV.23.3.

[92] Ibid.: οὐ χαλεπὸν αὐτῷ ἐγένετο.

The two themes present here are the military success despite the wound, in Curtius' remark that "nevertheless he took the town",[93] and the soldiers' devotion to Alexander, this time resulting in a massacre of the captured enemies by the Macedonians angered at Alexander's wounding.[94] (We shall encounter this turn of the story again at Alexander's last wound.)

The authors appear to invest more interest in the wound suffered by Alexander at the siege of Massaga in 327, an arrow wound to the leg - the ankle according to Arrian IV.26.4, who adds that it was not a serious wound, and the calf according to Curtius VIII.X.6. As with most of the others, this wound, too, is a consequence of Alexander's style of personal leadership and of his readiness to take risks, as he is hit when leading the troops up to the city walls,[95] and again we can see Alexander fighting on despite the wound. Thus, in Arrian's account,[96] Alexander is back leading the attack on the following days, especially on the third day, when he personally leads the hypaspists in the assault.

It is again Curtius who presents the most detailed and dramatic account of the event. He is the only author to mention the extraction,[97] without however going into further details, and he follows this up with a story very similar to that of the Gaza wound. Here again Alexander takes an attitude of command by ordering a horse to be brought up and, mounting it without having the wound bandaged, returns to his inspection of the city walls. (We are obviously meant to imagine Alexander having the arrow removed in the field, without even returning to his tent.)

In this case, too, the wound dries, swells, and the pain increases. This time, however, Alexander does not faint, and Curtius[98] quotes his reported comment that, although called a son of Zeus, he nevertheless felt the imperfection of an ailing body. This is presumably the occasion referred to by Plutarch in *Alex.* XXVIII.3, where Alexander, "hit by an arrow and in great pain", says to his friends that what is flowing from his wound is blood and not "*ichor* as it flows from the wounds of the happy gods".[99] The latter highlights Alexander's erudition and predilection for Homer, and both sayings demonstrate Alexander's ability to

---

[93] *cepit tamen oppidum* (VIII.X.6).
[94] Arr. IV.23.5.
[95] Arr. IV.26.4; Curt. VIII.X.28.
[96] IV.26.5f.
[97] VIII.X.28: "the point having been pulled out, ..." (*spiculo evolso*).
[98] VIII.X.29f.
[99] A quotation of *Iliad* V. 340: ἰχώρ, οἷος πέρ τε ῥέει μακάρεσσι θεοῖσιν.

deliver *bons mots* despite the pain of an arrow wound - which would appear to be one of the main points of these anecdotes. (The physical pain is explicitly mentioned in both stories.) Q. Curtius also stresses Alexander's endurance in the usual way: after being wounded Alexander does not return to the camp before having finished his reconnoitring of the fortifications and he is out again inspecting the siege works "his wound not yet covered by a scar".[100]

The examples discussed so far should make it obvious that all descriptions of wounding regarding Alexander contain at least one, if not several, of certain topoi. We can find all of those in the descriptions of Alexander's last and most dangerous wound and of the circumstances accompanying the wounding: Alexander's dynamic leadership, his daring and rashness, absence of fear of death (provided it was an honourable death), the men's devotion to Alexander, his active control of the situation, and, of course, his resistance to pain.

The episode features in all our authors and is obviously one of the dramatic highlights in the description of Alexander's life. It was also clearly a well-known story in antiquity, so that other writers could allude to it without having to go into detail. Thus, in Lucian's *Dialogues of the Dead* (397.5), Alexander quotes the incident at Philip as an example of his love of danger,[101] and when Strabo[102] speaks of the Mallians, he can distinguish them from other tribes by saying that it was in their country that "Alexander was in peril of death, having been wounded in the capture of some small town".[103] Both authors could obviously expect their audiences to be familiar with the story, not because it was a historical fact, but because it has many elements which made it attractive to popular imagination.

The events leading up to the wounding are yet another example - presumably the most famous one - of Alexander's impatience in leading an attack and his eagerness to take risks, as it is portrayed throughout the literature regarding him. It conforms with Plutarch's remark that Alexander held glory higher than his life and kingship.[104]

There is some disagreement among the authors as to whether the incident happened among the Mallians (Arrian, Diodorus and

---

[100] VIII.X.30f.: *nondum obducta vulneri cicatrice*.
[101] τὸ φιλοκίνδυνον.
[102] XV.1.33.
[103] ... ἀποθανεῖν ἐκινδύνευσεν Ἀλέξανδρος, τρωθεὶς ἐν ἁλώσει πολίχνης τινός, ...
[104] *Alex.* XLII.4.

Plutarch) or the Sudracae (Q. Curtius, Justin and Lucian, who calls them Oxydracae), but they generally agree that Alexander is the first to scale the walls of their stronghold - according to Arrian,[105] Curtius[106] and Diodorus,[107] pressing on in impatience at the soldiers' slowness. Curtius and Diodorus add the already familiar detail of the soothsayer predicting danger to the king's life.[108] There is a general rush to follow the king, the ladders break, Alexander is left on his own (or with two or three bodyguards) on top of the city wall, and decides to leap inside the citadel amongst the enemies.

Obviously it is not merely the sheer rashness of the decision that is of interest to the authors, but Arrian, Curtius and Diodorus also dwell on the thoughts crossing Alexander's mind. Thus Arrian's Alexander - "conspicuous by the splendour of his arms and by his extraordinary daring"[109] - realises that by remaining on the wall he is not only exposing himself to danger, but - and this seems more important - he will not achieve anything noteworthy. However, by leaping down within the citadel, even if it meant risking his life, he would "die not ignobly having done great deeds, worthy for coming generations to hear of".[110]

In Curtius,[111] Alexander's friends shout to him to leap down to them, but - for reasons not well defined - Alexander decides against it, although inside the city there is hardly hope for him to "die fighting and not unavenged".[112] Curtius points out (and presumably this is the point he wants to make) that this deed can be counted much more towards his reputation for rashness[113] than his glory. Curtius also uses the enemies' reaction as a means to emphasise Alexander's fame and courage; thus they do not dare approach him, but hurl missiles at him from a distance.[114]

Diodorus goes into more detail about Alexander's feelings and intentions: Alexander feels that to leap back to his men without accomplishing anything would be unworthy of him. He is determined to make this, the last deed of his life, the most

---

[105] VI.IX.3.
[106] IX.IV.30.
[107] XVII.98.4.
[108] Curt. IX.IV.27-30; D.S. XVII.98.3.
[109] δῆλος μὲν ἦν 'Αλέξανδρος ὢν τῶι τε ὅπλων τῇ λαμπρότητι καὶ ἀτόπῳ τῆς τόλμης, ...
[110] μεγάλα ἔργα καὶ τοῖς ἔπειτα πυθέσθαι ἄξια ἐργασάμενος οὐκ ἀσπουδεὶ ἀποθανεῖται (VI.9.5). The reference to Hector's thoughts - ἐσσομένοισι πυθέσθαι (Il. XXII.305) - is obvious.
[111] IX.V.1-3.
[112] *cum vix sperare posset dimicantem certe et non inultum esse moriturum.*
[113] Often presented as a facet of his courage.
[114] IX.V.5; ib.9.

glorious, showing "such courage as one would expect from a king who has achieved so much".[115] Thus all three authors use this part of the narrative to stress Alexander's rash daring, as well as his outstanding courage and desire to die a glorious death (greater than his desire to live). Pseudo-Callisthenes as well emphasises Alexander's courage in his brief remark that Alexander was wounded "fighting nobly".[116]

Another theme which one can find used here in order to express Alexander's special status and importance is the feelings of his men towards him - in particular the devotion shown by his bodyguard and the affection of the army in general. Again there is some disagreement about the names of the two or three bodyguards who are either with Alexander from the start or are the first to fight their way through to him, but all authors agree that they are ready to sacrifice themselves unsparingly for their king. (Pseudo-Callisthenes [II.15] also uses this dramatic element, saying that they valued their king's safety above their own.) One of them dies and the others are wounded, but still defend their wounded leader in truly Homeric style - reflected in Arrian's image of Peukestas standing astride the body,[117] holding the sacred shield from Troy over Alexander.

While the implications of the bodyguards' readiness to die for Alexander are only implicit in the other authors, Plutarch spells them out in *Fort. Al.* 344D-E, where he says that they risked their lives out of their good will and love for the king. "For", he continues the argument for *aretê* against chance, "it is not due to fortune that the companions of good kings die for them willingly and take risks for them ...".[118] It is therefore Alexander's virtue and outstanding qualities that make these men defend him rather than themselves. It is also for the same reasons that the Macedonian soldiers vent their anger on the enemy, and their sentiments about the incident are reflected in a massacre among the population and the destruction of the town.

The wound itself is described in some detail by most of the authors, and despite divergences all seem to agree that it was a deep chest wound made by an arrow. There is no doubt - although some of the aspects may be exaggerated in the

---

[115] τούτῳ τῷ θυμῷ παραστὰς ὡς ἄν τις βασιλεὺς τηλικούτων ἤδη ἀπειργασμένων ἀνδραγαθήσειε, τὴν ἐσχάτην τοῦ βίου καταστροφὴν εὐκλεεστάτην γενέσθαι φιλοτιμούμενος. (XVII.99.2).
[116] γενναίως ἀγωνιζόμενος (II.15).
[117] Πευκέστας δὲ περιβὰς (VI.X.2).
[118] οὐ γὰρ διὰ Τύχην ἀγαθῶν βασιλέων ἑταῖροι προαποθνήσκουσιν ἑκουσίως καὶ προκινδυνεύουσιν, ...

descriptions - that this was Alexander's most dangerous wound and that it could easily have been fatal. It would also appear that, of all the arrow wounds suffered by Alexander, this was the only case in which the arrow was barbed and had to be cut out rather than pulled out. This not only entailed an extremely painful operation, but also the danger of fatal haemorrhage following the enlargement of the wound.[119] It is self-evident that these facts alone make for dramatic narrative, and we find the authors describing the potential danger and Alexander's reaction and behaviour, thus making the most of the occasion to emphasise his courage and endurance, as well as in some descriptions his way of staying in control of the situation.

The latter is highlighted in Arrian, Curtius and Plutarch in particular, where Alexander, although desperately wounded, is still capable of telling others what to do. Thus Arrian[120] reports two versions of the treatment, one of them being that the bodyguard Perdikkas removes the arrow. He apparently does so by making an incision with his sword (*sic!*), no doctor being at hand, and he does this at Alexander's command.[121] This is, of course, again an entirely unrealistic story and must therefore have been created for a special effect. Not only is it highly improbable that, despite the number of doctors available to Alexander, a man without medical training or proper equipment should put the king's life at risk by inexpert treatment,[122] especially in the case of his most dangerous wound, but one would also expect the *philiatros* Alexander to know better than to give such an order. This may again be a deliberate imitation of the *Iliad*, where the heroes are often treated by their companions, but it may also be meant to show Alexander as taking the situation in hand.

The same is also the case in Plutarch's *Fort. Al.* (345A-B), when 'they' do not dare to saw off the shaft of the arrow,[123] and Alexander himself attempts to do so with his dagger. Failing to sever the shaft, he commands (ἐκέλευσεν) the others to do so, encouraging (θαρρύνων) them and railing at those who are in tears with concern for him. Again Alexander seems to be concerned much more with his reputation than with his life when he cries out to them that "it will not be believed that [he does] not

---

[119] Cf. Ch. 2.3.3.
[120] VI.XI.1.
[121] ἐγκελευσαμένου 'Αλεξάνδρου.
[122] One only has to think of the hesitation - even among the experts - to undertake treatment at the occasion of Alexander's illness in Cilicia.
[123] As the arrow has pierced the breastplate, the latter is effectively nailed to the body.

fear death if they fear for [his] death".[124] This story again contrasts the helpless, weeping, entourage with the fearless, unshaken Alexander. This aspect is stressed in particular in Curtius' narrative: although his Alexander fails to pull out the arrow because of his weakness,[125] he at least attempts to do so himself (although he has never attempted this with his earlier wounds and would know that it was a dangerous thing to do[126]).

It is in the description of the extraction in particular that the authors show Alexander in charge of the situation:[127] despite being of outstanding skill among the doctors (*inter medicos artis eximiae*),[128] the surgeon Critobulus[129] is terrified by the greatness of the danger and by the implications for himself if the extraction results in Alexander's death.[130] While Critobulus hesitates, pale with fear and concern and weeping, Alexander has to reassure him and convince him to undertake the operation. In Curtius' account Alexander himself seems convinced that he is fatally wounded and only asks for the removal of the arrow as a relief from pain before his certain death.[131] Thus we can again see the wounded Alexander in a better emotional state than those around him, ready to take his fate in his own hands.

The gravity of the wound, the extreme danger to Alexander's life, and the complications accompanying the extraction are emphasised in most accounts and these facts are a strong dramatic element, as well as the suffering implied for Alexander. The arrow has pierced the breastplate and the latter can only be removed by sawing off the shaft first,[132] with great care not to stir the point. According to Plutarch, this is done "with difficulty and painfully",[133] and he is more specific in *Fort. Al.* (loc.cit.), where he says that it was feared that the sawing might cause agonising pain and an internal haemorrhage.

---

[124] ἀπιστοῦμαι μὴ φοβεῖσθαι θάνατον, εἰ τὸν ἐμὸν φοβεῖσθ' ὑμεῖς.
[125] IX.V.10.
[126] Cf. Rufus, *Quaest. Med.* 51.
[127] Curt. IX.V.25-27 does so in the greatest detail.
[128] This is another example of what one could call the doctor's *aristeia*.
[129] Arrian (VI.11.1) calls him Kritodemos.
[130] This is not an unrealistic detail. His fears are not unfounded if one considers the fate awaiting Hephaistion's doctor after the former's death, when Alexander had him crucified (Plu. *Alex.* LXXII.2) or, according to Arrian's version (VII.14.4) hanged - an ignominious death in either case.
[131] IX.V.26: " ... and [why] do you not at least free me, who am about to die, from this pain?" (...*et non quam primum hoc dolore me saltem moriturum liberas?*)
[132] Curt. IX.V.22f.; Plu., *Alex.* LXIII.11; id., *Fort. Al.* 344F-345A.
[133] χαλεπῶς δὲ καὶ πολυπόνως (*Alex.*, loc.cit.).

The strong bleeding, both from the wound *per se* and at the extraction, is mentioned by most authors, as well as the loss of consciousness resulting from it, e.g. in Plutarch: "When it [sc. the point] had been taken out, he was brought very close to death by the repeated fainting."[134] According to Curtius - as usual furnishing the most theatrical description - the haemorrhage is almost impossible to check and only ceases at the last moment when everyone believes that Alexander is dying.[135] The continuous reference to the danger involved creates an image of Alexander's astonishing physical resistance.

The most explicit account of Alexander's resistance to pain is again in Curtius' version of the story:[136] Critobulus, who has at last "ended or concealed his fear", urges Alexander to "allow himself to be held down while he would extract the point" (as would be the normal procedure), since "even a slight movement of his body would be dangerous".[137] Given the picture of Alexander's character as it is presented in our sources, this is a rhetorical question, an unrealistic demand to which there could be only one answer. Hence the main purpose of this detail seems to be to draw attention to the pain involved and therefore to Alexander's courage. Needless to say, Alexander refuses and "having declared that there was no need of any to hold him, he offered his body motionless, as he had been enjoined'.[138] I shall not discuss the degree of realism or the plausibility of this story, but it is quite obviously a scene constructed to present Alexander as a superhuman hero endowed with extraordinary self-control and courage.

Alexander's resistance to pain and weakness is highlighted also in the remarks on how he refuses to rest long enough after his wound. This motif is coupled with that of the soldiers' affection for him, since it is the troops' fear that Alexander might have died from his wound which makes him decide to show himself to the army although not yet completely recovered.[139]

---

[134] ταῖς λιποθυμίαις ἔγγιστα θανάτου συνελαυνόμενος ἐξαιρουμένης αὐτῆς [sc. τῆς ἀκίδος] (*Alex.* LXIII.12). Cf. Ch. 2.2.1.4, where this passage is also quoted. According to Arrian (VI.11.2), the haemorrhage is checked by the fainting.
[135] IX.V.29.
[136] IX.V.27f.
[137] *At Critobulus vel finito vel dissimulato metu hortari eum coepit ut se continendum praeberet, dum spiculum evelleret: etiam levem corporis motum noxium fore.*
[138] *Rex, cum adfirmasset nihil opus esse iis, qui semet coninerent, sicut praeceptum erat, sine motu praebuit corpus.*
[139] Curt. IX.VI.1f.; Plu., *Alex.* LXIII.13.

As one can see, the same topoi appear again and again throughout the accounts regarding Alexander's wounds and one can say with some certainty that they play an important part in conveying the image of Alexander as a hero in ancient literature. Apart from his military exploits of hitherto unheard-of dimensions, several factors make Alexander the obvious figure for heroisation. His alleged emulation of Achilles is one of these, others being Alexander's youth and reported good looks - youth and beauty being essential attributes of the Homeric hero - and it is probably important that none of Alexander's wounds left him crippled or disfigured (unlike his father). Furthermore, all the wounds for which there is evidence, except for the blows to the neck, seem to have been in front. Clearly, if there were any records of wounds in the back, these were not included and presumably would not have been, since this would not have fitted into the heroic tradition concerning Alexander.

Whatever material our authors had to draw on, they clearly modified it to suit a certain image they sought to convey. As I have suggested earlier, the fact that Alexander did not die in battle may well have made the authors writing about Alexander feel that they needed to give visible proof of his heroism. Depicting Alexander's leadership in battle is certainly one of the ways of doing so, but the scenes of wounding prove to be a very useful means of highlighting certain aspects of Alexander's personality. Courage in bearing wounds would also be something more immediate and familiar for the audience, since many of them would have experience of being injured, but not of leading a battle. Scenes of wounding can therefore bring home the message in a readily understandable way whilst having all the connotations of epic heroism.

CHAPTER NINE

EPILOGUE

The *Iliad* and the material concerning Alexander the Great, which I have discussed in two preceding chapters, can be considered the two high points in ancient literature as far as heroism and the image of the hero are concerned. We have seen in the previous chapters that Homeric topoi in the description of death in battle, of wounds, and of wound treatment are frequently used in post-Homeric material and that - together with other Homeric references - they are particularly visible in the material about Alexander.

While these topoi continue to be popular in later Greek and Roman prose as well as poetry, much of the Alexander material itself becomes a source of literary topoi for later writers in their representation of the hero, in particular the heroic military commander. As we can see from frequent allusions to them in Greek and Roman authors, the stories relating Alexander's leadership, dashing courage and fortitude were very well known throughout later antiquity, and they appear to have influenced the expectations of our authors' audiences when it came to representations of the military leader as a hero. The purpose of this epilogue is to briefly examine the nature and use of the topoi as we find them in later authors.

There is a vast amount of (non-medical) literary material containing at least some kind of reference to wounds at our disposition, spanning the period from the first century BC to the fifth century AD. Among the authors relevant for this topic, those writing in Greek are: Diodorus Siculus, Dionysius of Halicarnassus, Plutarch, Appian, Dio Cassius, Lucian, Achilles Tatius, Quintus Smyrnaeus, Nonnos and Procopius. Among those writing in Latin are: Florus, Virgil, C. Nepos, Cicero, Ovid, Livy, Seneca, Frontinus, Lucan, Silius Italicus, Statius, Petronius, Valerius Maximus, Quintillian, Tacitus and Ammianus Marcellinus.[1] Some of these authors would merit far more detailed treatment than is possible here, but this section is intended merely as a general survey of the post-Alexandrian[2] evidence.

---

[1] Several of these authors have already been mentioned in earlier chapters.
[2] In the sense of 'after Alexander'.

For the majority of our authors compressing the material into a short chapter is justifiable, since the situation appears to be very similar for most of them. We shall see that Plutarch and, to a certain extent, Nonnos are in some ways exceptions. In most of the material one can find a varying number of recurrent motifs and literary topoi. Most of these are already familiar from the material dealing with Alexander and many from earlier sources, even Homer, and the main common feature of the material in question is that the descriptions of death in battle, wounding and wound treatment are largely topos-oriented, as should become evident.

This fact in itself, self-evident though it may seem at first sight, is worth mentioning and investigating, since the extent to which literary descriptions are dominated by the repetition of certain set topoi is often underestimated or deliberately understated by scholars who assume that its topos-guided nature would detract from the aesthetic or creative value of ancient literature. (I do not believe that this necessarily follows.)

Erbig's dissertation - *Topoi in den Schlachtenberichten römischer Dichter* (1931) - is a collection of such topoi, and, to my knowledge, the only one. However, even this is not complete and, as the title indicates, it is limited to Roman material (except for brief references to the *Iliad*). The necessity for an analysis of all battle scenes in Greek and Roman literature has also been recognised by Norden,[3] who states regretfully that even the ancient historiographers "have fallen prey to typology". Here we have had to limit ourselves to a brief investigation of topoi related to the image of the hero in narrative, but much research remains to be done in the field of literary motifs related to wars and battles.

F. Cairns,[4] who unfortunately has limited his work to poetry, strongly advocates what he calls generic analysis and sustains the theory that "the whole of classical poetry is written in accordance with the sets of rules of the various genres",[5] and these rules, he claims, are strongly linked to rhetoric and, in particular, the teaching of rhetoric. Of the generic formulae he says:

> They can be thought of, although ancient writers did not consider them in this mechanical fashion, as full lists of the primary elements and topoi of each genre. They could be used in all kinds of prose and poetry. The generic formulae were not confined to the narrow purposes

---

[3] (1915), p. 158.
[4] *Generic Composition in Roman Poetry* (1972).
[5] Ib., p. 31.

of rhetorical instruction but were part of the cultural and social heritage of all educated men in antiquity.

Cairns also argues for a high degree of continuity as far as motifs are concerned, from Homer onwards throughout antiquity,[6] and against exaggerated ideas of 'development' within literary genres. In his words: "... in a very real sense antiquity was in comparison with the nineteenth and twentieth centuries a time-free zone".[7]

In my own field I, too, believe that it is possible to demonstrate that there is considerable continuity in the topoi and motifs used in descriptions of death and wounding in battle as well as wound treatment, and that even in late antiquity we can still recognise topoi of Homeric origin.

It would also appear that whatsoever changes occurred in medical knowledge[8] or medical treatment found very little reflection in literary description of wounds and their treatment. (Admittedly, as far as wounds are concerned, there is little change in the treatment - except for the invention of arterial ligature, changing trends in which drugs or substances to apply to the wound, and probably the inventions of some new instruments.) This demonstrates how little the literary topoi depended on the reality of medical practice or on the author's experience.

Like Cairn, Erbig, too,[9] suggests that the dependence on topoi in literary descriptions may be due to the influence of rhetoric with its standard themes for practice pieces. It is very likely that this is the case, but we have also seen that a conscious choice of motifs is at work. Although some only appear to have been developed after Alexander, the majority of literary topoi can be traced back to Homer, some of them via the material regarding Alexander. There appears to be another group of topoi which are not Homeric, but are directly related to well-known stories about Alexander (or rather, the Alexander-myth). Thus Homer and the Alexander-mythology would seem to be the two major influences in literary imagery concerning heroism.

It is an important fact that these topoi are not limited to any particular literary genre (nor does Cairn deny this). It would appear that any differences in their use between, e.g., historical writing and poetry consist mainly in a difference in language and expression, but not in the basic topoi as such. Thus we can find

---

[6] Ib., p. 36.
[7] Ib., p. 32.
[8] Such as knowledge of anatomical structures, in particular the nature of the nerves or the vascular system.
[9] (1931), p. 5.

some of them in Cicero's or Seneca's works, incorporated into philosophical discourse, as well as in epic poetry or historiography. However, it has to be pointed out that the use of the same topoi by different authors does not imply a mere aping of literary conventions, and some authors show great originality in varying the choice and application of the topoi. The different ways in which such originality can be effected is again discussed by Cairns,[10] who claims that in antiquity originality in using set motifs was considered essential to a good style.

The most important of the topoi which we find in our authors are the following: glorious death in battle, wounds in front and consequently showing the scars of those wounds as a proof of courage; fighting on while the wounds are still fresh or not feeling the wounds; weakness from loss of blood, defending the dead or wounded (often by protecting them with one's own shield); enemies using long-range weapons, not daring to close in on the hero, and - a related motif - the inferiority of the archer. Others are: a warrior reusing the spear or arrow that has hit him to strike his enemy; the care for the casualties after the battle (often mentioned in connection with burying the dead) and the general or leader visiting them; the washing of the wound; the presence of medical 'specialists'; the physician's *aristeia*; and the contrast between the veteran soldier and the young recruit.

Given the topos-guided nature of the material, it seems to me that the most logical way to procede is to itemize the topoi and to discuss the relevant passages under those headings rather than treating the authors separately. This is therefore what I shall do, keeping the authors in chronological order - first the Greek, then the Roman authors - where possible. In most cases it is unnecessary to separate the Greek and Roman material, since the same topoi are used in both in a similar way.

The first topos on the list, the glory or beauty of death in battle, is one of the oldest and most popular of all. It is at least implicit in many authors describing wars or battles, and in many passages we find it explicitly stated. Since this is probably the most commonly used topos, a list of all its incidences would fill a book and a mere listing would also be pointless, so I have had to choose some representative examples from both Greek and Roman authors. Needless to say, no claim is made here that these passages in any way represent a particular author's own opinion on death in battle. They merely prove that he saw it fit to use this motif for one reason or another.

---

[10] (1972), p. 99.

There are several examples for the use of this topos in Diodorus Siculus. Two of them are related to the death of Epaminondas[11] in the battle of Mantineia, and in both of them the author speaks of Epaminondas dying as a hero: "he died heroically";[12] and: "He sustained a fatal wound in the chest while fighting heroically for victory".[13] At XV.80.5f. he uses very similar words for the death of Pelopidas. There is a strong similarity between this story and the death of Epaminondas: Pelopidas is "eager to decide the battle by his own courage",[14] he brings about the victory, but loses his own life, having sustained many wounds and "having heroically forfeited his life".[15]

Again, at XIII.79.2, Diodorus describes the state of mind of the Athenians and Mitylenians, fighting the Peloponnesians in 407 BC : seeing their only hope left in victory, they "strive to die nobly"[16] and "expose their bodies to danger without fear".[17] Very similar phrases are used in the depiction of the battle of Mantineia, such as "giving no heed to life",[18] or "they demonstrated their courage (*andragathia*) in danger".[19] Regardless of the risk, and in the desire to perform glorious deeds, each man "nobly took upon himself death for the sake of glory".[20]

The vocabulary used by Diodorus in passages describing death in battle is extremely standardised, repeating almost the same phrases and words. The expressions used obviously stress the heroic and noble character of death in battle, especially the recurrent terms *andragathia, andreia*, glory, 'nobly', 'heroically', etc.

The same motif of glorious death in battle also appears repeatedly in Plutarch's works as well as, compared to it, the shamefulness of fleeing the enemy, combined with praise for the disregard of danger for the sake of glory. The most famous example is presumably the anecdote about the Spartan mother who hands her son his shield telling him to come back "with it or on it".[21] (As mentioned in Ch. 7, the loss of a hoplite' s shield was

---

[11] Which apears to have been one of the most persistently popular stories throughout antiquity.
[12] ἡρωικῶς ἐτελεύτησεν (XV.79.2).
[13] ἡρωικῶς δ' ὑπὲρ τῆς νίκης ἀγωνισάμενος καιρίαν ἔλαβε πληγὴν εἰς τὸν θώρακα (XV.87.1).
[14] σπεύδων διὰ τῆς ἰδίας ἀνδρείας κρῖναι τὴν μάχην.
[15] τὸ ζῆν ἡρωικῶς προιέμενος.
[16] εὐγενῶς ἀποθνήσκειν ἔσπευδον.
[17] ἀφειδῶς τὰ σώματα τοῖς κινδύνοις παραριπτόντων (ib. 2-3).
[18] οὐδεμίαν φειδὼ ποιούμενοι τοῦ ζῆν (XV.86.2).
[19] τὰς ἐν τοῖς κινδύνοις ἀνδραγαθίας ἐπεδείξαντο (ib. 1).
[20] εὐγενῶς ἀνεδέχετο τὸν ὑπὲρ τῆς δόξης θάνατον.
[21] ἢ τὰν ἢ ἐπὶ τᾶς (*Mor.* 241F).

a code for ignominious flight.) In a story with a similar moral, a Spartan soldier claims that he will be of use in the phalanx despite his crippled leg, because "one must fight the opponents staying in place and not fleeing".[22] As usual, the only viable alternatives are victory or death.

The conviction that death in battle is a better death than dying of illness is exemplified by the story of Antigonos, who is dying from consumption. Rather than staying behind because of his illness, he decides to go into battle with the idea of "dying a more glorious death".[23] The concept is not explained in any way and the author obviously expects it to be familiar to the audience.

The worthiness of death in battle is also illustrated in Plutarch's passage about the centurion C. Crastinus, who rushes to the attack (and his death) shouting: "We will win gloriously, Caesar. You will praise me today, whether I be alive or dead".[24] Again the idea expressed here is that victory or glorious death are the only possible outcomes of a battle which make a man praiseworthy. There is no further point to this story, so we can assume that for the audience the interest lay in the centurion's deliberate choice of glory, even if it involved his own death. The fact that the story is told for the sake of this sole motif illustrates how popular this topos was.

The theme is particularly explicit in some passages in Qu. Smyrnaeus' *Fall of Troy* - as one would expect from a poet attempting to emulate Homer. It is most clearly expressed in Neoptolemos' exhortation to the Greeks: "But, come, take courage, for it is far better to die in war than to choose cowardly flight!"[25]
As could be expected, the idea of beautiful death in battle is present also in Virgil's *Aeneid*, where there is no doubt about the poet's heroising intentions. To cite but one example, Nisus, seeing his companion Euryalus taken captive by the Rutuli, ponders whether he should (as he finally will) risk certain death by attacking the captors: "... whether he should throw himself in the midst of the foes to die, and hasten a beautiful death through wounds".[26]

---

[22] ἀλλ' οὐ φεύγοντα, εἶπε, μένοντα δὲ δεῖ τοῖς ἀντιτεταγμένοις μάχεσθαι (*Mor.* 217).
[23] ὅσον ... εὐκλεέστερον ἀποθανεῖν (Plu., *Agis and Cleomenes*, XXX.1-2).
[24] νικήσομεν λαμπρῶς, ὦ Καῖσαρ. ἐμὲ δ' ἢ ζῶντα τήμερον ἢ τεθνηκότα ἐπαινέσεις (*Caesar*, 44.10).
[25] ἀλλ' ἄγε θέσθ' ἔνι θυμόν, ἐπεὶ πολὺ λώιόν ἐστι / τεθνάμεν ἐν πολέμῳ ἢ ἀνάλκιδα φύζαν ἑλέσθαι (XI.219f.).
[26] ... *an sese medios moriturus in hostis / inferat et pulchram properet per vulnera mortem* (IX.400f.).

The topos of heroic death is equally popular in Roman prose, and again I have had to choose only a few representative examples out of many. Thus, e.g., Florus uses the motif of beautiful death, limiting it, however, to death for the right cause (as I pointed out for earlier Greek material in Ch. 7): "Catilina was found far from his own men amidst the bodies of his enemies - a most beautiful death, if he had fallen thus for his country."[27]

In Cornelius Nepos' description of the death of Epaminondas the author stresses the already familiar notion that victory has to be valued beyond one's life. The words of Epaminondas, who is mortally wounded while fighting "most courageously" (*fortissime*), upon hearing the report of the Theban victory are: "I have lived long enough, for I die undefeated".[28]

In his discussion of fortitude in withstanding pain, in the *Tusculan Disputations*, Cicero refers to the same story, stating that for Epaminondas the renown gained by his victory was a sufficient compensation for the loss of his life. Two sentences earlier he makes a more explicit claim about the Decii, for whom "the excellence of their death and the glory alleviated all fear of wounds".[29] Thus even in a philosophical discourse we find the concept of honourable death, used as a given fact that needs no justification. Cicero seems to expect his audience to share these values without proffering further arguments to support them.

Not surprisingly, given the subject matter, examples can be found in Silius Italicus' *Punica*,[30] which by its nature is rich in popular topoi regarding battles and wounds, as well as in Statius' *Silvae*, which contains several passages in which the image of the wound is used as a metaphor for grief. Thus at II.IV.19-21 the poet depicts the image of the mortally wounded soldier advancing towards the enemy, obviously with the intention to die fighting: "... as when a dying soldier, aware of his deep wound, advances against the enemy".[31] In prose again, in two passages Tacitus[32] speaks of soldiers who have died facing the enemy rather than retreating.

Even these few examples show just how popular this particular topos was in both Greek and Roman literature, in prose as well as

---

[27] *Catilina longe a suis inter hostium cadavera repertus est, pulcherrima morte, si pro patria sic concidisset* (II.12.12).

[28] *'satis' inquit 'vixi: invictus enim morior'* (*Epam.* 9.2-4).

[29] *his levabat omnem vulnerum metum nobilitas mortis et gloria* (II.XXIV.59).

[30] E.g., "I saw the courage and death of the men and the vehement desire for glory." (*vidi animos mortesque virum decorisque furorem*; II.324).

[31] ... *sicut sibi conscius alti vulneris adversum moriens it miles in hostem.*

[32] *Hist.* III.LXXXIV and *Ann.* III.XX.

in poetry. Different passages stress different aspects of it, such as the glory of death in battle, the shame involved in running away, or the deliberate choice of death before dishonour, but the basic concept remains the same. As it is a very general topos, very little attention is paid to details which suggest the reality of being wounded in battle, such as pain or blood, but these aspects appear in other, more specific topoi.

It is also worth noting that the idea is never defended, and our authors apparently do not expect their audience to question the fact that death in battle *is* glorious. It is also important to realise, however, that some authors do not use the topos, although they are writing about wars and battles. (Thus, e.g., Procopius does not refer to the glory associated with death or wounds in battle, despite the fact that his work contains many passages about wounds or death.) Still, none of them overtly refutes the idea, and it appears to be more a case of not verbalising it in order to stress other points of interest or dramatic effects.

The second topos which appears in literature almost as frequently as the aforementioned is that of wounds in front being honourable wounds[33] and, because of this, the showing of one's scars to others, regarding them as a badge of honour. As with all the other topoi, it is not possible to examine all its occurrences in all Greek and Roman authors, and some typical examples will have to suffice. One of them is to be found in the description of the fighting prowess of Brasidas against the Athenians in Laconia, in 425 BC. Among several others of the motifs listed earlier on, the author also mentions that Brasidas sustained many wounds in front.[34] The word ἐναντίοις ('opposed', hence 'in front') is obviously a crucial detail in the narrative, since the objective of the story is to depict Brasidas' heroism as a warrior.

In the previous chapter I have already mentioned that Plutarch uses the motif of Alexander showing the scars of his wounds as "images ... of his virtue and courage",[35] and the same topos is used in some of his other works. Thus, for instance, in *M. Cato* we read that, even "when he was still a youth, his body was covered with [scars of] wounds in front".[36]

In the *Sertorius* we can again find the same attitude of regarding the scars of battle wounds as the visible signs of courage: Sertorius (who has lost one of his eyes in battle) claims that, while

---

[33] Familiar from the *Iliad*.
[34] πολλοῖς περιέπιπτεν ἐναντίοις τραύμασι (XII.62.3).
[35] εἰκόνας ... ἀρετῆς καὶ ἀνδραγαθίας (*Fort. Al.* 331C).
[36] ἔτι μειράκιον ὢν τραυμάτων τὸ σῶμα μεστὸν ἐναντίων εἶχε (I.5-6).

others have to take off their wreaths or other decorations received for gallantry, "the tokens of his valour are always present".[37] Thus, not only does Sertorius himself consider his wounds as such, but he also expects everybody else to see them that way. (This is more surprising in his case than in Alexander's, since the loss of an eye by a sword-cut would certainly entail some disfigurement.[38])

The shamefulness of being struck in the back is an essential element in the anecdote about the warrior, who has fallen on his face during a battle, and asks the enemy about to strike him to wait,[39] so that his lover will not find him wounded in the back.[40] This shows that the circumstances under which a man is hit in the back do not matter, since the warrior in question is not turning his back to run away. What matters is the fact that he is wounded in the back, which would be seen as a mark of cowardice. I have suggested earlier that wounds may have been regarded as proof of valour because there was no other way to check in a battle. The same line of thought may be valid here: if none of his fellow warriors had seen the man die and he was found dead with a wound in his back, he would automatically be considered a runaway coward.

An alleged custom for candidates for the consulship to go to the Forum wearing their toga but no tunic - for the purpose of showing their battle scars - is mentioned by Plutarch (*Coriol.* XIV.1-2). This custom may or may not have existed, but one can certainly say that the motif of displaying one's scars as a proof of courage is a popular one in Roman literature as well. It can be found, for example, in Livy: "... he bared his chest, distinguished by the scars he had received in war";[41] or in another passage: "... 'My body is distinguished by honourable scars, all received on the front of the body.' It is said that then he bared himself and related where and in which war he had sustained the wounds."[42]

In Quintilian, the defendant in a court case tears his garment and shows "the scars [of the wounds] which he sustained, on the front of his chest, for his country".[43] This corresponds exactly to

---

[37] αὐτῷ δὲ τῆς ἀνδραγαθίας παραμένειν τὰ γνωρίσματα (IV.2).

[38] Cf. Ch. 2.2.1.9: Tacitus (*Hist.* IV.XIII) and Aulus Gellius (II 27) call Sertorius' wound a 'blemish'.

[39] Presumably to give him time to turn over.

[40] Plu., *Mor.* 761C.

[41] *nudasse pectus insigne cicatricibus bello acceptis* (VI.XX.9).

[42] "... *insigne corpus honestis cicatricibus, omnibus adverso corpore exceptis, habeo.*" *Nudasse deinde se dicitur et, quo quaeque bello volnera accepta essent, rettulisse.* (XLV.XXXIX.16f.)

[43] ... *cicatrices, quas is pro patria pectore adverso suscepisset, ostendit* (II.XV.7).

what is said in Petronius' *Satyricon* of the *declamatores*, who shout: "These wounds I received for the common freedom".[44] As with the dishonourable back wound, it is the visual evidence that counts. What is required is the sight of the scars in the right places.

It is an important detail that almost all our material describing the showing of scars as a proof of courage is Roman. We can even find this custom ridiculed in comedy, where it is obviously presented as a typical habit of the vainglorious soldier. Thus in Terence's *Eunuchus*, the young Phaedria is compared favourably with the soldier Thraso: "... he neither tells about battles nor shows his scars".[45]

Although this hypothesis cannot be proved, I believe that the preponderance of Roman examples may well be related to the greater importance attributed to physical beauty and perfection in Greek culture by comparison with Rome. The pride in one's scars, even if they were disfiguring, figures well with the idea of Roman hardiness, which is often stressed by Roman authors in comparing their countrymen to the 'effeminate' Greeks.

Another topos which appears often in Greek and Roman literature is that of warriors not feeling their wounds, or continuing to fight while their wounds are still fresh. There is a realistic element in this motif in that the adrenalin in the bloodstream while the fighting was continued, as well as shock, may often have delayed the onset of pain. However, in literature this motif is certainly pushed beyond the point of realism in order to stress how for a brave man the thought of victory is more prominent on his mind than his own safety. This is also a topos which is already familiar both from the *Iliad* and from the material about Alexander.

Examples for this motif occur, for example, in Diodorus Siculus: "Some fought on, not feeling their wounds, as they were still warm."[46] Dio's remark at XLVII.44.3 that the pain of the wounds was forestalled by death appears to be based on a similar idea, and Statius uses the same motif in the *Thebaid*, when he speaks of a warrior whose thigh has been pierced by a spear: "... but he had not noticed it in his ardour, or he did not know it at the time ...".[47] The heroic aspect of this motif is definitely stressed in Cicero's statement that "brave men do not feel wounds in the

---

[44] *haec vulnera pro libertate publica excepi* (I.1f.).
[45] ... *neque pugnas narrat neque cicatrices suas ostendat* (482f.).
[46] τίνες δ' οὐκ αἰσθανόμενοι θερμῶν ἔτι τῶν πληγῶν οὐσῶν διηγωνίζοντο (XIII.79.3). Cf. also XVIII.31.5.
[47] ... *sed dissimulaverat ardens, sive ibi nescierat* (IX.203f.).

battle-line",⁴⁸ or - he elucidates - they do feel them, but prefer to die rather than retreat, because of the impulse of our souls towards true honour.

The weakness, or even fainting, caused by loss of blood - another basically realistic trait - is also used by authors. We have seen this motif used by various authors on the occasion of some of Alexander's wounds, and its popularity continues in post-Alexandrian material.

One of many examples for the use of this topos is to be found in Diodorus - again the aforementioned story of Brasidas fighting the Athenians on the coast of Laconia. Brasidas, who has sustained many wounds on the front of his body, finally faints from the loss of blood.⁴⁹ Although this is a very likely thing to happen, especially with multiple injuries, one could still see this description as more than just a realistic account. By telling the audience that a warrior is forced to stop fighting through the weakness caused by haemorrhage, the author implicitly highlights the severity of the wounds and the warrior's fortitude in supporting them so far.

The motif also appears, among others, in Dionysius of Halicarnassus (II.42.5), in connection with fatal wounds in the *Aeneid*,⁵⁰ and in Livy, e.g. XXX.XVIII.13, where Mago is carried from the battle, wounded and drained of blood.⁵¹

Defending the dead or wounded, often by protecting them with one's own shield, is another well-known Homeric topos, also used in the Alexander material,⁵² and it is present in later material as well. The readiness to give this kind of protection is one of the traditional virtues of the hero - as we have already seen in the *Iliad* - and it is important that defending a wounded man and defending a dead body rank equally high as a service given to another warrior.⁵³

We find instances of this topos for example in Diodorus, when the Messenian Kleonnis covers the king with his shield,⁵⁴ in Plutarch's *Alcibiades* VII.3 (Alcibiades saved by Socrates) and

---

⁴⁸ *non sentiunt viri fortes in acie vulnera* (*Tusc. Disp.* II.XXIV.58).

⁴⁹ ... διὰ τῶν τραυμάτων αἵματος ἐκχυθέντος πολλοῦ, καὶ διὰ τοῦτο λιποψυχήσαντος αὐτοῦ ... (XII.61.4).

⁵⁰ E.g. XI.818: "... he sank down, deprived of blood" (*labitur exsanguis*).

⁵¹ *postquam femine transfixo cadentem auferrique ex proelio prope exsanguem videre*.

⁵² The bodyguards covering Alexander's body when he was wounded in the Mallian stronghold (cf. Ch. 8).

⁵³ Cf. the injunction in the fourth-century BC oath, supposedly sworn by the Athenians before the battle of Plataea, not to leave the commander behind, be he alive or dead. (οὐκ ἀπολείψω τὸν ταξίλοχον οὐδὲ τὸν ἐνωμοτάρχην οὔτε ζῶντα οὔτε ἀποθανόντα, quoted in L. Robert [1938], p. 302.)

⁵⁴ ὑπερασπίσας τὸν βασιλέα πεπτωκότα (VIII.12).

Pelopidas IV.5-6, where Epaminondas bestrides the body of the grievously wounded Pelopidas.[55] In Lucian's *Anacharsis* (28), the Athenian claims that wrestling is a useful skill in war, because it enables a man to pick up and salvage a wounded friend.[56]

While Nonnos (XXX.54f.) uses the original Homeric version of the topos - a warrior bestriding another's body - Procopius (*Goth.* VI.XXVII.14f.) gives a different twist to the story. In an action reminiscent of Athena warding off the arrow aimed at Menelaos in the *Iliad* (IV.129ff.), a soldier saves the general Belisarius' life by thrusting his own hand in the way of the arrow. (This story is very much in the style of others reported by Procopius, which appear to be chosen for a common element of bizarre and unheard-of happenings rather than for aspects usually associated with scenes of wounding.)

The topos is equally popular in Roman literature, e.g. in Silius Italicus, IV.466ff. (Scipio saving his father), or V.348-51 (Hannibal saving his brother), and in Valerius Maximus, who writes of a certain L. Siccius Dentatus, who, among other exploits, had "saved fourteen citizens from certain death" in battle.[57]

Three other traditional topoi are linked to the use of long-range weapons, namely the enemies using missiles, not daring to close in on the hero, the cowardice or inferiority of the archer, and the motif of the wounded warrior pulling out a spear or arrow which has struck him and using it to strike an enemy. The first and second are familiar from the *Iliad* and also appear in the stories about Alexander, whereas the third appears to reflect a taste for the sensational and the gruesome, visible in particular in Roman material, e.g. Silius Italicus and Statius and especially Lucan.

The motif of the enemies not daring to approach appears, for instance, in the Diodorus passage about Brasidas (already quoted for other topoi), in the description of the death of the Goth leader Teias in Procopius (*Goth.* VIII.XXXV.24-30), in Virgil, *Aen.* X.715f., Silius Italicus V.442ff., or Valerius Maximus III.II.23. It is also implicitly present in the many cases in which the hero is wounded by a spear or an arrow rather than by a hand-held weapon, such as is the case with Epaminondas or Aeneas.

The contempt for the archer is best expressed in the passage in Plutarch's *Sayings of Spartans* (*Mor.* 234), in which the Spartan dying from an arrow wound regrets not the loss of his life, but that

---

[55] ὑπὲρ τοῦ σώματος καὶ τῶν ὅπλων ἔστη.
[56] ... εἰς τοὺς πολέμους καὶ χρήσιμα, εἰ δέοι φίλον τρωθέντα ῥᾳδίως ἀράμενον ὑπεξενεγκεῖν.
[57] *XIV cives ex media morte raptos servasse* (III.II.24).

he is killed "by a womanish archer".[58] As one would expect, this topos can also be found in Qu. Smyrnaeus (III.443-5), whose *Fall of Troy* follows Homeric patterns very closely.

The references to care for the wounded after the battle and to medical specialists have already been discussed in the chapter dealing with medical treatment in armies and some of this material, too, may well be based on realistic observations, but one has to keep in mind that these motifs form literary topoi as well. The motif of the leader of an army visiting casualties[59] is also situated in this context. This topos is not Homeric in origin and it may well have originated from the material describing Alexander visiting the wounded.

Washing the wound with water is also a motif which appears often in literature, e.g. *Aen.* IV.683f., ib.X.833f., ib.XII.420; Silius Italicus V.368, ib. VI.91; Statius, *Theb.* III.398. Although this, too, is a realistic detail as part of the treatment, it appears as a *pars-pro-toto* stylised representative wound treatment. This topos as well had Homeric connotations, since it would certainly conjure up images of Patroklos washing Eurypylos' wound with "tepid water" (XI.845f.).

As for another important topos, we have already seen examples of what one could call the physician's *aristeia*, namely Machaon's treatment of Menelaos' wound (*Il.* IV.208-19), Alexander's doctor Philippos administering a drug to cure Alexander's illness in Cilicia,[60] and Critobulus saving Alexander's life, in Q. Curtius' account (IX.V.22-30). One could also count Herodotus' story about Democedes treating the Persian king (III.129-30) under this category - despite Democedes' reluctance to play the part.

A passage in Appian's *Mithridatic War* (89) clearly shows the popularity and influence of the Alexander-material. The doctor Timotheos - mentioned by name for his achievement of finally stopping the bleeding from Mithridates' wound - lifts up his patient (*sic!*) in order to disperse the soldiers' fears, and the author compares the scene to the concern about Alexander's wound sustained at the Mallian stronghold. The passage has the characteristics of the *aristeia*, namely the mention of the protagonist by name and the associated difficulties which only he manages to master.

---

[58] ὑπὸ γύννιδος τοξότου.
[59] E.g. Plu., *Ant.* XLIII.1; Livy VIII.XXXVI.6f.; Lucan VII.566f.
[60] D.S. XVII.31.4-6; Justin XI.8; Plu., *Alex.* XIX.1-10; Arr. II.4.7-11; Q.C. III.V.1-VI.17.

Another such scene can be found (combined with an element of sensationalism) in Procopius:[61] Arzes, one of the bodyguards of Belisarius, is struck by an arrow between the nose and the right eye, and none of the unnamed *iatroi* dare treat his wound for fear of the consequences, Arzes being one of Belisarius' best men. In most of the cases this is an essential detail: the patient has to be the king, the leader, or at least somebody close to him. This sets the premises that the physician is taking a considerable risk by taking the treatment in hand, thus giving the story the desired touch of suspense. In the Procopius passage it is the physician Theoktistos (a Greek, to judge by his name) who decides to make a very unusual intervention by extracting the arrow from the back of the man's neck, as it has penetrated almost to the point of breaking the skin there.[62] The most essential element for this motif is - needless to say - the success of the treatment; we are not given detailed accounts of failures.

The association of prowess and daring with medical treatment occasionally appears in medical texts as well. Thus, in *Anat. Admin.*, Galen describes (as he frequently does) a successful treatment performed by himself: "No one dared excise the diseased bone [sc. the sternum] ... but I said I would cut it out."[63] In a similar vein he compares doctors with athletes in *De optimo medico* [*Opt. Med.*].[64] There appears to have been a trend in literature to depict the physician undertaking a risky treatment in a way faintly reminiscent of Homeric heroes.

As far as the casualty himself is concerned, the wounded warrior's courage and endurance are crucial elements in most descriptions, and this fact finds its reflection in a variety of topoi. One of them is the contrast between the raw recruit and the battle-hardened veteran.

The argument is that the recruit cannot yet bear the pain of wounds, whereas the veteran will show manful restraint. This topos not only stresses the importance of fortitude, but also reflects the belief that fortitude is a quality which can be acquired by training. Cicero and Seneca express this idea with particular clarity. Thus in *Tusc. Disp.* (II.XVI.38) Cicero claims that "habit teaches [men] to despise wounds".[65] One often sees wounded men carried out of the battle-line, he continues, "and some raw and untrained soldier

---

[61] *Goth.* VI.16-29. This passage has been mentioned in Ch. 2.2.1.9.
[62] In fact, a *diôsmos*, which is normally only used in leg and arm wounds.
[63] οὐδεὶς δ' ἐκκόπτειν ἐτόλμα τὸ πεπονθὸς ὀστοῦν· ... ἐγὼ δ' ἐκκόψειν μὲν ἔφην (II.632f. K).
[64] I.54-6 K, *passim*.
[65] *comtemnere vulnus consuetudo docet.*

will utter most disgraceful wails although only slightly wounded, whereas the trained, older, man (who is more brave for this very reason) only asks for a doctor to dress his wound".[66]

The same idea is expressed in Seneca's *Ad Helviam matrem de consolatione*, where the battle wound is used as a metaphor for his mother's grief:

> But, as slightly wounded recruits nevertheless scream and fear the doctors' hands more than the steel [i.e. the weapon], and veterans, although pierced through, suffer the treatment patiently and without a groan, as if it was another's body, thus you must now submit yourself bravely to the cure (3.1).[67]

These two passages give one a general idea of the prevailing attitude towards courage and the contempt for those who lack it. The aspect of courage and endurance was certainly the main attraction of stories such as that of Mucius Scaevola and that of Agesilaos, its Greek counterpart.[68] This aspect would appear to be the only reason for telling the story of Marius having his varicose veins operated without being bound,[69] as it is hardly an event of any historical importance.

The fortitude displayed by the hero also appears to be the point Virgil wants to make by adding the detail that Aeneas is standing, leaning on his spear, while the physician Iapex is attempting to extract the arrow from his thigh[70] - hardly a likely position for having a leg wound treated in real life. The same aspect is important in Aeneas' behaviour several lines before this passage, when he first (XII.387f.) tries to pull out the arrow himself (which turns out to be impossible because, as in the case of Eurypylos in the *Iliad*, the shaft has broken), and then (ib. 389f.) asks his companions to enlarge the wounds with a sword[71] and remove the arrow so that he can return to the battle. Like the Homeric heroes and, even more so Alexander, Aeneas is represented as undaunted

---

[66] *Quin etiam videmus ex acie efferri saepe saucios et quidem rudem illum et inexercitatum quamvis levi ictu ploratus turpissimos edere; at vero ille exercitatus et vetus ob eamque rem fortior, medicum modo requirens a quo obligetur.*

[67] *Sed quemadmodum tirones leviter saucii tamen vociferantur et manus medicorum magis quam ferrum horrent, at veterani, quamvis confossi, patienter ac sine gemitu velut aliena corpora exsaniari patiuntur: ita tu nunc debes fortiter praebere te curationi.*

[68] Plu., *Mor.* 306A; Val.Max. III.III.1; Plu., *Mor.* 305D-E.

[69] Plu., *Marius* VI.3; Cicero, *Tusc. Disp.* II.XXII.53.

[70] "He stood, ... leaning on his large spear" (*stabat ... ingentem nixus in hastam*; *Aen.*, XII.398). See Fig. 4.

[71] As Alexander does in Arrian's version of the Mallian incident (*An.* VI.XI.1).

by the pain of his wound and - again very much like Alexander - as unmoved amidst his distraught entourage.[72]

These stories reflect a certain fascination with fortitude in pain, another motif, which is also evident in Q. Curtius' account (discussed in Ch. 8) of Alexander refusing to be held down during the extraction of the Mallian arrow (IX.V.27-8). The vocabulary used also highlights this factor, as the accounts usually contain the topos of the man in question bearing the pain "without a movement" or "without a groan". Thus for example Plutarch says of Marius that he "neither moved nor groaned",[73] and he uses similar expressions for Scaevola and Agesilaos. Cicero, in the aforementioned passage, speaks of the disgraceful lamentations uttered by the recruit and postulates (equally in *Tusc. Disp.* II) that a man should not even groan with pain, let alone scream. As an example he cites Epaminondas, again in a way that makes it obvious that he expected his audience to know the story: "Do you think that Epaminondas groaned when he felt his life flow out together with his blood?"[74] In the passage quoted above, Seneca also uses the expression "without groaning" (*sine gemitu*), and according to Curtius, Alexander remains "motionless" (*sine motu*) while the arrow is cut out.

As we have seen, courage and fortitude, whether implicit or explicit, are essential components of accounts of fighting, wounding or wound treatment, and many of the literary topoi are related to these aspects. I have only discussed the major topoi here, but there are many more, which appear in various descriptions of wars and battles, such as, e.g., the ground covered with dead bodies, the effects of the sight of blood, or the re-opening of a wound (which has been dressed) as a means of suicide.

Two more aspects of the use of literary topoi have to be mentioned in this context. One is the fact that some of them show great medical exactness and detail, more than would actually be necessary for the literary appreciation of the respective passages. This is true in particular for some passages in Ovid's *Metamorphoses* as well as the *Remedia Amoris* (describing both actual wounds and wounds as a metaphor), and also for Nonnos' *Dionysiaca*. Thus at *Met.* IV.119-24, Ovid depicts the suicide of Pyramus, comparing the blood splashing from his wound to water

---

[72] *magno iuvenum et maerentis Iuli concursu, / lacrimis immobilis* (XII.399f.)

[73] οὐδὲν κινηθεὶς οὐδὲ στενάξας (*Marius* VI.3).

[74] *num ingemuisse Epaminondam putas, cum una cum sanguine vitam effluere sentiret?* (II.59).

spurting from a cracked water pipe, and Ovid's other works contain many passages using wounds as a metaphor for grief, e.g. *Rem. Am.* 101f.: "I saw a wound that had at first been curable take harm of the long delay by being deferred."[75] *Rem. Am.* 131f. in particular is an example of a detailed medical simile: "Medicine is more or less the art of time: wine given at the right time is beneficial and given at an unsuitable time it is harmful."[76] In Nonnos' *Dionysiaca*, the passage describing the excision of infected flesh around a wound (XVII.367ff.)[77] in particular gives an impression of greater medical detail than one would expect in a work of literature.

The first part of the treatment of Aeneas' arrow wound (before the divine intervention) should also be mentioned in this context. It is the only passage in Roman poetry describing the (attempted) extraction of an arrow by an expert, obviously following Homeric examples. Although, as we have seen, the passage shows strong elements of heroisation, it also contains some very realistic details. Thus the idea that the wound needs to be enlarged by cutting and, in particular, the detail of Iapex using a forceps ("he grasped the iron with a sturdy forceps"[78]), show that the poet had at least some knowledge of how wounds were treated in real life. Another realistic element is presumably intended as a clever variation on the wound treatment theme in order to build up the tension to the divine assistance: this is the only passage in non-medical literature in which a surgeon attempts to extract an arrow and fails.

One is tempted to see the poets' personal interest and knowledge reflected in these scenes, rather than a mere repetition of stock themes. It may, however, also be a desire to appear knowledgeable as a trend of fashion, since one can find more learned references in Hellenistic poetry (e.g. Callimachus) than in earlier works. As far as Plutarch is concerned, one could say that some of his descriptions are on the borderline between medical and non-medical literature, and we can assume that his medical knowledge went beyond that of the educated layman. (The topic

---

[75] *vidi ego, quod primo fuerat sanabile, vulnus / dilatum longae damnae tulisse morae.*

[76] *temporis ars medicina fere est: data tempore prosunt / et data non apto tempore vina nocent.*

[77] "He approached his hand to another, and cut the putrid edges of a wound smitten by a poisoned arrow with the knife, applying his fingers lightly, with [only] the very edge of the palm." (ἄλλῳ χεῖρα πέλασσε, καὶ ἕλκεος ἄκρα χαράξας / ἰῷ φαρμακόεντι σεσηπότα τάμνη μαχαίρῃ, / ἀκροτάτῃ παλάμῃ πεφιδημένα δάκτυλα βάλλων.)

[78] *prensatque tenaci forcipe ferrum* (XII.404).

of medical knowledge among laymen has been discussed in Ch.5.1.)

Another interesting aspect is the increasing gruesomeness of wounds described, in particular in some later Roman authors. This is especially true of Lucan and his epic poem, the *Pharsalia*, which abounds in scenes of the most striking goriness, e.g.:

> At the same time, his back and his chest are pierced by weapons thrown with equal strength; the iron [points] meet in the chest. And the blood stops, uncertain from which wound to flow, until a strong bleeding pushes out both spears at the same time, divides the soul and sheds death through the wounds. (III.587-91) [79]

Or, to cite another example, "a high flame lights his hair and cheeks; the fire hisses in his burning eyes".[80] The second example comes from what one could call the *aristeia* of the centurion Scaeva, which takes the topos of the warrior fighting on despite his wounds almost to the point of parody (Scaeva continues to fight with countless javelins and arrows stuck in his body). Again, in book IX, in the account of the army's march through the desert, Lucan describes in lurid detail the deaths of several soldiers from the bites of poisonous snakes such as (762-86) the *seps*, the bite of which makes the body dissolve instantaneously.

This gruesomeness and sensationalism, characteristic of Silver Latin, may stem from a desire to develop the standard topoi in an individual and original way, but also from a wish to outdo other poets and, in particular, to outdo Homer and Virgil. It is curious that this change in style coincides with the trend (mentioned in Ch. 3) towards polypharmacy and towards more and more elaborate and exotic remedies. One wonders therefore whether there is any relation between these two facts and whether external factors, such as the expansion of the empire, contributed to a certain baroqueness in attitude.

As has been said earlier, Nonnos is difficult to compare with the other authors, as he does not appear to use the same standards of heroic description. The wounds he describes have little or no heroic connotations, as the casualties are mainly female Bacchants. The wounding and treatment of the boy Hymenaeus are described in some detail, but again the setting is far from heroic (e.g., the boy looking up at Dionysus with tears in his eyes). It would

---

[79] *Terga simul pariter missis et pectora telis / transigitur: medio concurrit pectore ferrum. / Et stetit incertus, flueret quo volnere, sanguis, / donec ultrasque simul largus cruor expulit hastas / divisitque animam sparsitque in volnera letum.*

[80] *... alterius flamma crinesque genasque succendit: / strident oculis ardentibus ignes* (VI.178f.).

appear that Nonnos took a certain pleasure in inverting the heroic code for his poem and to create something like an antithesis to the *Iliad*.

Another factor which one can observe in the post-Alexandrian material is an increased interest in 'biography', containing more details on the protagonist's life (hence also his wounds?), and, in connection with this, a more pronounced representation of individual, rather than collective, heroism. Thus, for example, Hyperides' *Epitaphios*[81] begins with praise for the commander, mentioning him by name, a detail hitherto unheard of: "I shall begin first from the general, for that is just".[82] It may well be that the way in which the earlier - non-extant - sources depicted Alexander as a heroic leader contributed to a shift in focus and a more pronounced interest in the individual. We therefore appear to be faced with the paradox of authors writing more about the individual, but doing so in a series of set topoi and motifs.

In this section I hope to have given an idea of the material about wounds and heroism in the extant sources of the centuries after Alexander the Great. I believe that we can see the authors using a large set of topoi, prefabricated elements, so to speak, from which to build up their stories, and therefore even apparently realistic scenes should probably not be taken for such. Many of those elements can be traced back as far as the *Iliad*, but several are clearly influenced by the way in which Alexander was presented in literature, since he appears to have been the most influential and emulated hero figure in ancient literature. While there was obviously a large number of topoi to choose from for whatever purpose an author wanted to achieve, the choice and variation were left to the author, and this was where the author had the scope for stressing certain aspects of the story according to the effect he wanted to achieve. Thus despite the wide-spread use of topoi as building blocks for a story, there was still enough space for whatever individual twist an author chose to give to the material.

---

[81] Mentioned in Ch. 7.
[82] ἄρξομαι δὲ πρῶτον ἀπὸ τοῦ στρατηγοῦ· καὶ γὰρ δίκαιον.

PART THREE

NON-TEXTUAL MATERIAL

CHAPTER TEN

THE ARCHAEOLOGICAL EVIDENCE

In Parts I and II of this book I have discussed literary material exclusively,[1] but the written evidence is not all we have. In addition to it there is also a fairly large amount of archaeological evidence which can be extremely helpful for some aspects of our research. Although on its own this material would be open to numerous, contrasting, conjectures, it can be used along with the literary evidence and in comparison with it. Often the two groups of evidence will be mutually supportive, but occasionally - as we shall see in the case of surgical instruments - the archaeological material presents a picture which differs from the literary sources, and can be seen to support the claim that much of our medical literature is not the exact representation of an actual reality valid for any given point in time.

As for the nature of the evidence, the material can be divided into five major groups: 1) arms and armour; 2) skeletal remains; 3) architectural remains; 4) surgical instruments; and 5) artistic representation. All five groups would deserve a far more detailed study for purposes other than this, and by scholars who are experts in archaeology. However, for the present purpose I am using these groups as ancillary evidence for the sake of completeness, and Part III will only form a brief chapter. In general, the material tends to be ignored by scholars working on the literary evidence, but I believe that it is too important to be left out of the discussion altogether.

As was the case with the literary material - and perhaps to an even higher degree with this type of evidence - it is of course not possible to be comprehensive within the limits of this monograph (especially since the main argument of it is based on literary evidence). It is only possible to include a very selective discussion of all five groups of material, each in a short section, including some of the most relevant secondary literature in the respective fields.

---

[1] With the exception of the bas-relief from Trajan's Column, mentioned in Ch. 4.2.

1. *Arms and armour*

This group of artefacts is of interest for our topic for obvious reasons. The weapons are the tools by which battle wounds were made, and the armour not only gives us an idea of which parts of the body were protected, but occasionally the finds yield some information on the penetrability of armour by weapons.

Some of the most important contributions in this field are: A. M. Snodgrass, *Early Greek Armour and Weapons* (1964); id., *Arms and Armour of the Greeks* (1967); and P. Conolly, *Greece and Rome at War* (1988), which also contains much information on ancient tactics. P. H. Blyth's unpublished thesis, *Effectiveness of Greek Armour against Arrows in the Persian War (490-479 BC)* (1977), and the short article by D. Massey, 'Roman archery tested' (1994), are particularly relevant for the topic of war wounds as they examine the resistance of respectively Greek and Roman armour against arrows. Massey in particular provides fascinating insights into the practicalities of ancient warfare by employing practical experiments and actually shooting reconstructions of Roman and native British arrows at replicas of Roman armour. A. Hagemann's *Griechische Panzerung* (1919), long since out of print, is still an excellent source of information, especially for its frequent cross-references to literature.

One can deduce from the textual material that armour limited the vulnerable areas to some extent in hand-to-hand fighting and against missiles at a long range. It would seem that armour was not spear-proof and Blyth[2] suggests that the corselet was "designed primarily to resist a slashing blow, or as a second line of defence", and it certainly did not protect its wearer against javelins or arrows released at short range. There is no lack of literary evidence for armour being pierced on such occasions, e.g. in the case of Epaminondas (D.S. XV.87.1) or Alexander (Arr. II.26.2f; ib. IV.23.3; Qu. Curtius IV.VI.17f.; ib. IX.V.9 and Plu., *Alex.* LXIII.5). These descriptions, as well as those of a sword-cut splitting a helmet, could be dismissed as poetic exaggeration were it not for the archaeological evidence. Although the cause of damage is often difficult to ascertain, in several cases it can be said with some degree of certainty to be battle damage, such as a gash in a Corinthian helmet in the British Museum.[3] Blyth[4] records

---

[2] (1977), p. 194.
[3] 2819/1860.10-12.1.
[4] (1977) pp. 81ff.

battle damage, though in most cases not resulting in perforation, to forty-six pieces of armour examined by him in Olympia.

Massey (1994) describes the effect of various types of arrowheads, socketed as well as tanged, on three types of armour, namely ring mail (*lorica hamata*), scale armour (*lorica squamata*) and strip plate armour (*lorica segmentata*, worn by legionaries from the first century AD onwards). Not surprisingly, the *lorica hamata* proved to be the easiest to penetrate, followed by the *lorica squamata* and finally the *lorica segmentata* , in which none of the arrowheads penetrated to a depth sufficient to cause a fatal wound even at a range of seven metres. The experiments also showed that when an arrow had penetrated ring mail it would sometimes be locked into place by the damaged mail rings, thus making the arrow more difficult to extract.[5] It would also seem[6] that arrows often break upon impact, the breakage tending to occur immediately behind the socket in socketed arrows, tanged arrows being slightly less likely to break. This kind of stress breakage may be what we are meant to see in the case of Eurypylos[7] and Aeneas,[8] as in both cases the arrow appears to have broken.

Hand-held weapons were more or less homogeneous in their effects, except for the influence of fighting techniques - cf. Vegetius' description[9] of the advantages gained by the Roman style of sword-fighting, i.e. thrusting instead of slashing. Different types of arrows, on the other hand, would find their reflection in the size and gravity of the wound. It is clear from our finds that arrowheads came in an astonishing variety of shapes and sizes, the length of those in the British Museum collections varying between 5 and 85 mm. (Cf. Paul's description of the large variety of arrowheads known to him, VI.88.2/II.129.26-130.19.) The small hole in one arrowhead kept at the British Museum may well have held a separate piece of metal like the points described by Paul of Aegina[10] and Dio Cassius,[11] but so far no further evidence has been found either for those or for the hinged arrowheads mentioned by Paul.[12]

---

[5] (1994), p. 37.
[6] Ib., p. 39.
[7] *Il.* XI.584.
[8] *Aen.* XII.387.
[9] I.12, cited in Ch. 2.1.1.
[10] VI.88.2/II.130.13ff.; cf. Ch. 2.2.1.2.
[11] XXXVI.5; cf. ibid.
[12] Loc. cit.

The enormous variety in shapes and sizes of arrowheads again confirms the suspicion that the *kyathiskos*, or 'spoon of Diokles', was an impractical instrument for their extraction, since many of the arrowheads would not have fitted into it. It was presumably far more expedient for the surgeon to use a forceps or his fingers.

2. Skeletal remains

Palaeopathology is a field which had not attracted the attention of archaeologists until fairly recently and therefore only little work has been done on the subject of the traces of battle wounds on skeletons. Furthermore, most of the research that has been done regards periods earlier or later than the one discussed here or different geographical regions (e.g. the Middle East or North America).

However, there are some finds dating from Greek and Roman antiquity, namely the Spartan skeletons found in a grave in the Kerameikos (W. K. Pritchett, *The Greek State at War* [1985], vol.IV, pp.133f.; L. R. Van Hook, *AJA* XXXVI [1932], pp. 290f.); those found in the grave under the stone lion on the battlefield of Chaeronea - supposedly the Theban Sacred Band who died there fighting against Philip of Macedon in 338 BC - (Pritchett, op.cit., pp.136f.; *PAE* [1881], pp.16-20; E. Kastorchis, *Athenaion* 8 [1879], pp.486-91, ib.9 [1880], pp.157f.; L. Phytalis, *Athenaion* 9 [1880], pp.347-52+1 Plate); the skull found in one of the royal tombs at Vergina (A. J. N. W. Prag, 'Reconstructing King Philip II: the "nice" version' [1990]); the skeletons found in the Roman cemetery at Cirencester (A. Mc Whirr, L.Viner, C.Wells, *Romano-British Cemeteries at Cirencester*, 1982) and those found at Maiden Castle (R. M. Wheeler, 'Maiden Castle, Dorset' [1943]),

Van Hook's article[13] shows a photograph of four of the Spartan skeletons found in the Kerameikos: according to him as well as Pritchett,[14] these were the Spartans killed in an engagement near Piraeus in 403 BC.[15] In one of the skeletons a spear-head is clearly visible, still in place within the rib-cage. Judging from its position, the spear could either have pierced the breast-plate[16] or it could have entered downwards from the upper rim of the armour

---

[13] (1932), p. 291.
[14] (1985), p. 133.
[15] Xen., *Hell.* II.4.33.
[16] None of the dead were buried in their armour, but it seems reasonable to assume that they had been wearing it during the fighting.

(the throat being one of the main vulnerable targets on a hoplite), but in either case the thrust would have been nearly instantaneously fatal by either piercing the heart or slashing the aorta or the pulmonary artery. Van Hook[17] also mentions two bronze arrowheads embedded in the right leg of one of the other skeletons, but given the poor quality of the illustration, I have not been able to discern them.[18]

It is curious that neither the spear nor the arrows were removed prior to burial; this suggests that at least these two Spartans died immediately. Since the dead were not buried in haste as it might happen after a lost battle, it may well be that either the shaft was sawn off at skin level or that the point stayed in the wound when the weapon was pulled out. If it was the case that the weapons could not be removed without enlarging the wound, it is possible that it was considered improper to cut into a corpse, as this may have been perceived as mutilation, and that the iron points were left in place for that reason. The other surprising aspect of this find, namely the burial of Athen's enemies in the Kerameikos, the resting-place of Athen's heroic dead, may well represent a conscious show of Spartan power or a deliberate insult.

Documentation is particularly meagre when it comes to the potentially fascinating Chaeronea find, of which not a single photograph has been published. There is only a brief mention in Kastorchis' article[19] of many skeletons bearing the marks of wounds, but he provides no further details. Frustratingly, he refers to a site-report by Stamatakis which, however, does not appear to have been published – nor has the site been excavated since.

The only published Greek find other than the Kerameikos grave, the Vergina skull, is at the same time the most thoroughly documented and the most sensational - if controversial - find. The skull shows a healed fracture of the zygomatic bone, assumed to have been caused by an arrow or a similar missile striking from above. Given that the man was buried in one of the royal tombs and therefore had to be a member of the royal family of Macedon, the skull was identified by A. J. N. W. Prag on the basis of this injury as that of Philip II, the father of Alexander the Great.[20] The fracture would therefore indicate the wound

---

[17] (1932), p. 291.
[18] For the same reason it has not been possible to reproduce the photograph here. (On one of better quality, provided by the Deutsche Archäologische Institut in Athens, the spearhead had been removed.)
[19] (1880), p. 158.
[20] This supports the hypothesis put forward by the archaeologist who had excavated the tombs: see Andronikos (1984). Using the methods of forensic

sustained by Philip at the siege of Methone in 353 BC, where an arrow or ballista bolt, shot from the city walls, hit him, blinding his right eye.[21] (It has to be added, however, that this admittedly tempting hypothesis has not found universal acceptance and is contested by other scholars).

Among the material from Cirencester one can find several skulls bearing traces of wounds as well as the humerus cited in Ch. 2.1.2, n. 14, which bears two cuts on its medial surface.[22] All the wounds appear to be sword wounds.

The excavation of Maiden Castle also brought to light a number of skeletons. Several skulls show obviously fatal sword wounds (without any signs of healing)[23] and another what - judging by its shape - appears to be a hole made by a Roman ballista bolt.[24] Skeleton P7A from the same cemetery[25] has an iron arrowhead lodged in one of its vertebrae. Thus the two British sites have yielded the most illustrative examples for the efficacy of (presumably) Roman weapons, although we do not know what kind of armour, if any, these warriors were wearing. Given the continuity in military equipment throughout antiquity, we can probably assume the same effects for Greek weapons.

Our skeletal material can obviously not give us any clues on lesions to the soft tissues,[26] but it shows that sword-cuts would occasionally reach the bone (e.g. Cirencester, Inh. 21) and that arrows or spears would easily penetrate to, or even into, the bones (e.g. Maiden Castle skeleton P7A). This supports claims made in the texts, both medical and non-medical, about bone injuries, and as far as skeletal finds are concerned the literary and non-literary material are mutually supportive.

3. *Architectural remains*

Another group of archaeological finds should also be mentioned in this chapter, since they, too, contribute to our knowledge of ancient medicine. I am speaking of the remains of buildings,

---

science, Prag and J. Musgrave have also reconstructed Philip's (if that is who he was) features from the skull; see Prag (1990).

[21] Cf. Ch. 2.1.2.
[22] Mc Whirr, Viner and Wells (1982), p. 171.
[23] Wheeler (1943), pl. LIII.A-C.
[24] Ib., pl. LIII.D, skeleton P7.
[25] Ib., pl. LVIII.A.
[26] Mummy finds do provide that kind of information, and if the embalmed body of Alexander the Great should ever be found, we could perhaps verify the scars of all his wounds.

tombs and inscriptions with some kind of medical connection. Those of particular relevance for the topic of this monograph come mainly from a military medical context,[27] namely the remains of *valetudinaria* in Roman army camps and fortresses along the frontiers of the empire as well as the tombs of military doctors or votive inscriptions dedicated by them.

These have been discussed in Chapter 4.2, and *valetudinaria* are mentioned and described in numerous site reports as well as in a general overview in H. v. Petrikovits, *Die Innenbauten römischer Legionslager während der Prinzipatszeit* (1975).[28] M. Th. R. M. Dolmans' excellent discussion of all the available information regarding *valetudinaria*, his PhD thesis *Valetudinaria exercitus. Militaire hospitalen in de oudheid* (1993), is unfortunately as yet unpublished and there appears to be no monograph dealing exclusively with Roman military hospitals.

Occasionally, the excavations of *valetudinaria* have yielded more than merely the remains of buildings. Thus in some cases surgical instruments have come to light (especially the large find of Vindonissa[29]) and, in the case of Novaesium,[30] the charred remains of medicinal herbs, providing an invaluable insight into actual medical practice. The Novaesium find has been examined in detail in K.-H. Knörzer, *Römerzeitliche Pflanzenfunde aus Neuss* (1970), and the finds support the evidence of medical writings. Thus the plants include henbane[31] and centaury,[32] used as an analgesic/soporific and wound remedy respectively.[33]

As said in Chapter 4.2, a catalogue of all known inscriptions relating to the Roman army medical service can be found in J. C. Wilmanns, *Der Sanitätsdienst im Römischen Reich* (1995), and most of them also in the earlier A. v. Domaszewski, *Die Rangordnung des römischen Heeres* (1967).

This group of material differs from others insofar as the archaeological evidence is in fact our main source of information about doctors in the Roman army. Literary testimonies merely mention them, but never explain their rank, recruiting, training, etc. Thus here literature merely supports the archaeological material rather than vice versa.

---

[27] For buildings from a civilian context, cf. Eschebach (1984) about houses in Pompeii possibly inhabited by doctors.
[28] Pp. 98-102. The topic is dealt with also in Wilmanns (1995), pp. 103-16.
[29] See Fig. 5.
[30] Present-day Neuss in Germany.
[31] E.g. Celsus V.27.10/234.8.
[32] E.g. Pliny, *N.H.* XXV.66.
[33] Cf. Ch. 3.

For the Greek world, we have the various inscriptions concerning public doctors. Since inscriptions constitute the interface between different types of material, being both monument and text, I have preferred to treat them as written evidence and discuss them in Chapters 4 and 5. The Epidaurus inscriptions also belong to this group; although they do not come from a military context, they contain some war wounds. As I said in Ch. 1, these inscriptions have been published by Herzog (1931) and LiDonnici (1995).

4. *Surgical instruments*

This group of material has a particularly close relation with the practical, medical, side of the topic of this research, since we can assume that the surgical instruments that have been found had been used at some point in time or were at least intended for use. Until about two decades ago, this material had received only passing attention, e.g. in site reports or brief articles (e.g. in a medico-historical context, the article by K. Garnerus [1979]) - with the only exception of J. S. Milne's book *Surgical Instruments in Greek and Roman Times* (1907/1970). Milne's work still remains the standard reference work on the topic, correlating archaeological finds and relevant passages in the medical authors, although the author's medical training sometimes misleads him into drawing analogies from modern medical practice. The most recent and most useful literature in this field from an archaeologist's point of view is the work done by Ernst Künzl, whose publications provide a thorough coverage of all the finds of surgical instruments in Europe. A complete catalogue of secondary literature on the subject can be found in Künzl's contribution to *ANRW* 37.3 (1996).[34] Some very relevant research has also been done by Ralph Jackson, e.g. 'Roman doctors and their instruments; recent research into ancient practice' (1990), as well as Lawrence Bliquez, especially his catalogue of the surgical instruments in the Museo Nazionale Archeologico of Naples (1994).

As with all archaeological material, there is of course the problem whether what we have is at all a representative sample and not merely a collection of random finds, but this is a risk which always has to be taken when using archaeological evidence.

---

[34] Pp. 2473-536. It is followed by a bibliographical index by type of instrument.

The further limitation is that almost all the instruments that have come down to us are Roman, and we can only assume that they were largely similar to those used by the Greeks. There could be several reasons for this lack of evidence for classical Greece: it could be the difference in burial practices, chance (there must be many unexcavated sites throughout what used to be the Greek world) or a negligent attitude towards small finds. In countries such as Greece or Turkey, which possess a wealth of archaeological treasures, a few probes or cauteries may appear quite worthless.

There are a few bronze objects labelled 'surgical instruments' in the museum at Epidaurus, but most of them are not, or not unequivocally, medical. A set of instruments in the Meyer-Steineg collection - published in id. (1912) and containing the, as we now know, fake, *kyathiskos* - is supposed to be Greek, but very little detail is known about the provenance of these instruments. Most of our knowledge concerning Greek surgical instruments comes from depictions of cases containing such instruments on the tombstones of physicians.[35] The instruments look recognisably like their Roman equivalents, and the only difference suggested by the evidence is that the Greeks appear to have favoured flat rectangular (wooden?) cases with hinges that opened like a book rather than the rectangular metal boxes with sliding lids and the metal cylinders often found with sets of Roman instruments.

Because of a Roman custom, prevailing between the first and the third centuries AD, to bury doctors with their instruments (and members of other professions with the tools of their trade) we have better knowledge of this period of the later Empire as regards the surgical instruments in use than we have of any other period in antiquity. However, not all the finds of more or less complete sets of instruments are grave offerings. Thus, for example, we have the instruments found at Pompeii (kept in the Museo Nazionale Archeologico in Naples and now finally catalogued in Bliquez [1994]), including a portable set of instruments found with one of the bodies in the street. The most relevant find for our topic, since it comes from the site of a military camp, is the large number of instruments found at Vindonissa in Switzerland (most of them kept at the museum of Brugg and some in Zurich).[36]

---

[35] See, e.g., one depicted in Majno (1975), p. 357, fig. 9.9.
[36] See Fig. 5 for a selection. From left to right: bone or tooth forceps (copy of the original kept at the Vindonissa-Museum at Brugg); three pincettes; three awls/needles (possibly for stitching bandages); various types of probes and

It could be argued that we do not have a representative spectrum, as quite often the finds are of single instruments, seldom of complete sets, but it still seems relevant to investigate the percentage of different types of instruments. In a sample of about 1,300 instruments,[37] probes and spatulas take up approximately 60%, followed by pincettes (13%) and scalpels (11%), while only about 4% consist of highly specialised instruments such as specula or catheters. It has to be admitted that for probes, spatulas and tweezers it is hard to draw a line between implements for medical use and cosmetic or artists' tools and that cheaper instruments like probes were discarded more easily than the more costly ones when broken or bent, but there still remains a considerable bias in the percentage. This appears to confirm the suspicion which arises from the study of the texts, namely that the latter do not represent a realistic situation. With all probability most surgeons made do with a limited number of instruments, giving preference to those that could be applied for multiple purposes, and specialised instruments such as the *kyathiskos* were only mentioned by the authors for their novelty value - or perhaps as a show of knowledge intended to impress their audience.

5. *Artistic representation*

This type of material is the most closely related to literary representation of wounding and wound treatment, since both are forms of narrative in different media. Several of the literary topoi discussed in Part II are standard motifs in artistic representation as well, where they appear to be used with the same intentions and in order to create the same effect.

The parallel character of Greek and Roman literature on the one hand and art on the other had been largely ignored by classicists until very recently, and scholars tended to concentrate on either one of the two types of material to the exclusion of the other. There were some exceptions, however, notably: C. Dugas, *Tradition littéraire et tradition graphique* (1937); E. Keuls, *Plato and Greek Painting* (1978a) and id., 'Rhetoric and visual aids' (1978b); as well as some remarks in K. Weitzmann, 'Narration in early Christendom' (1957) and id., *Ancient Book Illumination*

---

spatulas; scalpel (the blade is a reconstruction with a blunt dissector at the other end.

[37] I am indebted to Dr Künzl, Römisch-Germanisches Zentralmuseum, Mainz, for granting me access to his extensive archive.

(1959). During the last five or six years the field has begun to attract attention, and some examples of this newly developed interest are: P. J. Holliday, ed., *Narrative and Event in Ancient Art* (1993); S. Goldhill and R. Osborne, eds., *Art and Text in Ancient Greek Culture* (1994); and J. Elsner, ed., *Art and Text in Roman Culture* (1996).

When speaking of artistic representation related to wounding, it is worth pointing out that originally there would have been two types of representation, distinct from each other by their purpose. One was the illustration of medical texts for didactic purposes, the other the representation of scenes of wounding or wound treatment in art as a form of narrative.

We do not know for certain whether any of the works in the Hippocratic Corpus were illustrated and none of them contain any references to illustrations, but we can take it for given that some medical texts were. In particular this would be the case for anatomical and surgical treatises because of the difficulties involved in written description, discussed in Ch. 5.2. It is likely that illustration became increasingly necessary in Alexandrian times, with the extensive development of anatomy and surgery and with, consequently, an increasing number of textbooks written on these subjects.

According to Bethe,[38] there is no doubt as to the presence of illustrations in treatises on mathematics, mechanics or poliorcetics, e.g. in Hippocrates of Chios (whose writings refer to diagrams), Hero or Philo of Alexandria, and this would appear to be true also for pharmacological and surgical works. Thus we read in Pliny[39] that Krateuas' work on pharmacology was illustrated, and Bethe[40] traces illustrations in medieval manuscripts of Nicander's *Theriaca* and *Alexipharmaca* back to at least the second or third century AD.

For our topic, the most relevant examples are two sets of illustrations related to surgery, namely the illustrations accompanying Apollonius of Kition's commentary on the Hippocratic *Art.*, and those pertaining to Soranus' *De fasciis*. Although both sets of illustrations are Byzantine, it is clear that they must go back to originals as old as the texts. (There is very little doubt that medical treatises such as Soranus' *Gynaecia* contained illustrations from the very beginning and that the illustrations found in medieval MSS of the latter are based on the

---

[38] (1954), p. 22.
[39] *H.N.* XXV.8.
[40] (1954), p. 24.

originals - in particular the different positions of the foetus within the uterus.)

Herrlinger[41] distinguishes between three co-existent types of medical illustration, i.e. schematic (diagrammatic sketches of organs), semi-schematic (full-figure drawings) and naturalistic illustrations of purely medical themes, such as the illustrations for *De fasciis*. According to him,[42] Alexandrian surgery, like anatomy, worked more with the first and second categories and less with naturalistic instructional illustrations. He supports this claim using the example of illustrations of cauterisation points - here again the claim is based on the assumption that later copies follow the earlier original closely.[43] However, we have to remember that our evidence only furnishes information on a minute fraction of whatever medical illustration was produced in antiquity.

Although obviously the material we have does not enable us to make any claims on what illustrations did not exist, we can draw some careful conclusions on what did exist. We can be quite certain that pharmacological manuals were illustrated,[44] and so were books such as Soranus', describing different types of bandages, some books on anatomy, and perhaps some on gynaecology. Full-figure drawings are likely to have been restricted to descriptions of the treatment for fractures and dislocations, where the correct body position - both the patient's and the doctor's - is crucial, but it is not impossible that they were occasionally used to illustrate general surgery. For the treatment of wounds this appears to be less probable, although it is possible (and even likely) that surgical instruments were sometimes represented by line drawings in the text or in the margin.[45]

Any medical illustration that may have existed in antiquity was created for the purpose of making the message conveyed in the text clearer and easier to understand They would therefore not contain a narrative element and hence would not follow the same conventions as artistic representation of scenes of wounding. The representation of scenes of wounding and wound treatment in art,

---

[41] (1967), p. 21.
[42] Ib., p. 16.
[43] The earliest examples appear in the eleventh-century Codex Laurentianus LXXIII.
[44] Cf. the lavishly illustrated sixth-century AD Vienna Dioscorides (Codex medicus graecus 1).
[45] For this practice there is evidence in the medieval Arabic writers, especially Abulcasis, who may have adopted it from the Greeks together with the texts - e.g. the instruments for operations on bones depicted in bk. II, ch. 86, Spink and Lewis (1973), pp. 565-75.

on the other hand, has an entirely different orientation and purpose, although these scenes, too, are 'illustrations' in Hermerén's sense of the word.[46] He applies the term 'to illustrate' to a relation between a work of art and a story -whether the story is written or not. Thus scenes of wounding in art could often be called illustrations inasfar as they illuminate or visualise a story.[47]

The intention of these narrative scenes is not to teach the viewer something - as the textbook illustration would - but to signal a message which is already familiar to the beholder. Given that artistic representation is the visual equivalent of literary description and narrative, it is only to be expected that these two ways of expression should be ruled by similar conventions.

In her article 'Art as communication in ancient Greece' (1978), C. M. Havelock stresses another aspect of Greek art in addition to the narrative, that is, its didactic function. The numerous representation of battles in Greek art, she claims,[48] served as a reminder of the fact that war was both inescapable and a way of life. According to her view, artistic representation of battles invited the beholder's imaginative participation: "In other words, his martial tendencies were encouraged and he was urged to fight as a hero." Although Havelock may be over-emphasising the intentionally didactic aspect of Greek art, the idea of the hero as role-model (in literature as well as in art) is very convincing. Thus some of the scenes of wounding and wound treatment in art may be meant to encourage emulation by presenting a good example.

As in literature, heroic death in battle is a very popular motif in both Greek and Roman art as well. While this is a well-known fact, it tends to pass unnoticed that there are numerous examples of scenes of wounding and wound treatment being made the object of artistic representation. The fact that such scenes are represented in art at all is in itself extraordinary, since the topic of blood and pain would not in itself be considered aesthetically pleasing. Just as in literature, this cannot be explained merely by stating that wounding in war was a common occurrence, as this is hardly a sufficient reason for a topic to appear in art. A brief survey of our material should provide us with some clues as to what people saw in those representations and why there was a market for them.

Among Greek and Roman works of art depicting the treatment of a wound, those most widely known nowadays (and most

---

[46] (1969), p. 55.
[47] It is a pity that the only monograph on the depiction of trauma in ancient art, Geroulanos and Bridler (1994), whilst containing beautiful illustrations, is a coffee-table book without scholarly aspirations.
[48] Ib., p. 106.

frequently used as illustrations in secondary literature about Greek and Roman medicine) are doubtless the cup by the Sosias painter, showing Achilles bandaging Patroklos' arm[49] and the wall-painting from Pompeii which depicts the surgeon Iapex in his attempt to extract an arrow from Aeneas' thigh - following Virgil, *Aen.* XII.391-404.[50] However, these are not the only examples to have come down to us. (Although for some others the exact age and provenance are not clear, it is still beyond doubt that they belong to Graeco-Roman antiquity.)

The healing of Telephos' wound, although not wound treatment in the usual sense, is a popular topic, containing the motif of the wound being healed by the man who struck it. Winckelmann (1821) claims that this scene is represented on a gem, then kept at the Royal Prussian Gem Collection in Berlin.[51] His line drawing of it[52] is indeed made to represent the scene in question, but it differs wildly from the illustration of supposedly the same gem in Overbeck.[53] The size and quality of the latter's illustration make it impossible to determine what kind of treatment is being undertaken, and therefore impossible to be certain about what it is meant to represent. I have nevertheless chosen Furtwängler's photograph rather than Winckelmann's or Overbeck's drawings; although the latter are much clearer, they are also more inventive and intrusive. Both artists have drawn in the details as they perceived or imagined them. Both Furtwängler[54] and Tœlken[55] explain the scene as Patroklos treating Eurypylos. If it is at all related to the *Iliad*, their suggestion seems the more plausible. However, as with several other representations, it is of course possible that it is either a scene thought up by the artist in order to represent some kind of heroic topos or that it is a scene the literary model of which has not survived.

The latter may be the case also with the gem in Fig. 6. It also shows a warrior having a leg wound treated; here the physician appears to be bandaging the leg. Again, though, Furtwängler's picture is not sufficiently clear and it is not evident whether the casualty is holding a staff or perhaps clutching an arrow stuck in his thigh. Furtwängler[56] interprets this scene, too, as Patroklos and

---

[49] Fig. 1.
[50] In particular XII.404: *sollicitat prensatque forcipe ferrum* (Fig. 4).
[51] Our Fig. 7a.
[52] (1821), II, no. 122.
[53] (1853), pl. XII, 13.
[54] (1900), II, p. 113.
[55] (1853), IV.3.254.
[56] (1900), II, p. 114.

Eurypylos (although the *Iliad* does not mention a bandage and Eurypylos would be lying down), but it is unlikely that the bearded man treating the wound represents the youthful Patroklos.

Furtwängler[57] sees Menelaos, Agamemnon and Machaon in a beautifully engraved gem now in the British Museum (Fig. 8), which depicts a young warrior struck in the thigh by an arrow or javelin, supported by one of his older, bearded comrades (they both appear to be warriors rather than surgeons), while the other reaches towards the weapon, presumably in order to pull it out. The Menelaos hypothesis is implausible because the casualty is a beardless youth, an unlikely appearance for the king Menelaos. If this is a scene from the *Iliad*, Sarpedon's wound would be a far more likely guess. As said above, it may of course be a scene that was instantly recognisable in antiquity but means nothing to us who no longer know the story it illustrates.

The group from Trajan's Column (Fig. 2) is fairly well known and often used in secondary literature as well. As I mentioned briefly in Ch. 4.2, Rossi[58] is the only scholar (to my knowledge) to have suggested the possible symbolic character of the different uniforms represented here. They may symbolize, he suggests, the unity of the Imperial Roman army despite its ethnic heterogeneity. I believe that Rossi's line of thought may be more fruitful than attempts to determine, e.g., the rank of the individual figures. One could argue along the same lines that many of the scenes on the Column appear to place great emphasis on unity, togetherness and *concordia* - e.g. legionaries lifting loads together, standing in close groups or touching each other. The scene in question may well be created with the specific intention of expressing such concepts. This may be the reason why the physical closeness between the figures is accentuated by the auxiliary leaning his hand on the shoulder of the man bandaging his leg and the legionary gently supporting his injured comrade.

Even a brief examination of our material immediately makes one point obvious: these are not realistic representations of wound treatment (although they do contain some realistic details), no more so than similar scenes in literature. The wound itself is hardly ever visible[59] and there is no expression of pain on the wounded man's face. The only exception, as far as facial expression is concerned, is the Sosias painter's cup. In a very life-

---

[57] Ib., p. 112.
[58] (1969), p. 540.
[59] Fatal wounds usually are; e.g. on the famous 'Dying Gaul'.

like movement Patroklos supports his wounded left arm with the other hand while Achilles is dressing it At the same time he turns his head away, baring his clenched teeth in a grimace of pain (admittedly a very stylised grimace that does not detract from his beauty).

In some cases the pain of the wound is hinted at by a contraction of the muscles, e.g. (on Trajan's Column) the cavalryman's hand clutching the rock he sits on while his left foot is contracted, pushing hard against the ground. The youth on the British Museum gem (Fig. 8) grips the arrow, but his face is serene, almost smiling, and Aeneas (Fig 2) gazes into the distance with an almost bored expression.

This is the same emphasis on the hero's endurance and contempt for pain as we have found in similar scenes in literature. The casualty's fortitude is expressed in another way as well. Since all artists appear to have adhered to this convention, it is so familiar that it passes unnoticed: again in a parallel to literature, none of the wounded warriors ever needs to be held down while having his wound treated, a situation not at all likely in real life, especially with the extraction of an arrow.

A further interesting motif is that the wounded man is always sitting, or even standing, sometimes leaning on his spear or a staff (e.g. Aeneas), never lying down, although the latter would often have been the case in reality - and even in the *Iliad* (XI.844) Patroklos makes Eurypylos lie down for cutting out the arrow. This detail as well serves to emphasise the casualty's fortitude, and it shows him in control of the situation, an aspect which we have encountered several times in literature, especially the literature about Alexander.

In addition to this, almost invariably the person treating the wound is physically on a lower level than the wounded man. On most representations the doctor - or whoever takes his place - is either sitting or stooping, or crouching, with his head bent. There are very few depictions in art of the treatment of ordinary illness or injury, with the exception of some votive reliefs showing cures effected by Asclepius,[60] but it seems that this style is never adopted. Thus there appears to be a conscious distinction between the representation of war wounds and that of illness, the wound

---

[60] But see, for example, the bas-relief from a physician's tomb in Holländer ([1912], p. 461). The doctor is seated, but he is larger than the patient standing in front of him whom he is examining. Again, the physician performing phlebotomy on a fifth-century BC red-figured aryballos now at the Louvre (see, e.g., E. D. Philips, *Aspects of Greek Medicine*, Philadelphia 1973, fig. 5) is also seated with the patient standing, but he is not in a subservient position.

being the 'nobler' and more heroic affliction, which makes the casualty superior to those who treat him - an attitude which is familiar from literature as well.

Incidentally, the aforementioned posture adopted by the attendant is the one which we also encounter in representations of midwives. They usually sit in front of the woman giving birth, but on a lower level with their heads bent or averted (as enjoined by Soranus). In the case of the midwife the representation does reflect an actual situation in reality, and we are left to wonder whether this similarity is a mere coincidence or whether there is some deeper analogy involved. This idea would seem far-fetched if we had not already come across it in connection with the *Iliad*. It would appear that the affinity was sometimes seen in the way that childbirth is for the woman what war (and wounding) is for the man,[61] and it is not impossible that this underlying idea of parallelism would lead to a similarity in representation. A further parallel is the single-sex character of the situation: a man surrounded and assisted by men, and a woman surrounded and assisted by women.

If Holländer[62] is correct - and it seems very likely that he is - in explaining the scene of Fig. 7b as one of childbirth, there is indeed a striking similarity in composition. The composition of the scene is almost identical with that of Fig. 7a, despite the fact that the posture of the wounded man in the latter is very unusual and elaborate. With his right arm he is leaning on his spear and his left arm is thrown back, his left hand holding on, as if for comfort, to the shoulder of the youth standing behind him, whose left hand supports the casualty's left flank in a protective gesture. We find exactly the same gestures again in the ivory carving, including a staff in place of the spear. The two artefacts constitute an extreme example of similar representation of wound treatment and childbirth and it would be interesting to know whether one of them could possibly have imitated the other or whether there was some common source for both.[63]

Another motif, familiar from literature, reappears in art as well, namely the sollicitude expressed either by the person treating the

---

[61] Cf. Loraux (1981b).
[62] (1912), p. 270.
[63] An intriguing possibility appears to be suggested by two Egyptian depictions of childbirth: one in Holländer (1912), p. 269, fig. 162, and the other in H. Ploß, *Das Weib in der Natur- und Völkerkunde*, eighth edn. (edited posthumously by M. Bartels), Leipzig 1905, p. 199, fig. 474. While the women are kneeling rather than sitting, the position of the arms is almost identical with the two depictions above.

wound (note the gentleness in Achilles' gestures and expression on Fig. 1) or by those surrounding the wounded warrior or supporting him (the legionary on Fig. 2 or the bearded warrior supporting the wounded man on Fig. 8). As in literature, this device highlights the casualty's importance seen through the eyes of others.

This importance is one of the meanings expressed in the motif of protecting a wounded warrior in a battle - which appears in art as well as in literature, e.g. on the so-called Fugger Sarcophagus (Fig. 3). More than on the wounded man himself, however, this gesture reflects on the warrior who covers the other with his shield in an expression of the warrior's *aretê*. Another aspect of this *aretê*, recovering the dead, is also often represented in art.

There is no space here to discuss all the representations of heroic death in battle, but even from the few examples of scenes of wounding and wound treatment we can see that artistic representation follows very much the same conventions as narrative in literature, and the same topoi appear in both forms of narrative. Scenes in art which focus on war wounds helpfully support and reinforce the impressions gained from a study of the relevant passages in literature. This parallelism also suggests that a differentiation between different types of evidence constitutes an artificial division.

CONCLUSION

Given the multi-disciplinary approach of this book, it is obviously impossible to provide an overall conclusion other than stating that the topic of wound treatment in antiquity is of far greater interest than most scholars assume. However, there are several points which I hope to have brought across.

One is that the frequency of wars made the treatment of trauma an important part of medical activity and - one can therefore assume - of medical training. The absence of extant works dealing exclusively with war wounds can be misleading, partly because information on wound treatment can be found throughout various kinds of medical writings and partly because much of the training would have been by practical apprenticeship without the need for textbooks.

It should also have become clear that the the practical aspect is not the only, or even the main, point of interest: more than any other type of medical treatment, army surgery is linked with a framework of associated ideas which go far beyond the limits of medicine. For ancient authors and their audiences wounding and the treatment of battle wounds was closely related to the concept of heroism, and consequently descriptions of wounds and their treatment are used with the purpose of highlighting this idea. This same intention is visible in artistic representations of such scenes, where the non-textual material supports conclusions drawn from the literary material.

To summarise the main findings of the examination of the textual material: these relate both to the interrelation between medical and lay literature in antiquity and to the stranglehold of topoi on ancient writing in general (more obvious and easier to demonstrate in non-medical literature). This study suggests the need to exercise extreme caution in respect to distinctions made between different genres. If we take the descriptions of war wounds in the Hippocratic *Epidemics* as an example, they are obviously 'medical' both in their subject matter and in their purpose, but the way in which the cases are presented does not differ from non-medical literature to the extent that the modern reader would expect. What makes them appear quite different at first sight is the style of which - lacking other comparable collections of 'case-histories' - we can only say that it is typical of the *Epidemics*. It would appear that the differences between medical and non-medical writings are mainly a matter of degree and of focusing more or less on medical aspects rather than a clean-cut distinction and that both groups are rhetorical, each in its distinct way. That is to say that each group had its own determined ways of presenting its message: a medical writer would not describe a wound in the same way as, e.g., a poet, but this need not mean that his account is any more factual or objective.

It has also been my intention to draw attention to another point. As I have already said in the Introduction, when scholars treat this topic at all, they single out certain aspects of it, such as surgical techniques or literary formulae. However, I find this approach methodologically mistaken and I believe that the only way of grasping how wounds and wound treatment were perceived by Greeks or Romans lies in examining as many different facets of the topic as possible. (The same is true for other aspects of Greek and Roman life as well). Only thus can one hope to gain some insight into Greek or Roman ways of thinking - which should after all still be the aim of classical scholarship.

BIBLIOGRAPHY

I. *Primary sources*

Achilles Tatius, *Clitophon and Leucippe*. Ed. S. Gaselee. London/Cambridge, Mass., 1969.
Aeschines, *Oratio in Timarchum*. Ed. F. Franke. Leipzig, 1893.
Aetius Amidenus, *Libri Medicinales*. Ed. Alexander Olivieri, 2 vols. *CMG* VIII.1, VIII.2. Leipzig/Berlin, 1935/1950.
Ammianus Marcellinus, *Rerum Gestarum Libri qui supersunt*. Ed. J. C. Rolfe, 3 vols. London/Cambridge, Mass., 1963 (4th edn., vols. 1, 2), 1958 (3rd ed. vol. 3).
Anonymi Byzantini vita Alexandri regis Macedonum. Ed. J. Trumpf. Stuttgart, 1974.
Appian, *Roman History*. Ed. Horace White, 4 vols. London/Cambridge, Mass, 1958-79.
Apollonius Rhodius, *Argonautica*. Ed. R. C. Seaton. London/Cambridge, Mass., 1980.
Aretaeus. Ed. Carolus Hude, *CMG* II. Leipzig/Berlin, 1923.
Aristotle, *Ars Rhetorica*. Ed. W. D. Ross. Oxford, 1959.
— , *De Arte Poetica*. Ed. Rudolfus Kassel. Oxford, 1965.
— , *Ethica Nicomachaea*. Ed. I. Bywater, (13th edn.). Oxford, 1959.
— , *Ethica Eudemia*. Ed. R. R. Walzer and J. M. Mingay. Oxford, 1991.
— , *Liber de Interpretatione*. Ed. L. Minio-Paluello. Oxford, 1949.
— , *Minor Works*. Ed. W. S. Hett. London/Cambridge, Mass., 1953.
— , *Problems*. Ed. W. S. Hett, 2 vols. London/Cambridge, Mass., 1936/7.
Arrian, *History of Alexander and Indica*. Ed. P. A. Brunt, 2 vols. London/Cambridge, Mass., 1976/83.
Asclepiodotus: *Asclépiodote, Traité de tactique*. Ed. Lucien Poznanski. Paris, 1992.
Bentham, Edward, ed., Θουκυδίδου, Πλάτωνος καὶ Λυσίου λόγοι ἐπιτάφιοι. Oxford, 1746.
Caelius Aurelianus: *Caelii Aureliani Celeres Passiones. Tardae Passiones*. Ed. G. Benz, tr. I. Pape. *CML* VI.1, 2 vols. Berlin 199xxx/93.
Caesar, *De Bello Gallico*. Ed. R. Du Pontet. Oxford, 1937.
A.Cornelii Celsi quae supersunt. Ed. Fridericus Marx, *CML* vol. I. Leipzig/Berlin, 1915.
Celsus, *De Medicina*. Ed. W. G. Spencer, 3 vols. London/ Cambridge, Mass., 1960/61.
Cicero, *Tusculan Disputations*. Ed. J. E. King. London/ Cambridge, Mass., 1971.

Cornelius Nepo, *Cornelii Nepotis Vitae cum fragmentis*. Ed. Peter K. Marshall. Leipzig, 1977.
Qu. Curtius, *History of Alexander*. Ed. J. C. Rolfe, 2 vols., London/ Cambridge, Mass., 1946.
Diels, Hermann, ed., *Die Fragmente der Vorsokratiker*, 7th ed. Berlin, 1954.
Dio, *Roman History*. Ed. Earnest Cary. 9 vols. 1914-27.
Diodorus Siculus. 12 vols., ed. C. H. Oldfather (I-VI), C. L. Sherman (VII), C. Bradford Welles (VIII), R. M. Geer (IX/X), F. R. Walton (XI/XII). London/ Cambridge, Mass., 1933-67.
Dionysius of Halicarnassus, *Roman Antiquities*. Ed. Earnest Cary. 7 vols. London/Cambridge, Mass., 1937-50.
-- , *The Critical Essays*. Ed. Stephen Usher. 2 vols. London/ Cambridge, Mass., 1974/85.
Dioscorides, *Pedanii Dioscoridis Anazarbei De Materia Medica*. Ed. Max Wellmann. 3 vols., 1907 (vol. 1), 1906 (vol. 2), 1914 (vol. 3). Berlin.
Erotian: *Erotiani Vocum Hippocraticarum Collectio cum Fragmentis*. Ed. Ernst Nachmanson. Göteborg/Upsala, 1918.
Euripides, *Hercules*. Ed. J. Diggle, (*Euripidis Fabulae*, vol. II). Oxford, 1981.
-- , *Hippolytus*. Ed. J. Diggle, (*Euripidis Fabulae*, vol. I). Oxford, 1984.
Frontinus: *Frontin, Kriegslisten*. Ed. Gerhard Bendz (Schriften u. Quellen der Alten Welt, 10). Berlin, 1963.
Galen, *Cl. Galeni Opera Omnia*. 22 vols. Ed. C. G. Kühn (facs. reprint of 1821 edition). Hildesheim, 1964-86.
A. Gellius, *Noctes Atticae*. 2 vols. Ed. P. K. Marshall. Oxford, 1990.
Gentili, Bruno and Prato, C., ed., *Poetae Elegiaci. Testimonia et Fragmenta*, Pars I. Leipzig, 1979.
Heraclitus, *Fragments*. Ed. T. M. Robinson (*The Phoenix Pre-Socratics*, vol. II). Toronto, 1987.
Herodotus: *Herodoti Historiae*. Ed. Carolus Hude. 2 vols. (repr.). Oxford, 1976.
Hippocratic Corpus, *Oeuvres complètes d'Hippocrate*. Ed. Émile Littré. 10 vols. Paris, 1839-61.
Hippocratis opera. Ed. Hugo Kühlewein. Leipzig, 1894.
Historia Alexandri Magni. Recensio g. (l.b. 2). Ed. H. Engelmann, *Der griechische Alexanderroman*. Meisenheim, 1963. In *Beitr. z. klass. Phil.* 12, 152-328.
Homer. *Homeri Opera*. Ed. David B. Monro and Thomas W. Allen. 4 vols. Oxford, 1978 (I, II), 1975/6.
Hyperides, *Epitaphius*. Ed. G. Schiassi. Florence, 1959.
M. Iunianus Iustinus, *Epitoma Historiarum Philippicarum*. Ed. O. Seel. Stuttgart, 1972.
Köchly, H. and Rüstow, W., eds. *Griechische Kriegsschriftsteller*. 3 vols.: Aeneias, Heron, Philon; Asclepiodotus, Aelianus; Anonymus Byzantinus. (Repr. of the 1853-55 edition.) Osnabrück, 1969.

T. Livius, *Ab Urbe Condita*. 5 vols., ed. R. Seymour Conway and C. Flamstead (I-III), R. Seymour Conway and S. Keymer Johnson (IV), Alexander Hugh McDonald (V). Oxford, 1914-74.

Lucan, *Pharsalia*. Ed. J. D. Duff. London/Cambridge, Mass., 1969.

Lucian, *Opera*. Ed. M. D. Macleod, 4 vols. Oxford, 1972/74/80/87.

Lycurgus, *Oratio in Leocratem. Cum Ceterarum Lycurgi orationum fragmentis*. Ed. Nicos C. Conomis. Leipzig, 1970.

Lysias, *Orationes*. Ed. Carolus Hude. 3rd edition, Oxford, 1946.

Menander, *Menandri Reliquiae Selectae*. Ed. F. H. Sandbach. Oxford, 1972.

Müller, Karl (1979), *The Fragments of the Lost Historians of Alexander the Great. Fragmenta Scriptorum de Rebus Alexandri Magni, Pseudo-Callisthenes, Itinerarium Alexandri* (facs. repr. of Paris 1846). Chicago.

Oribasius, *Collectionum Medicorum Reliquiae*. Ed. Ioannes Raeder, 5 vols.: *CMG* VI. 1.1, VI 1.2, VI 2.1, VI 2.2, VI 3. Leipzig, 1928/29/31/33/26.

Orphei Hymni. Ed. Guilelmus Quandt. Berlin, 1955.

Ovid, *Metamorphoses*. Ed. G. Lafaye, 2 vols. Paris, 1928.

— , *Amores, Medicamina Faciei Femineae, Ars Amatoria, Remedia Amoris*. Ed. E. J. Kenney. Oxford, 1961.

— , *Tristia, Ibis, Ex Ponto, Halieutica, Fragmenta*. Ed. S. G. Owen. Oxford, 1969 [1915].

Page, D. L., ed. *Epigrammata Graeca*. Oxford, 1975.

— , *Lyrica Graeca Selecta*. Oxford, 1976.

Paulus Aegineta. Ed. I. L. Heiberg, 2 vols. *CMG* IX.1, IX.2. Leipzig/Berlin, 1921/24.

Philo, *Mechanicae Syntaxis libri quartus et quintus*. Ed. R. Schoene. Berlin, 1891.

Philostratos, Περὶ γυμναστικῆς. Ed. Julius Jüthner. Leipzig/Berlin,

Philumenus, *De venenantis animalibus eorumque remediis*. Ed. Max Wellmann, *CMG* X. 1.1. Leipzig/Berlin, 1908.

Pindar, *Carmina*. Ed. C. M. Bowra. Reprint. Oxford 1968.

Plato, *Platonis Opera*. Ed. J. Burnet. 5 vols. Oxford, 1946/60.

— , *Res Publica*. Ed. J. Burnet. Oxford, 1902.

Plinius Secundus, *Historiae Naturalis libri XXXVII*, various eds., 10 vols., London/ Cambridge, Mass., 1938-62.

Plinii Secundi Iunioris qui feruntur de medicina libri tres. Ed. Alf Önnerfors (Academia Scientiarum Germanica Berolinensis). Berlin, 1964.

Plutarch, *Lives*. Ed. Bernadotte Perrin, 11 vols. London/ Cambridge, Mass., 1914-62.

— , *Moralia*. Various eds., 15 vols.. London/Cambridge, Mass., 1927-69.

Poetae Lyrici Graeci. Ed. Th. Bergk, 3 vols. Leipzig. 1882.

Polybius, *The Histories*. Ed. W. R. Paton, 6 vols. London/ Cambridge, Mass., 1922-7.

Procopius, *History of the Wars*. Ed. H. B. Dewing, 7 vols., London/Cambridge, Mass., 1914-28.

Pseudoapulei Herbarius. Ed. Ernestus Howald. Henricus E. Sigerist, *CML* IV. Leipzig/Berlin, 1927.

Quintus Serenus, *Liber Medicinalis*. Ed. Fridericus Vollmer, *CML* II.3. Leipzig/Berlin, 1916.

Reinesius, Thomas, *Syntagma Inscriptionum Antiquarum*. Leipzig/Frankfurt, 1682.

Rufus Ephesius: *Oeuvres de Rufus d'Éphèse*. Ed. Charles V. Daremberg (contd. by Charles Émile Ruelle). Amsterdam, 1962.

Scholia in Hippocratem et Galenum. Ed. F. R. Dietz, 2 vols. Königsberg, 1834.

Scholia Graeca in Homeri Iliadem (Scholia Vetera). Ed. H. Erbse, 6 vols. Berlin, 1969/71/74/75/77/83.

Scholia Graeca in Homeri Iliadem Townleyana. Ed. E. Maass, 2 vols. Oxford, 1887/88.

Seneca, *Epistulae Morales*. Ed. R. M. Gummere, 3 vols. London/Cambridge, Mass., 1920/25.

— , *Moral Essays*. Ed. J. W. Basore, 3 vols. London/Cambridge, Mass., 1928-35.

Silius Italicus, *Punica*. Ed. J. Volpilhac, P. Miniconi, G. Devallet, 3 vols. Paris, 1979/81/84.

Sophocles, *Fabulae*. Ed. A. C. Pearson. Oxford, 1924.

Soranus of Ephesus, *Gynaeciorum libri IV/ De signis fracturarum/De fasciis/ Vita Hippocratis secundum Soranum*. Ed. Ioannes Ilberg, *CMG* IV. Leipzig/Berlin, 1927.

Spengel, Leonardus, ed. *Rhetores Graeci*. 3 vols. Leipzig, 1854.

Statius, *Silvae. Thebaid. Achilleid*. Ed. J. H. Mozley, 2 vols. 3rd edition, Harvard/London 1961.

Tacitus, *Annalium Libri*. Ed. C. D. Fisher. Oxford, 1906.

— , *Historiarum Libri*. Ed. C. D. Fisher. Oxford, 1911.

Terence, *Comoediae*. Ed. W. M. Lindsay. Oxford, 1977[1926].

Theodorus Priscianus, *Euporiston*. Ed. Valentinus Rose. Leipzig, 1894.

Theognis, *Elegies*. Ed. Douglas Young. Leipzig, 1971.

Theophrastus, *Enquiry into Plants*. Ed. Sir Arthur Hort, 2 vols. London/Cambridge, Mass., 1916.

Theophylactus Simocatta, *Historiae*. Ed. Carolus De Boor. Stuttgart, 1972.

Thucydides, *Historiae*. Ed. Henry Stuart Jones, 2 vols. Oxford, 1974/6.

Valerius Flaccus, *Argonautica*. Ed. J. H. Mozley. London/ Cambridge, Mass., 1972.

Valerius Maximus, *Factorum et dictorum memorabilium libri novem*. Ed. Pierre Constat. Paris, 1963.

Vegetius, *Epitoma rei militaris*. Ed. Carolus Lang. Stuttgart, 1967.

Velleius Paterculus, *Ad M.Vinicium libri duo*. Ed. R. Ellis. Oxford, 1898.

Virgil, *Opera*. Ed. F. A. Hirtzel. Oxford, 1900.
Vitruvius, *De Architectura*. Ed. F. Granger, 2 vols. London/Cambridge, Mass., 1970.
Wellmann, Max, ed. *Fragmentensammlung der sikelischen Ärzte Akron, Philiston und Diokles von Karystos*. Berlin, 1901.
West, M. L., ed. *Delectus ex Iambis et Elegis Graecis*. Oxford, 1980.
Xenophon. Ed. E. C. Marchant, etc., 5 vols. Oxford, 1900-74.

II. *Secondary sources*

(The abbreviations are those used in *L'Année Philologique* where available.)

Adamson, P. B. (1973), 'The influence of Alexander the Great on the practice of medicine', *Episteme* 7: 222-30.
Adkins, Arthur W. H. (1960), *Merit and Responsibility: A Study in Greek Values*. Oxford.
— (1972), *Moral Values and Political Behaviour in Ancient Greece: From Homer to the end of the fifth century*. London.
Albarracin Teulón, Agustín (1971), 'La cirugia Homerica', *Episteme* 5: 83-97.
Althoff, Jochen (1993), 'Formen der Wissensvermittlung in der frühgriechischen Medizin'. In Kullmann and Althoff (1993), 211-23.
— (1998), 'Die aphoristisch stilisierten Schriften des Corpus Hippocraticum'. In Kullman, Althoff, and Asper (1998), 37-63.
Amundsen, Darrel W. (1973), 'The liability of the physician in Roman law'. In Karphus (1973), 17-31.
— (1974), 'Romanticizing the ancient medical profession: the characterization of the physician in the Graeco-Roman novel', *BHM* XLVIII, 3 (Fall 1974): 320-37.
Andorlini Marcone, Isabella (1993). 'L'apporto dei papiri alla conoscenza della scienza medica antica', *ANRW* II.37.1, 458-562.
Andronikos, M. (1984), Βέργινα. Οἱ βασιλικοὶ τάφοι καί οἱ ἄλλες ἀρχαιότητες. Athens.
Argoud, Gilbert (1978), 'Honneurs funèbres à Athènes au Ve et au IVe siècle avant J.-C.', *Mémoires Centre Jean-Palerne* I, 3-18.
Artelt, Walter (1968), *Studien zur Geschichte der Begriffe 'Heilmittel' und 'Gift'. Urzeit - Homer - Corpus Hippocraticum*. Darmstadt.
Baader, Gerhard (1970), 'Lo sviluppo del linguaggio medico nell' antichità e nel primo medioevo', *A&R* XV: 1-19.
— and Winau, Rolf (1989), *Die hippokratischen Epidemien. Theorie-Praxis-Tradition. Verhandlungen des Ve Colloque International Hippocratique, Berlin 10-15.9.1984*. Stuttgart.
Baron, W., ed. (1967), *Beiträge zur Methode der Wissenschaftsgeschichte*. Wiesbaden.

del Barrio Vega, Maria Luisa (1992), 'La medicina hipocrática y los *iamata* de Epidauro'. In López Férez (1992), 539-48.

Bartels, Klaus (1965), 'Der Begriff Techne bei Aristoteles'. In Flashar and Gaiser (1965), 275-87.

Baur, P. V. C. and Rostovtzeff, M. I. (1929-52), *The Excavations at Dura-Europos*. 10 vols. New Haven.

Baxandall, Michael (1985), *Patterns of Intention: On the historical explanation of pictures*. New Haven/London.

Beecher, Henry K. (1959), *Measurement of Subjective Responses: Quantitative effects of drugs*. New York.

Below, Karl-Heinz (1953), 'Der Arzt im römischen Recht', *MBP* 37: 1-136.

Bennike, Pia (1985), *Palaeopathology of Danish Skeletons: A comparative study of demography, disease and injury*. Copenhagen.

Bérard, Claude (1982), 'Récupérer la mort du prince: héroïsation et formation de la cité.' In Gnoli and Vernant (1982), 89-105.

Bertier, Janine (1989), 'A propos de quelques résurgences des épidémies dans les *Problemata* du corpus aristotelicien'. In Baader and Winau (1989), 251-9.

Bertolotti, Mario (1933), *La critica medica nella storia. Alessandro Magno*. Turin.

Berrettoni, Pierangiolo (1970), 'Il lessico tecnico del I e III libro delle Epidemie ippocratiche.' *ASNP*, Ser.II, 39: 27-106, 217-311.

Bethe, Erich (1914), *Homer.Dichtung und Sage. I: Ilias*. Leipzig/Berlin.

— (1945), *Buch und Bild im Altertum. Aus dem Nachlaß hrsg. v. Ernst Kirsten*. Leipzig/Wien.

Bliquez, Lawrence J. (1982), 'Roman surgical instruments in the Johns Hopkins University Institute of the History of Medicine', in *Bull. Hist. Med.* 56 (Summer 1982): 195-217.

— (1984), 'Two lists of Greek surgical instruments and the status of surgery in Byzantine times.' In J. Scarborough, ed. *Symposium on Byzantine Medicine* (Dumbarton Oaks Papers, 38), 187-204.

— (1994), *Roman Surgical Instruments and Other Minor Objects in the National Archaeological Museum of Naples*. With a catalogue of the surgical instruments in the "Antiquarium" at Pompeii by Ralph Jackson. Mainz.

— (1998), 'Two "sets" of Roman surgical tools from the Holy Land', *SJ* 49: 83-92.

Blyth, Philip Henry (1977), *The Effectiveness of Greek Armour against Arrows in the Persian War (490-479 B.C.): An inter-disciplinary enquiry*. Unpublished PhD-thesis, Dept. of Engineering and Cybernetics, Reading.

Boscherini, Silvano (1991), 'La metafora nei testi medici latini'. In Sabbah (1991), 188-93.

— (1993), 'Termini medici negli scritti di M. Porcio Catone'. In S. Boscherini, ed. *Studi di lessicologia medica antica. Opuscula Philologa* 6, Bologna, 31-43.

Boswinkel, E. (1956), 'La médecine et les médecins dans les papyrus', *Eos* 48, 1: 181-90.
Bosworth, A. B. (1988), *From Arrian to Alexander: Studies in historical interpretation.* Oxford.
Bouffartigue, Jean (1992), *L'Empereur Julien et la culture de son temps. Collection des Etudes Augustiniennes.* (Série Antiquité 133). Paris.
Bowie, Ewen L. (1990), 'Miles ludens? The problem of martial exhortation in early Greek lyric'. In O. Murray, ed. *Sympotica. A symposium on the Symposion*, Oxford, 221-9.
Bradeen, Donald W. (1969), 'The Athenian Casualty Lists', *CQ* 63: 145-59.
Brelich, Angelo (1958), *Gli eroi greci: Un problema storico-religioso.* Rome.
Briau, Renée (1866), *Du service de santé militaire chez les Romains.* Paris.
— (1874), 'Mémoire sur l'assistance médicale chez les Romains.' *Mémoires présentés par divers savants à l'Académie des Inscriptions et Belles-Lettres.* Prem. Série, VIII, 2ième partie. Paris.
Brisson, Luc (1982), *Platon: Les mots et les mythes.* Paris.
Brommer, Frank (1969), *Die Wahl des Augenblicks in der griechischen Kunst.* Munich.
Bruns, Ivo (1898), *Die Persönlichkeit in der Geschichtsschreibung der Alten: Untersuchungen zur Technik der antiken Historiographie.* Berlin.
Buess, H. (1956), 'Mediko-chirurgisches in Ilias und Odyssee', *Dtsche. Med. Wschr.* 81: 1818-22.
Bulanda, Edmund (1913), 'Bogen und Pfeil bei den Völkern des Alterums'. *Abh. d. Archäol.-epigr. Seminars d. Univ. Wien* 15 (Neue Folge II): 67-128.
Cadbury, Henry (1919), 'The style and literary method of Luke. I: The diction of Luke and Acts', *Harvard Theological Studies* VI.
Calame, Claude (1984), 'D'Hippocrate à Galien: trois recettes médicales sur papyrus (P. Aberd. 10)', *REG* 97: 206-13.
Callies, Horst (1968), 'Zur Stellung der medici im römischen Heer', *MHJ* 3: 18-27.
Capitani, Umberto (1974), 'Il recupero di un passo di Celso in un codice del *De medicina* conservato a Toledo', *Maia* 26.3: 161-212.
— (1975), 'A. C. Celso e la terminologia tecnica greca', *ASNP*, serie III, V.2: 449-518.
Cardona, Virginia D., ed. (1984), *Trauma Reference Manual.* Bowie, Maryland.
Casarini, Arturo (1929), 'La medicina militare nella leggenda e nella storia.' (Collana medico-militare, pubblicata dal Ministero della Guerra, XX). Rome.
Caton, Richard (1914), 'Notes on a group of medical and surgical instruments found near Kolophon.' *JHS* 34: 114-18 & Pls. X-XII.
Charlesworth, Dorothy (1976), 'The hospital, Housesteads.' *Archaeologia Aeliana*, Fifth Series, 4: 17-30.

Cobet, J. (1986), 'Herodotus and Thucydides on War.' In Moxon, Smart and Woodman (1986), 1-18.
Cohn-Haft, Louis (1956), *The Public Physicians of Ancient Greece* (Smith College Studies in History XLII). Northampton, Mass.
Colinge, N. E. (1962), 'Medical Terms and Clinical Attitudes in the Tragedians.' *BICS* 9: 43-55.
Connolly, Peter (1988 [1981]), *Greece and Rome at War*. London.
Croiset, Maurice (1910), *Histoire de la littérature grecque*, vol. I. Paris.
Daremberg, Charles Victor (1848), *Fragments du commentaire de Galien sur le Timée de Platon*. Paris.
— (1865), 'Études d'archéologie médicale sur Homère.' *RA*, N. S. 6, 12: 95-111, 248-67, 338-55.
— (1868/69), 'L'état de la médecine entre Homère et Hippocrate, 962-460, d'après les poètes et les historiens grecs.' *RA*, N. S. 18: 345-66; 19: 63-72, 199-212, 259-67.
Davie, Maurice R. (1929), *The Evolution of War: A study of its role in early societies*. New Haven/London.
Davies, Roy.W. (1969), 'The medici of the Roman armed forces.' *Epigr. St.* 8: 83-99.
— (1970), 'The Roman military medical service.' *SJ* XXVII: 84-104.
— (1972), 'Some more military medici.' *Epigr. St.* 9: 1-11.
Deichgräber, Karl (1933), 'Review of *Oribasii Collectionum Medicorum Reliquiae*, ed. Joannes Raeder, vol. III', *Gnomon* 9: 600-07.
— (1950), 'Professio Medici: zum Vorwort des Scribonius Largus.' *Ak. Wiss. Lit., Abh. d. Geistes-u. Sozialwiss. Kl.* (1950): 854-79.
Delbrück, Hans (1900), *Geschichte der Kriegskunst im Rahmen der politischen Geschichte*, vol. I. Berlin.
Demand, Nancy (1993), 'Medicine and philosophy: the Attic orators'. In Wittern and Pellegrin (1993), 91-9.
Detienne, Marcel (1967), *Les maîtres de vérité dans la Grèce archaïque*. Paris.
— (1968), 'La phalange: Problèmes et controverses.' In Vernant (1968), 119-42.
— (1972), *Les Jardins d'Adonis*. Paris.
— , ed. (1988), *Les savoirs de l'écriture en Grèce ancienne* (Cahiers de Philologie 14). Lille.
Di Benedetto, Vincenzo (1966), 'Tendenza e probabilità nell'antica medicina greca', *CS*, 5, 3: 315-68.
— (1986), *Il medico e la malattia: la scienza di Ippocrate*. Turin.
Diels, Hermann (1906), *Die Handschriften der antiken Ärzte. Griechische Abteilung*. Berlin.
Dierbach, Johann Heinrich (1969), *Die Arzneimittel des Hippokrates. Versuch einer systematischen Aufzählung der in allen hippokratischen Schriften*

vorkommenden Medikamenten (facs. repr. of Heidelberg 1824). Hildesheim.

Dihle, Albrecht (1956), 'Studien zur griechischen Biographie.' *Abh. Ak. Wiss. Göttingen, Philol.-hist. Kl.*, III.37:

Dirckx, John H. (1981), 'Virgil and medicine', *J. Am. Med. Ass.* 246.12: 1326-29.

Dolmans, Maarten (1993), *Valetudinaria Exercitus. Militaire hospitalen in de oudheid*. Unpublished PhD thesis, Leiden.

Domaszewski, Alexander von (1967), *Die Rangordnung des römischen Heeres*. With corrections and additions by B. Dobson. (Bonner Jahrbücher, Beiheft 14). Cologne.

Donlan, Walter (1980), *The Aristocratic Ideal in Ancient Greece: Attitudes of superiority from Homer to the end of the fifth century BC*. Lawrence, Kansas.

Dover, Sir Kenneth J. (1987), 'The Colloquial Stratum in Classical Attic Prose'. In id., *Greek and the Greeks: Collected Papers, Vol. 1*, Oxford, 1987, 16-30.

Drabkin, I. E. (1944), 'On Medical Education in Greece and Rome.' *BHM*, 15: 333-51.

Dugas, Charles (1937), 'Tradition littéraire et tradition graphique dans l'antiquité grecque.' *AC* 6: 5-26 & Pl. I-V.

Dumont, Louis (1975), 'On the comparative understanding of non-modern civilizations', *Daedalus* (Spring): 153-72.

Dumortier, Jean (1935), *Le Vocabulaire médical d'Eschyle et les écrits hippocratiques*. Paris.

Durling, Richard J. (1993), *A Dictionary of Medical Terms in Galen* (Studies in Ancient Medicine 5). Leiden.

Dutoit, Ernest (1948), 'Tite-Live s'est-il interessé à la médecine?', *MH* 5: 116-23.

Dyer, Robert (1974), 'The coming of night in Homer', *Glotta* 52: 31-6.

Easterling, P. E. (1985), 'Books and readers in the Greek world. The Hellenistic and Imperial periods'. In Easterling and Knox (1985), 16-41.

Easterling, P. E. and Knox, B. M. W., eds. (1985), *The Cambridge History of Classical Literature*, vol. I. Cambridge.

Edelstein, Emma J. and Ludwig (1945), *Asclepius: A collection and interpretation of the testimonies*. 2 vols. (I.Testimonies, II. Interpretation). Baltimore.

Edlow, Robert Blair (1977), *Galen on Language and Ambiguity (An English translation of Galen's 'De Captionibus', On Fallacies, with introduction, text, and commentary)*. Leiden.

Eijk, Philip J. van der, Horstmanshoff, H. F. J., and Schrijvers, P. H., eds. (1995), *Ancient Medicine in its Socio-Cultural Context. Papers read at the congress held at Leiden University, 13-15 April 1992* (Clio Medica 27, 28), 2 volumes. Amsterdam.

Ellis, E. S. (1946), *Ancient Anodynes: Primitive anaesthesia and allied conditions*. London.
Elsner, Jas (1996), *Art and Text in Roman Culture*. Cambridge.
Erbig, Franz (1931), *Topoi in den Schlachtenberichten römischer Dichter*. Inaugural-Dissertation. Würzburg.
Erdmann, Elisabeth (1973), 'Die sogenannten Marathonpfeilspitzen in Karlsruhe.' *AA* 88: 30-58.
Eschebach, Hans (1984), *Die Ärztehäuser in Pompeji*. (*Antike Welt*, Sondernummer).
Fantham, Elaine (1985), 'Caesar and the mutiny: Lucan's reshaping of the historical tradition in *De Bello Civili* 5, 237-373.' *CPh* 80: 119-31.
Fantuzzi, Marco (1980), 'Oralità, scrittura, auralità. Gli studi sulle tecniche della communicazione nella Grecia antica (1960-1980)', *L&S* 15: 593-612.
Fenik, Bernard (1968), *Typical battle scenes in the Iliad: Studies in the narrative techniques of Homeric battle description*. (Hermes Einzelschriften, 21).
de Filippis Cappai, Chiara (1993), *Medici e medicina in Roma antica*. Turin.
Fischer, Klaus-Dietrich (1982), 'Zu einigen medizinischen Fachwörtern auf Papyrus', *ZPE* 45: 121f.
Flashar, H. and Gaiser, K., eds. (1965), *Synusia. Festgabe für Wolfgang Schadewaldt zum 15 März 1965*. Pfullingen.
Fox, Robin Lane (1973), *Alexander the Great*. London.
-- (1980), *The Search for Alexander*. London.
Fraser, Paul M. (1972), *Ptolemaic Alexandria*. 3 vols. (I. Text, II. Notes, III. Indexes). Oxford.
Frege, Gottlob (1892), 'Über Sinn und Bedeutung', *Zeitschr. f. Philosophie u. philos. Kritik*, 100: 25-50.
Friedrich, Wolf Hartmut (1956), 'Verwundung und Tod in der Ilias: Homerische Darstellungsweisen.' *Abh. Ak. Wiss. Gött* 3 XXXVIII.
Frölich, Hermann (1879), *Die Militärmedicin Homers*. Stuttgart.
-- (1880a), 'Paulus von Aegina als Kriegschirurg', *Wr. Med. Wochenschrift* 45: 1241-43, 46, 1265-67.
-- (1880b), 'Ueber die Kriegschirurgie der alten Römer', *Archiv f. klin. Chirurgie* 25: 285-321.
Fuhrmann, Manfred (1960), *Das systematische Lehrbuch. Ein Beitrag zur Geschichte der Wissenschaften in der Antike*. Göttingen.
Furtwängler, Adolf (1900), *Die antiken Gemmen: Geschichte der Steinschneidekunst im klassischen Altertum*. 3 vols. Leipzig/Berlin.
Gardner, P. (1920), 'A Numismatic Note on the Lelantine War.' *CR* 34: 90f.
Garlan, Yvon (1972), *La guerre dans l'antiquité*. Paris.
Garnerus, Kurt (1979), 'Die Versorgung von Schußverletzungen bei der Römern.' *ROE*: 55-64 & Tafel 6-8.

Geroulanos, Stephanos and Bridler, René (1994), *Trauma. Wund-Entstehung und Wundpflege im antiken Griechenland.* (Kulturgeschichte der antiken Welt, 56). Naples.
Giannantonio, G. and Vegetti, M., eds. (1985), *La scienza ellenistica. Atti delle tre giornate di studio tenutesi a Padova dal 14 al 16 aprile 1982* (Elenchos, vol. 9). Naples.
Gibbins, David (1988), 'Surgical instruments from a Roman shipwreck off Sicily.' *Antiquity* 62, 235: 294-97.
Gil, Luis and Rodríguez Alfageme, Ignacio (1972), 'La figura del médico en la comedia ática.' *CFC* 3: 35-91.
Gilson, Andrew G. (1983), 'A group of Roman surgical and medical instruments from Cramond, Scotland', *MHJ* 18: 384-93.
Gnoli, Gherardo and Vernant, J.-P., eds. (1982), *La Mort, les morts dans les sociétés anciennes.* Cambridge/Paris.
Gómez-Royo, E. and Buigues-Oliver, G. (1990), 'Die Haftung der Ärzte in den klassischen und nachklassischen Quellen', *RIDA* 3rd S., 37: 167-96.
Gouldner, Alvin W. (1965), *Enter Plato: Classical Greece and the origins of social theory.* London.
Gourevitch, Danielle (1982), 'Les faux-amis dans les textes médicaux grecs et latins'. In G. Sabbah, ed. *Mémoires III, Centre Jean-Palerne*, Sainte-Étienne, 1982, 189-91.
Grasberger, Lorenz (1864/75/81), *Erziehung und Unterricht im klassischen Altertum mit besonderer Berücksichtigung auf die Bedürfnisse der Gegenwart.* 3 vols. Würzburg.
Green, Peter (1978), 'Caesar and Alexander: *Aemulatio, Imitatio, Comparatio.*' *AJAH* 3: 1-26.
Grensemann, H. (1968), *Der Arzt Polybus als Verfasser hippokratischer Schriften.* Wiesbaden.
Griffin, Jasper (1976), 'Homeric pathos and objectivity', *CQ* 26: 161-87.
— (1980), *Homer on Life and Death.* Oxford.
Grmek, Mirko D. (1983), *Les Maladies à l'aube de la civilisation occidentale. Recherches sur la réalité pathologique dans le monde grec préhistorique, archaïque et classique.* Paris.
— (1991), 'La dénomination latine des maladies considérées comme nouvelles par les auteurs antiques'. In Sabbah (1991), 196-214
— (1993), *Storia del pensiero medico occidentale. I: Antichità e Medioevo.* Bari.
— , ed. (1980) *Hippocratica: Actes du Colloque hippocratique de Paris,*
Guhl, Ernst and Koner, Wilhelm (1860), *Das Leben der Griechen und Römer nach antiken Bildwerken.* 2 vols. (I. Griechen, II. Römer). Berlin.
Gummerus, Herman (1932), 'Der Ärztestand im römischen Reiche nach den Inschriften.' *Soc. Scient. Fennica. Commentationes Humanarum Litterarum,* III. 6: 1-103.

Haberling, W. (1909), 'Die Militärlazarette im alten Rom.' *Deutsche Militärärztliche Zeitschrift*, 11: 441-67.
-- (1912), 'Die Entdeckung eines kriegschirurgischen Instruments des Altertums.' *Deutsche Militärärztliche Zeitschrift*, 17: 657-60.
Hadot, Ilsetraut (1984), *Arts libéraux et philosophie dans la pensée antique*. Paris.
Hagemann, Arnold (1919), *Griechische Panzerung. Eine entwicklungsgeschichtliche Studie zur antiken Bewaffnung. I. Der Metallharnisch*. Leipzig/Berlin.
Hammond, Nick G. L. (1983), *Three Historians of Alexander the Great*. Cambridge.
-- (1989), 'Casualties and reinforcements of citizen soldiers in Greece and Macedonia.' *JHS* 109: 56-68.
Hanfmann, George. M. A. (1957), 'Narration in Greek Art.' *AJA* 61: 71-78 & Pls. 27-29.
Hanson, Victor Davis (1989), *The Western Way of War: Infantry battle in classical Greece*. London.
Harig, Georg (1971), 'Zum Problem "Krankenhaus" in der Antike.' *Klio* 53: 179-95.
-- (1974), *Bestimmung der Intensität im medizinischen System Galens. Ein Beitrag zur theoretischen Pharmakologie, Nosologie und Therapie in der Galenischen Medizin*. Berlin.
-- (1980), 'Anfänge der theoretischen Pharmakologie im Corpus Hippocraticum'. In M. D. Grmek, ed. *Hippocratica: Actes du Colloque hippocratique de Paris (4-9 septembre 1978)*, Paris, 1980, 223-45.
Havelock, Christine M. (1978), 'Art as communication in ancient Greece.' In E. A. Havelock and J. P. Hershbell, eds. *Communication Arts in the Ancient World*, New York, 1978, 95-118.
Havelock, Eric A. (1982), *The Literate Revolution in Greece and its Cultural Consequences*. Princeton.
Hellweg, Rainer (1985), *Stilistische Untersuchungen zu den Krankengeschichten der Epidemienbücher I und III des Corpus Hippocraticum*. (Habelts Dissertationsdrucke. Reihe Klassische Philologie, 35). Bonn.
Hermerén, Göran (1969), *Representation and Meaning in the Visual Arts: A study in the methodology of iconography and iconology*. Lund.
Hernández Muñoz, Felipe (1992), 'Demóstenes y el vocabulario hipocrático'. In López Férez (1992), 527-37.
Herrlinger, Robert (1967), *Geschichte der medizinischen Abbildung. I. Von der Antike bis um 1600*. Munich.
Herter, Hans (1963), 'Die Treffkunst des Arztes in hippokratischer und platonischer Sicht', *AGM* 47: 247-90.

Herzog, Rudolf (1903), 'Vorläufiger Bericht über die archäologische Expedition auf der Insel Kos im Jahre 1902.' *Arch. Anz., Beiblatt z. Jahrb. d. Arch. Inst.* XVIII: 1-13.

— (1931), 'Die Wunderheilungen von Epidauros: ein Beitrag zur Geschichte der Medizin und der Religion.' *Philologus*, Suppl. XXII, III.

Hibbs, Vivian A. (1991), 'Roman surgical and medical instruments from la Cañada Honda (Gandul)', *AEA* 64: 111-34.

Himmelmann-Wildschütz, Nikolaus (1967), 'Erzählung und Figur in der archaischen Kunst.' *Abh. Ak. Wiss. Lit. Mainz*, 2: 69-100.

— (1976), *Utopische Vergangenheit: Archäologie und moderne Kultur*. Berlin.

Hirsch, Eric D., Jr. (1967), *Validity in Interpretation*. New Haven/London.

Hoffmann, Martin (1914), *Die ethische Terminologie bei Homer, Hesiod und den alten Elegikern und Jambographen*. Tübingen.

Holländer, Eugen (1912), *Plastik und Medizin*. Stuttgart.

Holliday, Peter J. (1993), *Narrative and Event in Ancient Art*. Cambridge.

Humphreys, S.C. (1981), 'Death and Time.' In Humphreys and King (1981), 261-83.

— and King, Helen, eds. (1981), *Mortality and Immortality: The anthropology and archaeology of death*. London/New York,

Ieraci Bio, Anna Maria (1991), 'Sulla concezione del medico pepaideuménos in Galeno e nel tardoantico'. In López-Férez (1991), 133-51.

Ilberg, Johannes (1887), 'Zur Ueberlieferung des Hippokratischen Corpus', *Rh. M.*, N. F. 42: 436-61.

— (1888), 'De Galeni vocum Hippocraticarum glossario'. In *Commentationes philologae quibus Ottoni Ribbeckio praeceptori inlustri sexagensimum aetatis magisterii Lipsiensis decimum annum exactum congratulantur discipuli lipsienses*, Leipzig, 1888, 327-54.

— (1930), 'Rufus von Ephesos: ein griechischer Arzt in Trajanischer Zeit.' *Abh. Sächs. Ak. Wiss., Philol.-hist. Kl.* 41.1: 1-53.

Inghirami, Francesco (1821-26), *Monumenti etruschi (o di etrusco nome)*. 2 vols. of text & 3 vols. of plates. Fiesole.

— (1831-36), *Galleria Omerica*. 3 vols. in 2 of text & 3 vols. of plates. Fiesole.

Ireland, S. and Steel, F. L. D. (1975), 'Φρένες as an anatomical organ in the works of Homer', *Glotta* 53: 183-95.

Irigoin, Jean (1980), 'La formation du vocabulaire de l'anatomie en grec: du mycénien aux principaux traités de la collection hippocratique.' In Grmek (1980), 247-56.

Irmer, Dieter (1980), 'Die Bezeichnung der Knochen in Fract. und Art.' In Grmek (1980), 265-83.

Jackson, A.H. (1987), 'An early Corinthian helmet in the Museum of the British School at Athens.' *ABSAA*, 82: 107-14, Pl.17, 18.

Jackson, Henry (1910), 'Aristotle's lecture-room and lectures', *Journal of Philology* 35: 191-200.
Jackson, Ralph (1986), 'A set of Roman medical instruments from Italy.' *Britannia* XVII: 119-67.
— (1987), 'A set of surgical instruments from Italy.' *Archéologie et Médecine*. VIIièmes Rencontres Internationales d'Archéologie et d'Histoire, Antibes, Oct. 1986.
— (1990), 'Roman doctors and their instruments: recent research into ancient practice.' *J.Rom.Arch.* 3: 1-27.
— (1991), 'Roman bivalve dilatators and Celsus' "instrument like a Greek letter" (*De med.* VII.5, 2B)'. In Sabbah (1991), 101-09.
Jacob, O. (1932), 'Les cités grecques et les blessés de guerre.' In *Mélanges Gustave Glotz* (Festschrift), II: 461-81. Paris.
— (1933), 'Le service de santé dans les armées romains', *AC* 2: 313-31.
Jaeger, Werner (1932), 'Tyrtaios über die wahre ἀρετή.' *SAW, Phil.-hist. Kl.*: 537-68.
— (1934/44/47), *Paideia: Die Formung des griechischen Menschen*. 3 vols. Berlin/Leipzig.
— (1938), 'Vergessene Fragmente des Peripatetikers Diokles von Karistos.' *APAW, Phil.-hist. Kl.*, 3: 1-46.
— (1957), 'Aristotle's use of medicine as model of method in his ethics', *JHS* 77: 54-61.
— (1965), 'Ideas of immortality.' In O. Cullmann, H. A. Wolfson and W. Jaeger, eds., *Immortality and Resurrection*. New York, 1965.
Jetter, Dieter (1966), *Geschichte des Hospitals*. Vol. I. (*AGM*, Beiheft 5). Wiesbaden.
Joly, Robert (1969), 'Esclaves et médecins dans la Grèce antique', *AGM* 53: 1-14.
Jouanna, Jacques (1984), 'Rhétorique et médecine dans la Collection hippocratique', *REG* 97, 26-44.
Justesen, P. Th. (1928), *Les principes psychologiques d'Homère*. Copenhagen.
Karphus, H., ed. (1973), *International Symposium on Society, Medicine and Law. Jerusalem, March 1972*. Amsterdam.
Kastorchis, E. (1879/1880), 'Report on the Theban grave at Chaironeia.' *Athenaion* 8: 486-91/9, 157f.
Kellett, Anthony (1982), *Combat Motivation: The behavior of soldiers in battle*. Boston/The Hague.
Kerkhoff, A. H. M. (1975), 'La médecine dans Homère', *Janus* 62: 43-9.
Keuls, Eva C. (1978a), *Plato and Greek Painting*. Leiden.
— (1978b), 'Rhetorical and visual aids in Greece and Rome.' In E. A. Havelock and J. P. Hershbell, eds. *Communication Arts in the Ancient World*, New York, 1978, 121-34.

Kislinger, Ewald (1986), 'Der kranke Justin II und die ärztliche Haftung bei Operationen in Byzanz', *JÖByz* 36, 39-44.
Knörzer, Karl-Heinz (1970), *Römerzeitliche Pflanzenfunde aus Neuss.* (Limesforschungen 10. Römisch-Germanische Kommission d. Deutschen Arch. Instituts.) Berlin.
Knox, Bernard M. W. (1985), 'Books and readers in the Greek world. From the beginnings to Alexandria'. In Easterling and Knox (1985), 1-16.
Koelbing, Huldrych M. (1989), 'Therapeutischer Optimismus und therapeutische Zurückhaltung in der hippokratischen Medizin'. In Baader and Winau (1989), 338-46.
Koller, H. (1954), *Die Mimesis in der Antike: Nachahmung, Darstellung, Ausdruck.* Bern.
— (1967), 'Haima.' *Glotta* 15: 149-55.
Kollesch, Jutta (1991), 'Darstellungsformen der medizinischen Literatur im 5. und 4. Jahrhundert v. Chr.', *Philologus* 135, 177-83.
— (1992), 'Zur Mündlichkeit hippokratischer Schriften'. In López Férez (1992), 355-42.
Koumanoudis, S. (1881), Untitled report on excavations at Chaironeia, given at the annual meeting of the Society, *PAE*: 16-20.
Krafft, Fritz (1967), 'Die Anfänge einer theoretischen Mechanik'. In Baron (1967), 12-33.
Krentz, Peter (1985), 'Casualties in hoplite battles.' *GRBS* 26: 13-20.
Kripke, Saul A. (1980), *Naming and Necessity.* 2nd edition. Oxford.
Kromayer, Johannes and Veith, Georg (1928), *Heerwesen und Kriegführung der Griechen und Römer.* Munich.
Kudlien, Fridolf (1961), 'Wissenschaftlicher und instrumenteller Fortschritt der antiken Chirurgie', *AGM* 45: 329-33.
— (1964), *Untersuchungen zu Aretaios von Kappadokien.* (Ak. d. Wiss. u. d. Lit., Abh. d. geistes- u. sozialwissensch. Kl., 1963 xi). Wiesbaden.
— (1965), 'Zum Thema "Homer und die Medizin".' *RhM*, N. F., 108: 293-9.
— (1967), *Der Beginn des medizinischen Denkens bei den Griechen: Von Homer bis Hippokrates.* Zurich/Stuttgart.
— (1968), 'Early Greek primitive medicine.' *CM* 3: 305-36.
— (1968), *Die Sklaven in der griechischen Medizin der klassischen und hellenistischen Zeit* (Forschungen zur antiken Sklaverei 2). Wiesbaden.
— (1970), 'Medical education in classical antiquity'. In O'Malley (1970), 3-37.
— (1974), 'Cynicism and medicine', *BHM* XLVIII, 3 (Fall 1974): 305-19.
— and Durling, R. J., eds. (1991), *Galen's Method of Healing. Proceedings of the 1982 Galen Symposium.* Leiden.
Kühnert, Friedmar (1961), *Allgemeinbildung und Fachbildung in der Antike.* (Deutsche Ak. d. Wiss. zu Berlin. Schriften d. Sektion f. Altertumswiss. 30). Berlin.

Kullmann, Wolfgang and Althoff, Jochen, eds. (1993), *Vermittlung und Tradierung von Wissen in der griechischen Kultur*, Tübingen.
— and Asper, Markus, eds. (1998), *Gattungen wissenschaftlicher Literatur in der Antike*. ScriptOralia 95. Tübingen.
Künzl, Ernst (1983), *Medizinische Instrumente aus Sepulkralfunden der römischen Kaiserzeit*. Cologne.
— (1984a), *Ein Beitrag zur Typologie römischer chirurgischer Skalpelle*. (Typescript).
— (1984b), 'Einige Bemerkungen zu den Herstellern der römischen medizinischen Instrumente.' *Alba Regia* XXI: 59-65.
— (1984c), *Medizinische Instrumente der Römerzeit aus Trier und Umgebung im Rheinischen Landesmuseum Trier*. Trier
— (1986), 'Operationsräume in römischen Thermen.' *BJ* 186: 491-509.
— (1988), 'Archäologische Beiträge zur Medizingeschichte. Methoden, Ergebnisse, Ziele'. In Sabbah (1988), 61-79.
— (1991), 'Die medizinische Versorgung der römischen Armee zur Zeit des Kaisers Augustus und die Reaktion der Römer auf die Situation bei den Kelten und Germanen'. In B. Trier, ed., *Die römische Okkupation nördlich der Alpen zur Zeit des Augustus*. Münster, 1991, 185-202.
— (1996), 'Forschungsbericht zu den antiken medizinischen Instrumenten', *ANRW* II, 37.3: 2433-639.
— (1998), 'Zur Typologie von Klammern und Pinzetten', *SJ* 49: 76-82.
Kutsch, Ferdinand (1913), 'Attische Heilgötter und Heilheroen (Religionsgeschichtliche Versuche u. Vorarbeiten, 12). Gießen.
Laín Entralgo, Pedro (1987), *La curación por la palabra en la Antigüedad clásica* (Autores, textos y temas. Antropología 13). Barcelona.
Lammert, Friedrich (1953), 'Alexanders Verwundung in der Stadt der Maller und die damalige Heilkunde.' *Gymnasium* 60: 1.-7.
Lanata, Giuliana (1968), 'Linguaggio scientifico e linguaggio poetico: note al lessico del "de morbo sacro".' *QUCC* 5: 22-36.
Langholf, Volker (1989), 'Generalisationen und Aphorismen in den Epidemienbüchern'. In Baader and Winau (1989), 131-43.
— (1990), *Medical Theories in Hippocrates. Early texts and the 'Epidemics'*. Berlin.
— (1993), 'Nachrichten bei Platon über die Kommunikation zwischen Ärzten und Patienten'. In Wittern and Pellegrin (1993), 113-42.
Langslow, David R. (1991), 'The development of Latin medical terminology: some working hypotheses', *PCPhS* 37: 106-30.
— (1994), 'Celsus and the makings of a Latin medical terminology'. In Sabbah and Mudry (1994), 297-318.
Lanza, Diego (1972), '"Scientificità" della lingua e lingua della scienza in Grecia', *Belfagor* 27, 4 (July): 392-429.
— (1979), *Lingua e discorso nell' Atene delle professioni*. Naples.

-- (1981), 'Quelques remarques sur le travail linguistique du médecin.' In Lasserre and Mudry (1981), 181-5.
Lara Nava, Dolores (1991), 'Aspectos lexicográficos del Glosario de Galeno a Hipócrates'. In López Férez (1991), 119-31.
Laser, Siegfried (1983), *Medizin und Körperpflege*. (Archaeologia Homerica). Göttingen.
Lasserre, François and Mudry, Philippe (1983), *Formes de pensée dans la collection hippocratique*. Actes du Colloque International Hippocratique. Geneva.
Leander Touati, Anne-Marie (1987), 'The great Trajanic frieze. The study of a monument and of the mechanisms of message transmission in Roman art.' (Skrifter Utgivna av Svenska Institutet i Rom, 40, XLV). Stockholm.
Lehmann, Y. (1982), 'Varron et la médecine'. In Sabbah (1982), 67-72.
Leschhorn, Ilona-Eva (1985), *Der Gesundheits- und Krankheitsbegriff in der griechischen Antike von Homer bis Demokrit*. Unpublished PhD thesis. Aachen.
Leumann, Manu (1950), *Homerische Wörter*. (Schweizer. Beitr. z. Altertumswissenschaft, 3). Basle.
Lewis, David M. (1968), 'Dedications of Phialai at Athens.' *Hesperia* 37: 368-80 & Pl. 110-12.
Lewis, Walter H. and Elvin-Lewis, Memory P. F. (1977), *Medical Botany: Plants affecting man's health*. New York/London.
LiDonnici, Lynn R. (1992), 'Compositional background of the Epidaurian 'IAMATA', *AJPh* 113, 25-41.
-- (1995), *The Epidaurian Miracle Inscriptions. Text, Translation and Commentary* (Texts and Translations 36). Georgia.
Lloyd, Sir Geoffrey E. R., ed. (1983), *Hippocratic Writings*. Harmondsworth, Middlesex.
-- (1983), *Science, Folklore and Ideology*. Cambridge.
-- (1987), *The Revolutions of Wisdom: Studies in the claims and practice of ancient Greek science*. Berkeley.
Lonie, Iain M. (1983), 'Literacy and the development of Hippocratic medicine'. In Lasserre and Mudry (1983), 145-61.
López Férez, J. A.(1991a), 'Acerca del comentario de Galeno a los Aforismos hipocráticos.' In López Férez (1991b), 161-203.
-- , ed. (1991b), *Galeno: Obra, pensamiento e influencia* (Coloquio internacional celebrado en Madrid, 22-25 de Marzo de 1988). Madrid.
-- (1992), *Tratados Hipocráticos (Estudios acerca de su contenido, forma e influencia)*. Actas del VIIe Colloque International Hippocratique (Madrid, 24-29 de septiembre de 1990). Madrid.
Loraux, Nicole (1973), '"Marathon" ou l'histoire idéologique.' *REA* 75: 13-42.
-- (1974), 'Socrate, contrepoison de l'oraison funèbre: Enjeu et signification du *Ménexène*.' *AC* 42: 172-211.

—— (1975), 'HBH et ANDREIA: Deux versions de la mort du combattant athénien.' *Anc. Soc.* 6: 1-31.
—— (1981a), *L'invention d'Athènes: Histoire de l'oraison funèbre dans la cité classique*. Paris.
—— (1981b), 'Le lit, la guerre.' *L'Homme* 21 (I): 37-67.
—— (1982), 'Mourir devant Troie, tomber pour Athènes: de la gloire du héros à l'idée de la cité.' In Gnoli and Vernant (1982).
—— (1985), *Façons tragiques de tuer une femme* Paris.
—— (1986), 'Le corps vulnérable d'Arès.' *Le temps de la réflexion* 7: 335-54.
—— (1989a), 'Blessures de virilité.' In id., *Les expériences de Tirésias: Le féminin et l'homme grec*, 108-23 (notes 334-36).
—— (1989b), 'Crainte et tremblement du guerrier.' Ib. 92-107.
Lorimer, H. L. (1947), 'The hoplite phalanx, with special reference to the poems of Archilochus and Tyrtaeus.' *ABSA* 42: 76-138; Pls. 18A, 19.
Lossau, Manfred (1989), '"Strategische" Wundheilung in der Ilias', *Hermes* 117: 390-402.
Louis, Pierre (1956), 'Observations sur le vocabulaire technique d'Aristote.' In *Mélanges de philosophie grècque offerts à Mgr. Diès*, 141-49. Paris.
Lowenstam, Steven (1981), *The Death of Patroklos*. (Beitr. Kl. Philol. 133).
Mac Cary, W. Thomas (1982), *Childlike Achilles: Ontogeny and phylogeny in the Iliad*. New York.
Mac Intyre, Alasdair (1967), *A Short History of Ethics: A history of moral philosophy from the Homeric age to the twentieth century*. London/New York.
Mai, Angelo (1819), *Iliadis fragmenta antiquissima cum picturis item scholia vetera ad Odysseam*. Milan.
Majno, Guido (1975), *The Healing Hand: Man and wound in the ancient world*. Cambridge, Mass.
Maloney, Gilles and Savoie, R. (1982), *Cinq cents ans de bibliographie hippocratique. 1473 - 1982*. Quebec.
Manchester, Keith (1983), *The Archaeology of Disease*. Bradford.
Mann, Ronald D. (1988), *The History of the Management of Pain. From Early Principles to Present Practice*. Carnforth.
Manuli, Paola (1985), 'Lo stile del commento. Galeno e la tradizione ippocratica'. In Giannantonio and Vegetti (1985), 375-94.
Marasco, Gabriele (1995), 'L'introduction de la médecine grecque à Rome: une dissension politique et idéologique'. In van der Eijk, Horstmanshoff and Schrijvers (1995), 35-48.
Marcillet-Joubert, Jean (1982), 'Un médecin de cohorte auxiliaire'. In Sabbah (1982), 73-80.
Marg, Walter (1976), 'Kampf und Tod in der Ilias.' *WJA*, N. F., 2: 7-19.
Marganne, Marie-Hélène (1981), *Inventaire analytique des papyrus grecs de médecine* (Hautes Etudes du Monde Gréco-Romain 12). Geneva.

—— (1982), 'Nouvelles perspectives dans l'étude des sources de Dioscoride'. In Sabbah (1982), 81-4.
Marrou, Henri-Irénée (1965), *Histoire de l'éducation dans l' antiquité*. Paris.
Marsden, E. W. (1969/1971), *Greek and Roman Artillery*. 2 vols.: *I. Historical Development, II. Technical Treatises*. Oxford.
Massey, Duncan (1994), 'Roman archery tested', *Military Illustrated* 74: 36-9.
Mawet, Francine (1979), *Recherches sur les oppositions fonctionelles dans le vocabulaire homérique de la douleur (autour de πῆμα-ἄλγος)*. (Ac. Roy. de Belgique, Mémoires de la Classe des Lettres, 2e série, 63, 4).
Mazzini, Innocenzo (1978), 'Il greco nella lingua tecnica medica latina', *Ann. Fac. Lett. Filos. Univ. Macerata* II: 543-56.
—— (1991), 'Il lessico medico antico: caratteri e strumenti della sua differenziazione'. In Sabbah (1991), 175-85.
—— (1994), 'La chirurgia celsiana nella storia della chirurgia greco-romana'. In Sabbah and Mudry (1994b), 135-66.
Mc Lleod, Wallace (1965), 'The range of the ancient bow.' *Phoenix*, 19. 1: 1-14.
Meinecke, Bruno (1941), 'Aulus Cornelius Celsus, plagiarist or *artifex medicinae*?' *BHM* 10: 288-98.
Melzack, Ronald (1961), 'The Perception of Pain.' *Scient. Am.* 204, 2 (Feb.): 41-9.
—— (1973), *The Puzzle of Pain*. Harmondsworth.
de Meo, Cesidio (1986), *Lingue tecniche del latino*. 2nd edition. Bologna.
Merbs, Charles F. (1989), 'Trauma'. In M. Y. Iscan and K. A. R. Kennedy, eds. *Reconstruction of Life from the Skeleton*. New York, 161-89.
Meyerhof, Max (1929), 'Autobiographische Bruchstücke Galens aus arabischen Quellen.' *AGM*, 22: 72-86.
—— and Schacht, J. (1931), 'Galen, Über die medizinischen Namen. Arabisch/Deutsch.' *APAW, Philos.-hist. Kl.*, 3: 1-53.
Meyer-Steineg, Theodor (1912), *Chirurgische Instrumente des Altertums*. (Jenaer medizin-historische Beiträge, 1).
Meyboom, P. G. P. (1978), 'Some observations on narration in Greek art.' *MNIR* XL, N.S. 5:
Michler, Markwart (1970), 'Die Palpation im Corpus Hippocraticum', *Janus* 57: 261-
Miniconi, Pierre-Jean (1951), *Étude des thèmes 'guerriers' de la poésie épique gréco-romaine*. Paris.
Miller, Harold W. (1944), 'Medical terminology in tragedy.' *TAPhS* 75: 156-67.
—— (1945), 'Aristophanes and medical language.' *TAPhS* 76: 74-84.
Milne, John S. (1970), *Surgical Instruments in Greek and Roman Times*. New York (facs. repr. of the 1907 edn.).
Misch, Georg (1907), *Geschichte der Autobiographie. Vol. I: Das Altertum*. Leipzig.
Mitchell, W. J. T., ed. (1980), *The Language of Images*. Chicago/London.

Mitropoulos, K. (1962), "Ομήρου Ιατρικά', *Platon* 14: 145-76.
— (1978), Γλωσσάριον 'Ιπποκράτους ('Ιδία κατ' 'Ερωτιανὸν καὶ Γαληνὸν). Τιμητικὴ διάκρισις 'Ακαδημίας 'Αθηνῶν. Athens.
Momigliano, Arnaldo (1966), 'Time in ancient historiography.' *H&T*, Beiheft 6.
Mollière, Humbert (1888), 'Le service de santé militaire chez les Grecs et les Romains (1).' *Lyon Médical* 58: 402-08.
Moreuz, S., ed. (1950), *Aus Antike und Orient. Festschrift Wilhelm Schubart zum 75. Geburtstag.* Leipzig.
Morris, David B. (1991), *The Culture of Pain.* Berkeley.
Moulin, Daniel de (1974), 'A historical-phenomenological study of bodily pain in western man', *BHM* 48.4 (Winter 1974): 540-70.
Moxon, I. S., Smart, J. D. and Woodman, A. J., eds. *Past Perspectives*: 1-18. Cambridge.
Mudry, Philippe (1980), '*Medicus amicus*. Un trait romain dans la médecine antique', *Gesnerus* 37: 17-20.
— (1982), *La Préface du 'De Medicina' de Celse. Texte, traduction et commentaire.* (Bibliotheca Helvetica Romana XIX). Rome.
— (1991), 'Saisons et maladies. Essai sur la constitution d'une langue médicale à Rome.' In Sabbah (1991), 257-69.
Müller, Carl W. (1989), 'Der schöne Tod des Polisbürgers, oder "Ehrenvoll ist es, für das Vaterland zu sterben"', *Gymnasium* 96.4: 317-40.
Nachmanson, Ernst (1918), *Erotiani Vocum Hippocraticorum Collectio cum fragmentis* (Collectio Scriptorum Veterum Upsaliensis). Göteborg.
Nagy, Gregory (1979), *The Best of the Achaeans: Concepts of the Hero in Archaic Greek Poetry.* Baltimore/London.
Neumann, Alfred (1965), 'Disciplina militaris'. *RE* Suppl. X: 142-78.
Nieddu, Gian Franco (1984), 'Testo, scrittura, libri nella Grecia arcaica e classica: note e osservazioni sulla prosa scientifico-filosofica', *S&C* 8: 213-62.
— (1993), 'Neue Wissensformen, Kommunikationstechniken und schriftliche Ausdrucksformen in Griechenland im sechsten und fünften Jahrhundert v. Chr: Einige Beobachtungen'. In Kullmann and Althoff (1993), 151-65.
Nijhuis, Karin (1995), 'Greek doctors and Roman patients: a medical anthropological approach'. In van der Eijk, Horstmanshoff and Schrijvers (1995), 49-67.
Norden, Eduard (1915), *Ennius und Vergilius: Kriegsbilder aus Roms großer Zeit.* Leipzig/Berlin.
Nutton, Vivian (1968), 'A Greek doctor at Chester.' *J. Chester Archaeol. Soc.*, 55: 7-13.
— (1969), 'Medicine and the Roman army: a further reconsideration' *MH* 13: 260-70.
— (1977), 'Archiatri and the medical profession in antiquity.' *Papers Brit. School Rome*, 45: 191-226 & Pls.XXXI-XXXII.

—— (1988a), 'Murders and miracles: lay attitudes towards medicine in classical antiquity.' In id., *From Democedes to Harvey: Studies in the history of medicine.* London, VIII.
—— (1988b), 'The Seeds of Disease: an explanation of contagion and infection from the Greeks to the Renaissance.' Ib., XI.
—— (1991), 'Style and context in the method of healing'. In Kudlien and Durling (1991), 1-25.
Ollero Granados, Dionisio (1973), 'Dos nuevos capitulos de A. Cornelio Celso', *Emerita* 41: 99-108.
O'Malley, C. D., ed. (1970), *The History of Medical Education.* Berkeley.
Onians, Richard Broxton (1951), *The Origins of European Thought: About the body, the mind, the soul, the world, time and fate.* Cambridge.
Oppenheimer, Heinrich (1928), *Medical and Allied Topics in Latin Poetry.* London.
Overbeck, Johannes (1853), *Gallerie heroischer Bildwerke der alten Kunst.* 2 vols. & *Abbildungen zur Gallerie heroischer Bildwerke der alten Kunst* (plates). Brunswick.
Panofsky, Erwin (1960), *Idea: Ein Beitrag zur Begriffsgeschichte der älteren Kunsttheorie.* Berlin.
Paribeni, R. and Romanelli, P. (1914), 'Studi e ricerche archeologiche nell'Anatolia meridionale.' *MonA* 73: 1-274.
Parry, Adam (1969), 'The language of Thucydides' description of the plague,' *BICS* 16: 106-18.
Pauly, Alphonse (1874), *Bibliographie des sciences médicales.* Paris.
Peek, Werner (1960), *Griechische Grabgedichte.* Berlin.
Penn, R. G. (1964), 'Medical Services of the Roman Army.' *J. Roy. Army Med. Corps* (1964): 253-58.
Pereira, Maria Luisa Veiga Silva (1990), 'Instrumentos cirúrgicos de Balsa (Quinta da Torre de Ares)', *Conimbriga* 29: 107-27.
Perelli, Antonella (1989), 'Problemi dell' esegesi virgiliana', *GIF* 41: 317-26.
Petrikovits, Harald v. (1975), *Die Innenbauten römischer Legionslager während der Prinzipatszeit.* (Abh. d. Rhein.-Westfäl. Ak. d. Wiss., 56). Opladen.
Pezzi, Domenico (1894), *Saggi d'indici sistematici illustrati con note per lo studio dell' espressione metaforica di concetti psicologici nella lingua greca antica.* (Memorie della Reale Academia delle Scienze di Torino. Serie seconda, XLVI).
Pfohl, Gerhard (1977), *Inschriften der Griechen: Epigraphische Quellen zur Geschichte der antiken Medizin.* Darmstadt.
Phytalis, Lazaros (1880), 'Ἐρευναί ἐν τῷ πολυανδρίῳ Χαιρωνείας.' *Athenaion* 9: 347-52.
Pigeaud, Jackie (1988), 'Le style d'Hippocrate ou l'écriture fondatrice de la médecine'. In Detienne (1988), 305-29.
Pope, Saxton T. (1930), *A Study of Bows and Arrows.* Berkeley.

Potterton, David, ed. (1983), *Culpeper's Colour Herbal*. London.
Prag, A. J. N. W. (1990), 'Reconstructing King Philip II: The "nice" version.' *AJA* 94: 237-47.
Pritchett, W. Kendrick (1985), *The Greek State at War*. 4 vols. Berkeley.
Proff, Peter (1992), 'Lesungswege zur funktionellen Deutung griechisch-römischer medizinischer Instrumente', *AGM* 76, 2: 179-90.
Psichari, Jean (1908), 'Sophocle et Hippocrate: à propos du Philoctète à Lemnos.' *RPh*, N. S. 32: 95-128.
Pugliese Carratelli, Giovanni (1991), 'La norma etica degli Asklapiadai di Cos', *PP* 46: 81-94.
Quine, Willard Van Orman (1960), *Word and Object*. Cambridge, Mass.
Raffaelli, Renato (1987), *Rappresentazioni della morte*. Urbino.
Redfield, James M. (1975), *Nature and Culture in the Iliad: The tragedy of Hector*. Chicago/London.
— (1985), 'Herodotus the tourist.' *CPh*, 80: 97-118.
Redondo, Jordi (1992), 'Niveles retóricos en el *Corpus Hippocraticum*'. In López Férez (1992), 409-19.
Rehounek, Vàclav (1981), *Grundzüge frühgriechischer Wundbehandlung*. Unpublished med. diss. Kiel.
Richardson, F. M. (1978), *Fighting Spirit: A Study of Psychological Factors in War*. London.
Richmond, I. A. (1952), 'The Roman army medical service.' *Univ. Durham Med. Gazette*, June 1952: 2-6.
Riddle, John M. (1985), *Dioscorides on Pharmacy and Medicine*. Austin, Texas.
Riginos, Alice Swift (1994), 'The wounding of Philip II of Macedon: fact and fabrication', *JHS* 114: 103-19.
Robert, Carl (1919), *Archaeologische Hermeneutik: Anleitung zur Deutung klassischer Bildwerke*. Berlin.
Robert, Fernand (1973), 'La bataille de Délos', *BCH*, Suppl. I: 427-33.
— (1989), 'Médecine d'équipe dans les Epidémies V'. In Baader and Winau (1989), 20-7.
Robert, Louis (1938), *Études épigraphiques et philologiques* (Bibliothèque des Hautes Études, 272). Paris.
— (1940), *Les Gladiateurs dans l'orient grec* (Ib., 278). Paris.
Roberts, C.H. (1950), 'An army doctor in Alexandria'. In Moreuz (1950), 112-15.
Robinson, H.Russell (1975), *The Armour of Imperial Rome*. London.
Rodriguez Fernandez, Perfecto (1973), 'La terminologia médica en Seneca', *Durius* (1973): 301-08.
Rollet, J. (1877), *Des caractères particuliers et du traitement de la blessure d'Alexandre le Grand reçue dans le combat contre les Malliens*. Lyon.
Romilly, Jacqueline de (1979), *La Douceur dans la pensée grecque*. Paris.

— (1984), *'Patience, mon coeur!' L'essor de la psychologie dans la littérature grecque classique*. Paris.
Roselli, Amneris (1975), *La chirurgia ippocratica*. Florence.
Rosenthal, Franz (1973), 'An eleventh-century list of the works of Hippocrates', *JHM* 28 (April 1973): 156-65.
Rossi, Lino (1966), 'L'exercitus nella colonna Traiana: criteri generali ed elementi nuovi di studio su legionari ed auxilia.' *Epigraphica* 28: 150-5.
— (1969), 'Il corpo sanitario dell'armata romana nel medio impero.' *Physis* 11: 534-51.
— (1977), 'La medicina dei Daci nelle guerre Traianee', *Physis* 19: 161-71.
Roura, Carlos (1972), 'Aproximaciones al lenguaje cientifico de la Colección hipocratica', *Emerita* 40, 2: 319-27.
Ruffalo, Cesare, ed. (1996), *La medicina in Roma antica. Il 'Liber medicinalis' di Quinto Sereno Sammonico*. Turin.
Sabbah, G., ed. (1982), *Médecins et médecine dans l'antiquité*. (Mém. Centre Jean-Palerne III). Saint-Étienne.
— (1988), *Études de médecine romaine*. (Mém. C. J.-P. VIII). Saint-Étienne.
— (1991), *Le Latin médical. La Constitution d'un langage scientifique. Réalités et langage de la médecine dans le monde romain. Actes du IIIe Colloque international Textes médicaux latins antiques (Saint-Ét., 11-13 sept. 1989)*. (Mém. C. J.-P. X). Saint-Étienne.
— and Mudry, P. (1994a), 'La médecine de Celse' (Introduction to Mém. C. J.-P. XIII). Saint-Étienne.
— —, eds. (1994b), *La Médecine de Celse. Aspects historiques, scientifiques et littéraires* (Mém.C. J.-P. XIII). Saint-Étienne.
Salazar, Christine F. (1997), 'Fragments of lost Hippocratic writings in Galen's Glossary', *CQ* 47.ii, 543-7.
— (1998a), 'Die Verwundetenfürsorge in Heeren des griechischen Altertums', *AGM* 82.1: 92-7.
— (1998b), 'Getting the point: Paul of Aegina on arrow wounds', *AGM* 82. 2: 170-87.
Sander, Erich (1959), 'Zur Rangordnung des römischen Heeres: Der Duplicarius.' *Historia* 8: 239-47.
Scarborough, John (1968), 'Roman medicine and the legions: a reconsideration.' *MH* 12: 254-61.
— (1969), *Roman Medicine*. London.
— (1971), 'Galen and the gladiators.' *Episteme* 5: 98-111.
— — (1981), 'Theoretical assumptions in Hippocratic pharmacology'. In Lasserre and Mudry (1981), 307-25.
Schadewaldt, Wolfgang (1938), *Iliasstudien. ASG* 43.
Schmiedeberg, Oswald (1918), *Über die Pharmaka in der Ilias und Odyssee* (Schriften d. Wiss. Ges. in Straßburg, 36).
Schöne, Hermann, (1909), 'Aus der antiken Kriegschirurgie', *B. Jb.* 118: 1-11.

— (1927), Review of I. L. Heiberg, ed. *Paulus Aegineta*. In *Gnomon* 3 129-38.
Schöne, Hermann, ed. (1896), *Apollonius von Kitium: Illustrierter Kommentar zu der hippokratischen Schrift* Περὶ ἄρθρων. Leipzig.
Schultze, Clemence (1986), 'Dionysius of Halicarnassus and his audience.' In Moxon, Smart and Woodman (1986), 121-41.
Schultze, Rudolf (1934), 'Die römischen Legionslazarette in Vetera und anderen Legionslagern.' *Bonn. Jb.* 139: 54-63.
Schwenk, Cynthia J. (1985), *Athens in the Age of Alexander. The dated laws and decrees of 'The Lykourgan Era', 338-322 BC*. Chicago.
Sconocchia, Sergio (1993), 'Alcuni rimedi nella letteratura medica latina del 1 sec. d. C.: *emplastra, malagmata, pastilli, acopa*'. In Boscherini (1993), 133-59.
— (1994), 'Osservazioni sull' lessico e sulla sintassi del *De medicina* di Celso'. In Sabbah and Mudry (1994b), 319-41.
Senn, G. (1929), 'Über Herkunft und Stil der Beschreibungen von Experimenten im Corpus Hippocraticum.' *AGM*, 22: 217-89.
Setaioli, Aldo (1983), 'Seneca e il greco della medicina', *Vichiana*, n.s., 12: 293-303.
Shibles, Warren, ed. (1972), *Essays on Metaphor*. Whitewater, Wisconsin.
Simpson, Sir James Y. (1872), 'Was the Roman army provided with medical officers?' In id., *Archaeological Essays*, vol. II, 197-227. Edinburgh.
Skoda, Françoise (1988), *Médecine ancienne et métaphore. Le vocabulaire de l'anatomie et de la pathologie en grec ancien*. Paris.
Smith, Gertrude (1919), 'Athenian casualty lists.' *CPh* XIV: 351-64.
Snell, Bruno (1965), *Dichtung und Gesellschaft: Studien zum Einfluß der Dichter auf das soziale Denken und Verhalten im alten Griechenland*. Hamburg.
Snodgrass, Anthony M. (1964), *Early Greek Armour and Weapons: From the end of the Bronze Age to 600 BC*. Edinburgh.
— (1967), *Arms and Armour of the Greeks*. London.
— (1982), 'Narration and allusion in archaic Greek art.' The eleventh J. L. Myres Memorial Lecture, delivered at Oxford 1981. London.
— (1999), *Homer and the Artists. Text and picture in early Greek art*. Cambridge.
Sokoloff, Th. (1904), 'Zur Geschichte des dritten vorchristlichen Jahrhunderts. 2. Der Antiochos der Inschriften von Ilion', *Klio* IV: 101-10.
Spink, M. S. and Lewis, G. L., eds. (1973), *Abulcasis on Surgery and Instruments*. Berkeley.
Spivey, Nigel (1997), *Understanding Greek Sculpture: Ancient meanings, modern readings*. London.
Staden, Heinrich von (1994), 'Celsus, the "Rationalists", and Erasistratus'. In Sabbah and Mudry (1994b), 77-101.
— (1995), 'Anatomy as rhetoric: Galen on dissection and persuasion', *JHM* 50: 47-66.

Stadter, Philip A. (1980), *Arrian of Nicomedia*. Chapel Hill.
Stanford, William B. (1942), *Aeschylus in His Style: A study in language and personality*. Dublin.
Stannard, Jerry (1961), 'Hippocratic pharmacology', *BHM* 35: 497-518.
Steckerl, Fritz (1945), 'Plato, Hippocrates and the Menon Papyrus.' *CPh* 40: 166-80.
Stella, Luigia Achillea (1934), 'L'ideale della morte eroica nella Grecia del V secolo.' *A&R*, Ser.III, 2: 313-24.
Stenzel, Julius (1921), 'Über den Einfluß der griechischen Sprache auf die philosophische Begriffsbildung.' *NJA*, 47: 152-64.
Strömberg, Reinhold (1940), 'Griechische Pflanzennamen.' *GHA* 46: 1-190.
— (1945), *Griechische Wortstudien: Untersuchungen zur Benennung von Tieren, Pflanzen, Körperteilen und Krankheiten*. Göteborg.
Stückelberger, Alfred (1993), 'Aristoteles illustratus. Anschauungshilfsmittel in der Schule des Peripatos', *MH* 50: 131-41.
— (1994), *Bild und Wort. Das illustrierte Fachbuch in der antiken Naturwissenschaft, Medizin und Technik* (Kulturgeschichte der Antiken Welt, 62). Mainz.
Sudhoff, Karl (1929), 'Aus der Vergangenheit der Verwundetenfürsorge.' *AGM*, 21: 261-72. (Reprinted from *Jahresk. f. ärztl. Fortbildg.*, 1915, VI: 32-40).
Temkin, Owsei (1977), *The Double Face of Janus and Other Essays in the History of Medicine*. Baltimore/London.
Thomas, Rosalind (1991), *Oral Traditions and Written Record in Classical Athens*. (Cambridge Studies in Oral and Literate Culture 18). Cambridge.
— (1992), *Literacy and Orality in Ancient Greece*. Cambridge.
Throuvalas, Antonios (1970), "Η ιατρική ἐν Ἑλλάδι κατὰ τοὺς Ὁμηρικοὺς χρόνους.' In *International Homeric Symposium 1963. The Communications*. Athens.
Toledo-Pereyra, Luis H. (1973), 'Galen's contribution to surgery', *JHM* 28 (Oct. 1973): 357-75.
Usener, Knut (1990), '"Schreiben" im Corpus Hippocraticum'. In W. Kullmann and M. Reichel, eds., *Der Übergang von der Mündlichkeit zur Literatur bei den Griechen*. (ScriptOralia 30). Tübingen, 291-9.
Van Hook, La Rue (1932), 'On the Lacedaemonians buried in the Kerameikos.' *AJA* 36: 290-92.
Van de Waal, H. (1977), *Iconclass: An iconographic classification system*. Amsterdam.
Vazquez Buján, Manuel Enrique (1988), 'Réception latine de quelques concepts médicaux grecs'. In Sabbah (1988), 167-78.
Vegetti, Mario (1967-69), 'La medicina in Platone', *RSF*, I.21 (1966): 3-39; II.22 (1967): 251-70; III.23 (1968): 251-67; IV.24 (1969): 3-22.
Vermeule, Emily (1979), *Aspects of Death in Early Greek Art and Poetry* (Sather Classical Lectures, vol. 46). Berkeley.

Vernant, Jean-Pierre, ed. (1968), *Problèmes de la guerre en Grèce ancienne*. Paris/The Hague.
—— (1980), 'La belle mort et le cadavre outragé.' *J. de psychologie normale et pathologique*, 77: 209-41. Repr. in Gnoli and Vernant (1982), 45-76.
—— (1981), 'Death with two faces', transl. J. Lloyd. In Humphreys and King (1981), 285-91.
—— (1989), *L'Individu, la mort, l'amour: soi-même et l'autre en Grèce ancienne*. Paris.
Vivante, Paolo (1970), *The Homeric Imagination: A study of Homer's poetic perception of reality*. Bloomington.
Vogel, Virgil J. (1970), *American Indian Medicine*. Norman, Oklahoma.
Walsh, John (1937), 'Galen's writings and influences inspiring them', *Am. Med. Hist*. n.s. 9: 34-61.
Watson, Peter (1978), *War on the Mind: The military uses and abuses of psychology*. London.
Wear, Andrew (1985), 'Historical and cultural aspects of pain. Perceptions of pain in seventeenth-century England', *Bull. Soc. Social Hist. Med*. 36: 7-9.
Wehrli, Fritz (1951a), 'Zur Vorgeschichte der aristotelischen Mesonlehre', *MH* 8: 36-62.
—— (1951b), 'Der Arztvergleich bei Platon', *MH* 8: 177-84.
Weitzmann, Kurt (1957), 'Narration in Early Christendom.' *AJA* 61: 83-91 & Pls. 33-36.
—— (1959), *Ancient Book Illumination* (Martin Classical Lectures, XVI). Cambridge, Mass.
—— (1970), *Illustrations in Roll and Codex: A study in the origin of text illustration*. Princeton.
Welcker, F.G. (1850), 'Wundheilkunst der Heroen bei Homer.' In id., *Kleine Schriften*, III, 27-32. Bonn.
Wellmann, Max (1913), 'A. Cornelius Celsus: Eine Quellenuntersuchung.' *Philol. Untersuchungen* 23: 1-136.
—— (1931), 'Hippokratesglossare.' *QGNMed*. 2: 1-88.
Wenkebach, Ernst (1933), 'Der hippokratische Arzt als das Ideal Galens. Neue Textgestaltung seiner Schrift "Ὅτι ὁ ἄριστος ἰατρὸς καὶ φιλόσοφος.' *QGNMed*, 3: 156-75.
West, Martin L. (1973), *Textual Criticism and Editorial Technique applicable to Greek and Latin Texts*. Stuttgart.
Whatley, N. (1964), 'Reconstructing Marathon.' *JHS* 84: 119-39.
Wheeler, R. E. M. (1943), *Maiden Castle, Dorset*. (Reports of the Research Committee of the Society of Antiquaries of London, No. XII). Oxford.
Whitman, Cedric H. (1958), *Homer and the Heroic Tradition*. Cambridge, Mass./London.
Wichmann, Ottomar (1960), 'Platons Verhältnis zur Medizin seiner Zeit', *F&F* 34: 14-18.

Wickert, Lothar (1930), 'Homerisches und Römisches im Kriegswesen der Aeneis', *Philologus* 85: 285-302, 437-62.
Wilamowitz- Moellendorf, Ulrich v. (1912), 'Die griechische Literatur und Sprache.' In P. Hinneberg, ed. *Die Kultur der Gegenwart. Ihre Entwicklung, ihre Ziele.* Leipzig/Berlin.
Wilmanns, Juliane C. (1995), *Der Sanitätsdienst im Römischen Reich* (Medizin der Antike 2). Zurich.
Wilson, Pearl Cleveland (1952), 'Battle Scenes in the Iliad.' *CJ* 47: 269-74 & 299.
Winckelmann, Johann Joachim (1821), *Monumenti antichi inediti.* 2 vols., 1 of text & 1 vol. of plates. Rome.
Withington, E. T. (1920), 'Some Greek Medical Terms with Reference to St. Luke and "Liddell and Scott".' *Proc. Roy. Soc. Med. (Sect. Hist. Med.)*, 13: 122-32.
Wittern, Renate (1998), 'Gattungen im Corpus Hippocraticum'. In Kullmann, Althoff and Asper (1998), 17-36.
—— and Pellegrin, Pierre, eds. (1996), *Hippokratische Medizin und antike Philosophie. Verhandlungen des VIII. Internationalen Hippokrates-Kolloquiums in Kloster Banz/Staffelstein vom 23. bis 28. September 1993* (Medizin der Antike 1). Hildesheim.
Wöhrle, Georg (1991), 'Zur metaphorischen Verwendung von ΕΛΚΟΣ und *ulcus* in der antiken Literatur', *Mnemosyne* s. IV, XLIV: 1-16.
Wolff, B. Berthold and Langley, Sarah (1977), 'Cultural factors and the response to pain'. In David Landy, ed. *Culture, Disease, and Healing.* New York, 1977, 313-19.
Wood, S. (1931), 'Homer's surgeons', *Lancet* 1: 892-5; 947-8.
Wunderer, Carl (1989), *Polybios-Forschungen: Beiträge zur Sprach- und Kulturgeschichte.* 2 vols. Leipzig.
Zimmermann, Bernhard (1992), 'Hippokratisches in den Komödien des Aristophanes'. In López Férez (1992), 513-25.

INDEX LOCORUM

ACHILLES TATIUS
Cleitophon and Leucippe
   IV.10   72

AELIANUS
Tact.
   II.2   74 n. 25

AENEAS TACTICUS
   XXXI.4   52
   XXXI.16   47

AESCHYLUS
Th.
   1005-25   173
   1009ff.   173

AETIUS OF AMIDA
        (ed. Zervos)
   XII, XV   38
   XV/p. 19 Z   21, 64
   XV/p. 57 Z   29

ALEXANDER TRALLIANUS
   I.14   46 n. 145

AMMIANUS MARCELLINUS
   XVI.8.2   93
   XVIII.8.11   47, 74 n. 26, 83, 92
   XIX.2.9   83, 93
   XIX.2.15   83, 93
   XXV.3.6-23   93
   XXX.6.3-6   93
   XXXI.15.1   18
   XXXV.3.6   93
   XXXV.3.23   93

APPIAN
Mith.
   XIII.88   76
   89   221

ARCHILOCHUS
   5   165 n. 28
   13.8   173
   13.10   173

ARETAEUS
   I.VI/5.14-7.23   31 n. 89

ARISTOPHANES
Ach.
   1190f.   174
   1205   174

ARISTOTLE
EE
   1216b   182, 183

EN
   1103b   182
   1104a   182
   1104b   182
   1116a   182
   1181b2ff.   105 n.102

Int.
   16a20f.   118

PA
   639a   97
   672b   114

PO.
   1452b   174 n. 64

Pol.
1282a	98

Rh.
1404b	119

ARRIAN
An.
I.8.3	197 n. 66
I.12.1	185 n. 3
I.15.7	13, 193 n.43
I.16.5	91 n. 34
II.4.7-11	221 n. 60
II.4.8	191
II.4.11	192 n. 31
II.11.6	194 n. 47
II.12.1	70 n. 10, 194 n. 46
II.26	195 n. 52
II.26.2f.	231
II.27.1f.	195 n. 53
II.27.2	197 n. 64
II.27.3	197 n. 65
III.15.2	198 n. 67
III.30.11	198 n. 71, 199 n. 75
IV.3.3	199 n. 78
IV.19.5f.	185 n. 6
IV.23.3	200 nn. 91 and 92, 231
IV.23.5	201 n. 94
IV.26.4	201 n. 95
IV.26.5f.	201 n. 96
VI.9.3	203 n. 105
VI.9.5	203 n. 110
VI.10.1-11.2	15
VI.10.2	204 n. 117
VI.11.1	70 n. 8, 72 n. 18, 191 n. 24, 205 n. 120, 206 n. 129, 223 n. 71
VI.11.2	44, 207 n. 134
VI.13.4	194 n. 49
VII.10.1-2	187 n. 11
VII.11.1	191
VII.14.4	185, 206 n. 130
VII.16.8	185 n. 4

ASCLEPIODOTUS TACTICUS
I.1	74 n. 25

CAELIUS AURELIANUS
Acut.
II.80/I.180.12	10 n. 6

Tard.
IX.186	44

JULIUS CAESAR
B.G.
I.26.5	77
VIII.48	82

CALLINUS
1.7	163
1.9-11	163
1.12f.	164
1.14f.	164
1.17f.	164
1.18f.	164
1.19	164
1.21	164

CELSUS, *De medicina*
II.1.12/47.20-3	30
III.18.15/125.15-17	63
IV.6.1/156.10-16	31 n. 84
V.1/190.25	57 n. 13
V.2/191/1	57 n. 17
V.2/191.3	57 n. 18
V.2/191.11	58 n. 28

INDEX LOCORUM

V.6/192.1	59 n. 34	V.26.26B/	
V.6/192.9	59 n. 34	223.29	25
V.7/192.13f.	59 n. 35	V.26.28A/	
V.8/192.20f.	59 n. 36	224.22f.	35
V.14/193.15f.	59 n. 33	V.26.28D/	
V.25.1/		225.11-13	32
212.10-13	61, 61 n. 41	V.26.29/225.16	59 n. 31
V.26.1C/		V.26.30B/225.31	11, 62 n. 49
215.17-20	39	V.26.31A/	
V.26.1C/		226.12-14	32
215.21-3	40	V.26.31B/	
V.26.2f./215.28-		226.15	32
216.3	20, 39 n. 111	V.27.3C/232.5-8	30 n. 78
V.26.3A/		V.27.10/234.8	236 n 31
216.9f.	18	V.28.3B/	
V.26.3B.5/		237.28-30	33 n. 92
216.12-15	11	V.28.12B/	
V.26.3B/		243.7f.	11 n. 11
216.15f.	9	V.28.12C-E/	
V.26.20/		243.18-27	20 n. 36
218.32-219.28	26	VI.6.38/274.16f.	103
V.26.21/		VI.18.1/290.19f.	91
219.21-220.18	43	VI.18.4/	
V.26.21A/		293.15-17	33 n. 92
219.29-31	26	VII.3.2/305.2f.	23
V.26.21C/		VII.5.1A-3B/	
220.15-18	43	308.6-310.28	4 n. 20, 47
V.26.22/		VII.5.5/310.34f.	29
220.20-22	26	VII *prooem.*	
V.26.23B/		4/302.2-5	64 n. 54
221.7f.	51	VII.5.2A-B/	
V.26.23C/		309.3-10	143
221.12	27	VII.5.2/309.6	144
V.26.23D/		VII.5.2B/309.6f.	102
221.20-22	27	VII.5.3B/	
V.26.25A/223.8	70 n. 11	309.20f.	102
V.26.25A/		VII.5.4A/310.4f.	17 n. 32
223.10f.	25	VII.7.10/318.17	108
V.26.25/		VII.8.3f./	
223.10-16	194 n. 48	324.27-325.7	35
V.26.26A/		VII.9.1-5/	
223.22f.	25		

325.8-326.15	35	III.V.6-8	191
VII.15.1/		III.V.10	191 n. 27
332.17ff.	11 n. 11	III.V.16-VI.2	192 n. 34
VII.16.4f./		III.V.16-VI.16	72 n. 18
333.24-334.7	52	III.VI.4	192 n. 28
VII.16.4f./		III.XII.1-3	94 n. 47
333.26-334.2	104	IV.VI.11-13	195 n. 52
VII.18.3/335.25	123	IV.VI.17	72 n.18,
VII.18.7/336.17	123		195 n. 51
VII.33.1/361.8f.	23		195 n. 54
VIII.3/376.6f.	46 n. 144,	IV.VI.17f.	231
	46 n. 145	IV.VI.17-20	195 n. 56
VIII.4/		IV.VI.18	195 n. 57
377.14-382.16	45	IV.VI.18f.	191 n. 23
		IV.VI.20	21
CICERO		IV.VI.21	197 n. 62
Att.		IV.VI.24	197 n. 63
XVI.I.1	97	IV.XVI.31f.	187 n. 14
		IV.XVI.31ff.	198 n. 68
Fam.		V.V.10-16	35
XVI.I.1	97	VI.VI.22	199 n. 82
XVI.IX	78	VII.VI.3	199 nn.
			73 and 74
Off.		VII.VI.8f.	199 n. 77
I.XLII.150f.	98 n. 72	VII.VI.23	200 n. 87,
			200 n. 89
Tusc.		VII.VII.5	200
II.XXIV.59	224 n. 74	VII.VIII.4f.	200 n. 90
II.XV.35	123	VII.VIII.19	200 n. 88
II.XVI.38	78, 222	VIII.X.6	201 n. 93
II.XXII.53	223 n. 69	VIII.X.28	201 nn.
II.XXIV.58	219 n. 48		95, 97
II.XXIV.59	215 n. 29	VIII.X.29f.	201 n. 98
		VIII.X.30f.	202 n. 100
CIL		IX.IV.27-30	203 n. 108
III.4279	79	IX.IV.30	203 n. 106
III.5959	79	IX.V.1-3	203 n. 111
VII.690	81	IX.V.5	203 n. 114
		IX.V.9	203 n. 114
CLEMENT OF ALEXANDRIA			231
Strom.		IX.V.9-30	15
IV.14.4	169	IX.V.10	206 n. 125
		IX.V.22f.	13,
Q. CURTIUS RUFUS			
III.V.1-VI.17	221		

	206 n. 132	XVII.31.5f.	192 n. 36
IX.V.22-30	221	XVII.34.5f.	193 n. 44
IX.V.23	48	XVII.37.2	194 n. 47
IX.V.25	72 n. 18	XVII.61.3	198 n. 69
IX.V.25-7	191 n. 26,	XVII.98.3	203 n. 108
	206 n. 127	XVII.98.4	203 n. 107
IX.V.26	206 n. 131	XVII.99.2	204 n. 115
IX.V.27f.	207 n. 136,	XVIII.31.5	218 n. 46
	224		
IX.V.29	207 n. 135	DIONYSIUS OF	
IX.VI.1f.	207 n. 139	HALICARNASSUS	
IX.VIII.20	28	II.42.1	77 n. 36
		II.42.5	219
DIGEST		V.36.3	76
L6	80	VIII.86.1	82
L7	80	XI.26.1	82
L13.13	87		
		DIOSCORIDES	
DIO CASSIUS		praef.4	3 n. 19
XXXVI.5	19, 28, 232	I.54	59 n. 30
XLVII.44.3	218	I.72.5	58 n. 28
LXVIII.14	82	I.73	57 n. 15
		I.107	57 n. 11
DIODORUS SICULUS		I.160	66 n. 62
IV.2.6	43	II.63	57 n. 12
VIII.12	186 n. 9,	II.165	117 n. 142
	219 n. 54	II.166 [RV]	117 n. 143
XII.61.4	21, 219 n. 49	II.178	58 n. 20
XII.62.3	216 n. 34	III.80.5	58 n. 26
XIII.79.2	213	III.128	58 n. 26
XIII.79.2-3	213 n. 17	IV.36	58 n. 22
XIII.79.3	218 n. 46	IV.64.3	61 n. 41
XV.79.2	213 n. 12	IV.75.5	60, 61 n. 40
XV.80.5f.	213	V.80	58 n. 21,
XV.86.1	213 n.19		66 n. 63
XV.86.2	213 n. 18	V.85	59 n. 33
XV.87.1	213 n. 13, 231	V.94	66 n. 63
XV.87.5	70 n. 8, 72	V.96	66 n. 63
XVI.34	14 n. 21		
XVII.17.3	185 n. 3	EPIDAURIAN *IAMATA*	
XVII.20	193 n. 43	(ed. Herzog)	
XVII.20.6	13	XXX	16
XVII.31.4-6	221 n. 60		

EROTIAN (ed. Nachmanson)
    31/p.4   115
    46/p.113   116
    47/p.113   113
    /p.136   3 n. 17

EURIPIDES
  HF
    161   172
    191f.   172

FLORUS
  II.12.12   215 n. 27

GALEN
  (*Without indication of the work*)
    I.239 K   113 n. 125
    VII.416 K   100
    VII.417f. K   108
    VIII.396 K   109
    VIII.678 K   105
    XI.415f. K   56
    XI.794 K   55
    XII.30 K   57 n. 19
    XII.118 K   58 n. 26
    XII.208 K   56
    XII.557 K   73
    XIII.668 K   113 n. 125
    XIV.254f. K   100
    XVIII.A.28 K   47 n. 146
    XVIII.548 K   113 n. 125
    XVIII.568 K   113 n. 125
    XVIII.B.694-700 K   104
    XIX.439 K   108
  De Anat. Admin.
    II.228f. K   40
    II.280 K   89
    II.282 K   95
    II.2/II.283f. K   4 n. 22, 47
    III/II.345 K   4 n. 23, 119
    II.349 K   109
    III.9/II.393 K   1 n. 2, 112
    III/II.394f. K   47
    II.628 K   103
    II.632f. K   222 n. 63
    II.633 K   122
    VIII/II.682 K   107, 110, 118
    VIII/II.682f. K   102
    II.780 K   109
  Ant.
    I/XIV.1 K   122
    II/XIV.138 K   61
  Capt. (ed. Edlow)
    p. 35   119
    p. 92   95
  Comp. Med. Gen.
    III/XIII.573 K   106 n. 108
    III/XIII.598 K   38
    III/XIII.599 K   4 n. 24, 11
    IV.4/XIII.759 K   58 n.28
  Comp. Med. Loc.
    9/XIII.104 K   87
    XIII.204 K   87
    XIII.259 K   87
    XIII.267ff. K   60 n. 37, 66 n. 64
    XIII.294 K   87
  Fasc.
    XVIII.A.773 K   52

INDEX LOCORUM

XVIII.A.774ff. K	53		35	120
			95	119
Glauc.			106v	100
II/XI.114 K	22, 62			
			MM	
In Hipp. Aph.			II.1-7/	
I.XLI/			X.318f. K	43
XVIII.B.105 K	26		V/X.320 K	51
VI.18/			V/X.323 K	43
XVIII.A.27-31 K	20		V/X.324 K	44
VI/XVIII.A.28 K			X.327 K	44
	3 n. 17		V/X.345 K	16
VI/XVIII.A.30 K	3 n. 17		VI/X.410-	
VI/XVIII.B.790 K	31		23 K	16
XIX/			VI/X.413ff. K	51 n. 161
XVII.B.491 K	36			51 n. 162
XVII.B.802 K	22		X.423f. K	122
XVIII.B.785f. K	116		X.424 K	111
			VI.6/X.447 K	46
In Hipp. Art.			VI.6/	
XVIII.A.688 K	33		X.448ff. K	45
XVIII.A.722f. K	37			
			Morb. Temp.	
In Hipp. Off.			IV/VII.414 K	107
XVIII.B.686 K	22, 41		IV/VII.417f. K	106
I/XVIII.B.707 K	41		IV/VII.418 K	120
In Pl. Ti.			*Nat. Fac.*	
10 (p. 8)	119		II.1f. K	119
			II.31 K	122
Intr.			II.53 K	59
XIV.783 K	46			
			Opt. Med.	
Libr. Propr.			I.54-6 K	222 n. 64
XIX.48 K	107			
			Oss.	
Ling. Expl.			II.739 K	10
XIX.62-157 K	3 n. 18		II.745 K	112
XIX.116 K	3 n. 17			
			PHP	
Loc. Aff.			I/V.195 K	115
VIII.92 K	111		V.715 K	113
VIII.414 K	122			
			Simpl.	
Med. N. (ed. Meyerhof)			XI.829 K	58 n. 24
14	120		XI.838 K	57 n. 14
17	122			

XI.885 K	58 n. 25	*Aff.*	
XII.25 K	57 n. 11	1/VI.208 L	84
X/XII.256	66 n. 62	38/VI.246f. L	55
		38/VI.248 L	58 n. 23, 67
Simul.			
XIX.1ff. K	100	45/VI.254 L	84, 88, 100
XIX.7 K	24		
		Aff. Int.	
Ther.		I/VII.166 L	103
XIV.244f. K	28, 29		
		Aph.	
Tum.		V.2/IV.532 L	113
VII.726 K	33	V.6/IV.534 L	31
		V.18/IV.538 L	31 n. 83
U. Puls.		V.20/IV.538 L	31 n. 83
V.160 K	44	V.20/IV.539 L	30
		V.23/IV.540 L	43 n. 127
Ven. Sect.		V.65/IV.558 L	113, 177
XI.289 K	23	V.65/IV.560 L	113
		VI.8/IV.564 L	113
AULUS GELLIUS		VI.18/	
II.27	34	IV.566f. L	20, 39 n. 111
XVIII.X.8	95	VII.44/	
		IV.590 L	26
HERACLITUS		VII.45/	
24D	169	IV.590 L	26, 113
47D	169		
136D	169	*Art.*	
		9/IV.100 L	40 n. 119, 55
HERODOTUS			
III.78.2	14	IV.106 L	34
III.129-30	221	11/IV.110 L	10
VI.114	170	12/IV.112f. L	40 n. 119, 55
VI.136	122		
VII.104	176	33/IV.148 L	101
VII.104.4f.	171	35/IV.158 L	52
VII.181.1	171	IV.170 L	55
VII.228	169 n. 45	68/IV.282 L	22
IX.71	171	69/IV.282 L	33 n. 91, 43 n. 127
IX.72	172		
		69/IV.284 L	22
HIPPOCRATIC CORPUS			
Acut.			
II.236f. L	122		

Coac.
   IV.XXIX.494ff./
      V.696f. L   10
   IV.XXIX.499/
      V.698 L   20, 39 n. 111
   IV.xxix/500/
      V.698 L   14

Epid. II
   3/V.20 L   177
   14/V.114f. L   44

Epid. IV
   39/V.180 L   33 n. 91

Epid. V
   21/V.220 L   15 n. 26, 71 n. 15
   27/V.226 L   15
   46/V.234 l   71 n. 15
   47/V.234 L   71 n. 15, 177
   49/V.236 L   14, 71 n. 15
   60/V.240 L   15 n. 25
   61/V.240 L   15 n. 26
   95/V.254 L   15 n. 26, 16, 48, 60, 71
   98/V.256 L   15 n. 26, 26
   99/V.256 L   15 n. 26

Epid. VI
   VII.2/V.336f.   44

Epid. VII
   29/V.400 L   15 n. 26, 71 n. 15
   30/V.400 L   15 n. 26, 71 n. 15
   31/V.400 L   71 n. 15
   32/V.400f. L   15 n. 25, 71 n. 15
   33/V.402 L   15 n. 26, 26, 71 n. 15
   34/V.402 L   71 n. 15
   121/V.466 L   15 n. 26, 16, 48, 60, 71, 71 n. 15

Flat.
   VI.90 L   100

Fract.
   III.428 L   55
   9/III.448 L   118
   III.486 L   55
   III.496 L   55
   III.510 L   55
   III.526 L   24, 25
   11/III.545 L   33 n. 91

Haem.
   2/VI.438 L   64
   VI.440 L   104

Int.
   52/VII.298 L   31

Liqu.
   2/VI.124 L   10

Loc. Hom.
   4/VI.285 L   31
   39/VI.328 L   64
   45/VI.340 L   55

Medic.
   4/IX.210 L   52
   11/IX.216 L   118
   14/IX.220 L   73, 86

Mochl.
   IV/376 L   43 n 127
   33/IV.376 L   117
   38/IV.384f. L   102

Morb.
I.3/VI.142f. L	20, 39 n. 111
I.8/VI.156 L	40
I.21/VI.180 L	15
II.33/VII.50 L	117
II.47/VII.72 L	103
II.49/VII.74 L	103
III/VII.146 L	103

Morb. Sacr.
VI.370 L	113
VI.392 L	114

Nat. Hom.
VI.44 L	18

Off.
III.278-82 L	104
6/III.288 L	64
11/III.310 L	25

Praec.
IX.266f. L	96

Prog.
II.122 L	117
II.138 L	117

Prorrh.
II.12/IX.32 L	25
II.12/IX.34 L	62
II.12/IX.34f. L	39, 39 n. 111
II.15/IX.40f. L	40 n. 119

Ulc.
I/VI.400 L	26, 27
VI.400ff. L (*passim*)	25
I/VI.402 L	26
2/VI.402 L	27
3/VI.404 L	52
8/VI.406 L	26
11/VI.410-26 L	55, 66
12/VI.414 L	58 n. 29
13/VI.416 L	59
15/VI.418 L	59 n. 33

VC
III.182-261 L	45
4-8/III.194-210 L	14
9/III.210 L	46
13.42-7/III.234 L	45
14.43-7/III.238 L	21, 45 n. 135
14.47f./III.240 L	46 n. 138
19/III.250-4 L	20, 40

VM
2/I.572 L	85
2.13-25/I.572f. L	99
19/I.616 L	114
22/I.634 L	114

HOMER
Il.
I.364	152
II.235	153
II.265-9	147
II.269	147
II.270	147
II.721-4	19 n. 7
II.729-33	137 n. 57
II.732	137
III.39	135
IV.12	138
IV.129ff.	220
IV.132-8	150
IV.140	113
IV.148f.	149
IV.150	150
IV.151	141
IV.154	154
IV.184-7	150

IV.190f.	150	V.798	146, 147
IV.208-19	221	V.815-24	148
IV.214	142	V.859	157
IV.217	153	V.899-904	135
IV.218f.	139	V.900	135
IV.450f.	152	VII.96	153
V.40f.	114	VIII.64f.	152
V.45f.	147	VIII.94f.	157
V.55f.	147	VIII.163	153
V.65f.	147	VIII.174	134
V.68	152	VIII.258f.	114
V.100	144	VIII.329	147
V.103	146	VIII.332f.	152
V.112	139, 143	VIII.513ff.	128
V.112f.	147	IX.16	152
V.113	148, 151	IX.701f.	146 n. 87
V.115-20	148	XI.28	140
V.118f.	148 n. 93	XI.145	130
V.121-32	135	XI.252-72	152
V.122	135	XI.254	150, 152
V.147	130	XI.266	113
V.306	119, 130	XI.267	113
V.310	147	XI.267f.	152
V.340	201 n. 99	XI.268-72	152
V.343	157	XI.273	139
V.393	141	XI.273f.	152
V.401	135	XI.284	153
V.414	146	XI.287	134
V.416f.	135	XI.309	139
V.393	141	XI.356	147
V.445-8	135	XI.385	156
V.445-50	135	XI.390	156
V.430	133	XI.396f.	154
V.529	134	XI.397f.	140, 14⌐, 147
V.530	134		
V.532	134	XI.398	151
V.550f.	133	XI.400	151
V.585ff.	130	XI.404-10	154
V.660ff.	142	XI.435ff.	154
V.694	142	XI.439	154
V.694f.	139	XI.446ff.	147
V.696	147	XI.456f.	140
V.794-8	135	XI.458	154

XI.474-81	152	XIV.6f.	141
XI.478	152 n. 107	XIV.85ff.	131
XI.487f.	139	XIV.428-32	139, 152
XI.506	138	XIV.438f.	147
XI.507	141	XV.235-70	135
XI.514	138	XV.242	136
XI.514f.	xi, 137	XV.251f.	136
XI.583f.	155	XV.262	136
XI.584	232	XV.295ff.	149
XI.810-13	155	XV.390-94	145
XI.813	155	XVI.7-10	153 n. 114
XI.830	155	XVI.20	152
XI.830ff.	139	XVI.28	136
XI.831	140	XVI.28f.	136
XI.833-6	137	XVI.492-	
XI.844	245	501	128 n. 6
XI.844f.	144	XVI.504	114
XI.844-8	139	XVI.510	146
XI.845f.	145, 200	XVI.511	113
XI.847f.	145	XVI.514	165
XII.42	156	XVI.514-26	148
XII.310-29	132	XVI.517-21	148
XII.388f.	141	XVI.523f.	148
XIII.210-14	136	XVI.527-31	135
XIII.213	136	XVI.528f.	136
XIII.275-94	133	XVI.791	157
XIII.277	133,	XVI.806f.	114, 157
	133 n. 32	XVI.844-54	128 n. 6
XIII.288ff.	157	XVI.850	157
XIII.421ff.	139	XVI.857	134
XIII.442f.	130	XVI.862	113
XIII.533-9	139	XVII.51f.	134
XIII.538f.	151	XVII.142	135
XIII.567-70	147	XVII.588	151 n. 102
XIII.568f.	130	XX.482f.	130
XIII.598	139, 141	XXI.108	134
XIII.599f.	145	XXI.110	134
XIII.618	147,	XXI.160	149 n. 98
	147 n. 91	XXI.180f.	130
XIII.663-72	131	XXI.273-87	132
XIII.669f.	131	XXI.274	132 n. 26
XIII.670	132	XXI.281	132 n. 27
XIII.671	132	XXII.65-76	133

XXII.66	134	JUSTIN		
XXII.71	166 n. 31	VII.VI	14 n. 21	
XXII.73	133 n. 36	XI.VIII	221 n. 60	
XXII.297	132	XI.VIII.5	192 n. 37	
XXII.305	203 n. 110	XII.X.3	28	
XXII.325	129			
XXII.328f.	129	LIVY		
XXII.338-43	128 n. 6	II.23	187 n. 11	
		II.47.12	75	
XXII.363	134	IV.XXVIII.7f.	13 n. 17	
XXII.370	134 n. 43	VI.XX.9	217 n. 41	
XXII.402f.	134 n. 44	VIII.		
XXIV.6	134	XXXVI.6-8	78, 221 n. 59	
XXIV.420	113	XXX.XVIII.13	219	
		XLV.		
Od.		XXXIX.16f.	217 n. 42	
i.261f.	28			
ix.301	114	LUCAN		
xvii.383ff.	137	Phars.		
		III.587-91	226	
HYGINUS		VI.178f.	226 n. 80	
Mun. Castr.		VII.566f.	221 n. 59	
4	81	IX.614f.	30	
		IX.762-86	226	
HYPERIDES		IX.923-37	30 n. 78	
Epit.				
I	227	LUCIAN		
		Abd.		
I. CRET.		7	99	
I.8.7	69 n. 5			
IV.168	69 n. 5	Anach.		
		28	220	
IG				
II2 304	69	DMort.		
II2 604	69	397.5	202	
ILS		Hist. Conscr.		
VI.20	79	16	90	
2092	79			
2432	79	Tox.		
2438	80	60	35	
9182	79			
		MENANDER		
		Georg.		
		60ff.	94	

CORNELIUS NEPOS
Epam.
   9.2-4   215 n. 28

NONNOS
D.
   XVII.359   67
   XVII.367ff.   93, 225
   XVII.371   67
   XXIX.155   67
   XXIX.270   67
   XXIX.274   67
   XXX.54f.   220

ONASANDER
   I.13-15   74 n. 25

ORIBASIUS
Ad Eun.
   III.14/407.20-4   60
   III.36.1-3/416.23-31   43
   IV.135/496.18-20   60 n. 37

Coll. Med.
   XIV.22/II.199.13   61 n. 45
   XV.12.19f./
     II.264.31f.   61 n. 41
   XLVI.7-21/III.26-32   45
   XLVIII.20-69/
     III.273-91   52
   XLVIII.27/III.276   53 n. 166
   L.50/IV.68   24, 25
   L.51/IV.68   37

Ecl. Med.
   87.10/IV.265.12-31   11

Syn.
   VII.1.12/212.19-24   60
   VII.20.1-7/223.16-224.10   43

OVID
Met.
   I.190f.   93 n. 44
   IV.119-24   224
   VI.252f.   93
   VII.848f.   93

Rem. Am.
   101f.   225
   131f.   225

PAUL OF AEGINA
   prooemium/I.3   5, 41 n. 120
   III.20.1/I.168.14-17   30
   III.22.5/I.17.3f.   41
   III.22.5/I.174   67
   III.22.24/I.181   67
   III.22.24/I.181.19f.   41
   III.64.1/I.280.34   36 n. 101
   III.70.1/I.288.8ff.   36 n. 101
   IV.37/I.358.2   57 n. 16
   IV.39/I.359.18   58 n. 27
   IV.54/I.376-80   11
   V.13/II.16.9   21
   V.53/I.373.20-376.15   43
   V.53.1/I.373.24-374.9   43
   V.53.2/I.374.22-5   42
   VI.40.5/II.80.25f.   44
   VI.52.5/II.93.18ff.   37
   VI.88.1/II.129.21   19
   VI.88.2/II.129.26-130.19   232
   VI.88.2/II.130.13ff.   18, 232 n. 10
   VI.88.3/II.130.25f.   141
   VI.88.3/II.131.1   37
   VI.88.3/II.131.1-4   143
   VI.88.3/II.131.3   10, 11
   VI.88.3/II.131.20   50, 102
   VI.88.3-9/II.130.25-135.5   47
   VI.88.4/II.131.23f.   48
   VI.88.4/II.131.25-132.1   50
   VI.88.4/II.132f.   51

VI.88.4/II.132.7-9	70 n. 9	155e	86
VI.88.4/II.132.8.f.	25	*Grg.*	
VI.88.4/II.132.11-13	29, 70 n. 9	456b	41
VI.88.4/II.132.13-16	28	*La.*	
VI.88.5/II.131.5	11	190e	181
VI.88.5/II.132.23-133.9	20	191b	181
VI.88.5/II.132.27f.	39	197b	181
VI.88.6-7/II.133.10-134.5	39 n. 111	*Lg.*	
VI.88.6/II.133.21	130	625e	xi
VI.88.9/II.134f.	117	633b	182
VI.88.9/II.134.24f.	17 n. 32	639b	182
VI.90/II.136.4-143.6	14, 45	691e	121
VI.90.3/II.138.5	46	720a	85
VI.90.5/II.139.11f.	46	720b	85
VI.98.1/II.151.12-15	37	943c	182
VII.11.14/II.300.16-19	60 n. 37	944a	21
		944d	182

PETRONIUS
 Satyricon
  I.1f.   218 n. 44

PHILO
 Bel.
  V.94.12-24 (Schoene)/
   VII.94.45 (D.--S.)   73
  V.96.15-19 (Schoene)/
   VII.96.72 (D.--S.)   73
  V.96.21-26 (Schoene)   73

PHILOSTRATUS
 Gym.
  14   88

PLATO
 Amat.
  136c   89 n. 25
  138d   89 n. 25

 Chrm.
  155b   86

Phdr.
 268b-c   89
 268c   94
 270c   2 n. 5

Plt.
 298c   85

Prt.
 311b   2 n. 5
 312a   97
 351b   180
 360d   181

R.
 399a   182
 426b   86, 89 n. 25
 525c   85
 564b   120
 564c-d   89 n. 25
 599c   99

Smp.
 185e-188e   97
 219d-221c   181
 220e   181

292 INDEX LOCORUM

221b-c	181	XIX.4	192 n. 29
		XX.8f.	194 n. 45
Ti.		XXV.4	195 n. 52
69e	119	XXVIII.3	201
70a	114	XLI	90
84e	32 n. 86	XLII.4	202 n. 104
		XLV.5	199 n. 52
PLINY THE ELDER		XLV.6	199 n. 76
H.N.		LXIII.5	231
VII.37.37	34	LXIII.5-13	15
XX.LXXVI	61 n. 41	LXIII.11	16, 206
XX.LXXVI.200	61		nn. 132, 133
XX.LXXXI	29 n. 74, 60	LXIII.12	23, 207 n. 134
XXI.CV.180	61	LXIII.13	207 n. 139
XXIV.XIII	29 n. 75	LXXII.2	206 n. 130
XXV.8	240 n. 39	LXXII.4	185 n. 5
XXV.66	236 n. 32	LXXV.5	186 n. 7
XXVI.			
LXXXVII.142	59	*Alc.*	
XXIX.6	77	VII.3	219
XXXV.94	61 n. 40		
		Ant.	
PLINY THE YOUNGER		XXVIII	97 n. 65
De Medicina		XLIII.1	221 n. 59
proleg.	91		
		Art.	
PLUTARCH		VI.6	90
Ages.			
XXXVII.2	23	*Caes.*	
		44.10	214 n. 24
Agis		45.2-4	35
XXX.1-2	214 n. 23		
		Cat. Ma.	
Aem.		I.5-6	216 n. 36
XIX.5	12 n. 14		
		Cat. Mi.	
Alex.		LXX.5f.	15 n. 28
VII.9	95		
VIII.1	90	*Cor.*	
VIII.2	184	XIV.1f.	187 n. 11, 217
XV.8	185 n. 3		
XVI.9f.	13	*Crass.*	
XVI.10	193 n. 42	XV.5	121
XIX.1-10	221 n. 60		
XIX.3f.	192 n. 38	*Dio.*	
		XXXIV.4f.	100

Fort. Al.	
327A	190 n. 19, 193, 199 n. 72
327A-B	187 n. 12
331C	216 n. 35
341B	193 n. 72, 199 n. 81
341C	15
344D-E	204
344F	15
344F-45A	17, 206 n. 132
345A-B	191 n. 25, 205, 206

Mar.
VI.3	223 n. 69, 224 n. 73

Mor.
158A-B	99
187C	187 n. 11
217	214 n. 22
220A	161 n. 3
234	220
241E-F	187 n. 11
241F	213 n. 21
305D-E	223 n. 68
306A	223 n. 68
698D	97 n. 64
761C	217 n. 40

Pel.
IV.5f.	15 n. 27, 184, 220

Publ.
XVI.7	34, 35

Sert.
IV.2	187 n. 11, 217 n. 37

POLYBIUS
III.66.9	79
XV.14.3	82

IULIUS POLYDEUCES
Index
IV.171	107

PROCOPIUS OF CAESAREA
Goth.
V.XXIII.27	77 n. 36
VI.I.26f.	13
VI.II.14-33	34
VI.II.16-29	222 n. 61
VI.II.25	71
VI.II.30-32	27
VI.II.31	121
VI.IV.15	35
VI.XXVII.14f.	35, 220
VII.XXIV.15	77 n. 36
VIII.XXV.24-30	220

Vand.
III.XXII.18	35

PSEUDO-ARISTOTLE
Mir.
86	28

Pr.
I.32-6/863a-b	7 n. 36

PSEUDO-CALLISTHENES
II.8 (rec. ref.)	191, 192 n. 33
II.15	204 n. 116

QUINTILIAN
II.XV.7	217 n. 42

RUFUS OF EPHESUS
Anat.
15	114

Onom.
208	10

Quaest. Med.
50ff.	28, 29
51	47, 206 n. 126
55	45 n. 135, 74, 83
55-62	45

SCHOLIA IN HOMERI ILIADEM
 ad IV.214 (Nic., A)   142
 ad IV.218 (AT)   141
 ad V.112 (b, Nic.)   143
 ad V.115ff. (Did.)   148
 ad V.193 (Aristonicus)   138
 ad XI.439 (Did., b)   154
 ad XI.515 (BT)   138
 ad XI.813 (T)   155
 ad XI.830 (a)   145
 ad XI.830 (b, T)   145
 ad XI.830 (c, T)   155 n. 122

SCRIBONIUS LARGUS
 Comp.
  XII   92
  CCVI   123
  CCXL   103

SEG
 III, 184   96 n. 61
 III, 416   96 n. 59

SENECA
 Cons. Helv.
  3.1   223, 224
 Ep.
  L.I.6   93 n. 43
  XCV.15   66 n. 64, 76
 Q.N.
  L.IV.13.11   93 n. 43

SILIUS ITALICUS
 Punica
  I.322   28
  II.324   215 n. 30
  III.272f.   28
  IV.466ff.   220
  V.348-51   220
  V.368   221
  V.442ff.   220

 VI.74-100   92, 94
 VI.91   221

SIMONIDES
 92 (Hdt. VII.228)   169 n. 45
 121 (Strabo 9.425)   169
 124 (Plu., *Hdt. Mal.* 39)   169
 126 (*Anth. Pal.* VII.251)   168
 127 (*Anth. Pal.* VII.253)   168
 130 (*Anth. Pal.* VII.442)   169
 133 (*Anth. Pal.* VII.443)   168
 135 (*Anth. Pal.* VII.254)   168

QU. SMYRNAEUS
 The Fall of Troy
  III.443-5   221
  XI.219f.   214 n. 25

SOPHOCLES
 Tr.
  1062   175
  1070-75   173
  1075   173
  1259-63   174

SORANUS
 Fract.
  24/158.22-5   36, 37
 Gyn.
  I.3.6/6.13   114
  I.18.1/12.19   118
  II.11/58.19ff.   37
  II.41/120.13   38
  II.42/121.29-31   93 n. 42
  II.49/88.22ff.   36
  III.22/107.17f.   36, 36 n. 101
  IV.9/140.6f.   37
  IV.15/145.14ff.   37, 38 n. 108

STATIUS			II.42.3	177
Silv.			II.47-51	90
II.IV.19-21	215		IV.34.3	13
Theb.			VII.15.1	106
III.398	221		TYRTAEUS	
IX.203f.	218 n. 47		6.1	163, 167
			6.2	163
STRABO			6.3-10	164
X.1.12	172		7.1	163
XV.1.33	202 n. 102		7.1-4	162
			7.23	166
TACITUS			7.26	166
Ann.			7.27-30	166
III.20	215 n. 32		7.31f.	163
IV.63	76		8.5f.	165
			8.13	165, 182
Hist.			8.14	164
II.45.3	78		8.19f.	167
III.84	215 n. 32		8.21f.	163
IV.13	34, 217 n. 38		8.38	153
			9.14	156
TERENCE			9.15	151 n. 4
Eun.			9.27f.	164
482f.	218 n. 45		9.27-32	165
			9.27-42	164
THEOGNIS			9.32	164
I.209f.	167		9.33f.	163
I.555	168		9.35-42	165
I.699f.	167			
I.885f.	167		VALERIUS MAXIMUS	
I.889f.	167		II.II.24	187 n. 11
			III.II.23	220
THEOPHRASTUS			III.II.24	220 n. 57
HP			III.III.1	223 n. 68
IX.VIII.2	66 n. 61			
IX.XVI.1	59		VEGETIUS	
IX.XVI.5	58 n. 24		*Mil.*	
			I.12	11f., 232
			II.10	80
THUCYDIDES				
II.40.3	179		VELLEIUS PATERCULUS	
II.41.5	176		II.114.2	83

VIRGIL
Aen.

IV.683f.	221	
IX.400f.	214 n. 26	
X.715f.	220	
X.833f.	221	
XI.818	219 n. 50	
XII.387	232 n. 8	
XII.387f.	223	
XII.380ff.	13 n. 17	
XII.389f.	223	
XII.391-404	243	
XII.398	223 n. 70	
XII.399f.	224 n. 72	
XII.404	225 n. 78, 243 n. 50	
XII.412	67	
XII.420	221	

VITRUVIUS
De architectura

I.10	98

XENOPHON
An.

I.VIII.26	90, 178
II.V.33	178
III.IV.30f.	69, 85 n. 10, 178 n. 79
III.IV.32	72
IV.II.28	18

Cyr.

V.IV.17f.	70 n. 10

HG

II.4.33	233 n. 15
IV.II.20	178

Lac.

XIII.7	71

Mem.

III.1	87
III.9	180
IV.2.10	94
IV.2.17	91 n. 34
IV.6	181

GENERAL INDEX

abdominal suture 51f., 104
abdominal wounds 15f., 15 n. 26
Achilles 129, 132, 134, 139, 146, 149, 153 n. 14, 175, 184f., 194, 198, 243, 245, 247
Aeneas 130, 223f., 225, 232, 243, 245
Agesilaos 178f.
Alexander the Great 15, 17, 23, 28, 48, 63, 64, 74, 90, 91 n. 34, 184-208 *passim*, 209, 211, 221, 223f., 227, 245
amputation, surgical 21f.
    traumatic 12f.
anaesthetics, absence of 63ff.
analgesics 59-63
andragathia 177, 213
andreia 134, 179-82, 213
archaeological evidence 7, 230-47
Archagathus 77
archer, inferiority of 156, 212
aretê 165, 167, 171, 180, 204, 247
aristeia 135, 138, 176, 212, 221
aristoi 149, 154
armour 16f., 82, 231f.
arrow, extraction of 18ff., 47, 139f., 147, 151
arrowhead, types of 18f., 50, 232f.
art, wounds in 239-47
artêria 9f., 115
Athens 159, 180

back, wounds in the 156f., 177f., 217
bandage 52f., 145, 195
barbs 18, 48f., 141f., 205
beautiful death 159-83, 214
beauty 35, 134f., 166, 208, 245
bleeding, counteracts inflammation 27
blood, symbolism of 18
bone injuries 13, 198f.

camp, doctors present in 71-4 82
capsarius 82
cauterisation 43, 86, 123, 241
Celsus 3, 9, 65, 91, 111; *see also* Index locorum
Chaeronea, battle of 69, 233f.
chest wounds 15f., 204ff.
childbirth as simile 153f., 346, 346 n. 63
citizen as warrior 160ff.
comedy, wounding in 6, 174, 218
Cos 1f., 69, 69 n. 4
courage 158, 163, 179-82, 191, 196, 207, 216f., 222
Critobulus *see* Kritodemos

death in battle 126, 131, 160, 169, 171, 210, 213f., 216
diagnosis 17, 39f.
Diocles, 'spoon' of 49, 102, 117, 238f.
diôsmos 48f., 141, 143
disablement 34f.
disfigurement 34f., 217
drugs 54-67, 236

emprosthotonos 31
Epaminondas 15, 72 n. 19, 215, 224
Epidaurus 6, 16, 237
epideixis 90
Erasistratus 61
extraction *see* arrow
eye wounds 14, 216, 235

faculty (of a drug) 55ff.
fainting 20-4, 147, 196, 219
fever 25, 59
flesh wounds 9-12
forceps 50, 225
fracture 13f., 45f., 122
funeral oration 170, 175ff.

Galen 4, 97; *see also* Index locorum

gangraina 32f.
gangrene 44
gladiators 4, 4 n. 23, 16
gods 135f., 225
Gorgias 41

haemorrhage 17f., 37, 48, 196, 207, 219
haemostasis 42-5, 195
head wounds 13ff.; treatment of 45f.
hedra 14, 46
helkos 2 n. 12, 112f.
helmet 13f., 231
helots 71
Hephaistion 185, 198, 206 n. 130
Heracles 43, 173ff.
heroism 126, 128, 146, 158, 160, 187, 242
Herophilus 109f.
Hippocrates 1f., 115
Hippocratic Corpus 12, 52, 86, 94, 96, 109f., 115f., 240; for individual works, *see* Index locorum
hoplite 160f., 167, 172

iatros xv, 69, 84ff., 98ff., 222
idiôtês 84f., 99f.
inflammation 24-8, 51
inscriptions 6, 69, 79ff., 96, 236f.
instruments, surgical 102, 117f., 237ff.

Julian the Apostate 5, 92f.

Kritodemos, doctor of Alexander the Great 72 n.18, 206

layman, medical knowledge of 84-101
lectures on medicine 96
ligature 44f.
literacy 105

Machaon 137-40, 145, 221
medicus xv, 78ff.
mercenaries, medical treatment for 73, 86

neuron, -a 9ff., 112f., 115

opisthotonos 31, 32 n. 86, 58 n. 26, 177
Oribasius 5, 92; *see also* Index Locorum

pain perception 65
Patroklos 21, 114, 134, 139f., 145f., 151, 153 n. 114, 155, 157, 185, 198, 243ff.
phalanx 160f.
pharmaka 54, 58f., 61, 145
Philip of Macedon 14, 184, 233ff.
Philippos, doctor of Alexander the Great 72 n.18, 190-3, 195
poisoned arrows 28ff., 70 n. 9
probe/probing 19f., 20 n. 36, 48, 50, 239
prognosis 17, 39f.
promachoi 158, 163
pus, 'good' and 'bad' 26

rhetoric, use in medicine 41, 90
Roman army, medical services 77-83, 244

scars, showing of 186f., 187 n. 11, 216ff.
self-control 156, 173f., 178f., 207, 223f.
sêpsis 32f.
shaft of arrow 48, 119, 223
shield, loss of 165, 213f.; protecting another warrior with 154, 154 n. 120, 204, 212, 219, 247
shock 23f., 218
siege, preparations for 73
Sparta/Spartans 71, 169, 180, 213, 233f.
spear wounds 15f., 142
sphakelos 32f., 122
suppuration 24-8
suture 50ff., 70 n. 9
sword wounds 11, 193
sympatheia 36ff.

technê 90
terminology, medical 101-24

tetanus 30ff., 58, 177
textbooks 94f.; illustrations in 240ff.
tragedy, wounding and death in 6, 173ff., 174 n. 64
Trajan's Column 82, 244f., 230 n. 1
treatment, surgical 42-53; pharmacological 54-67

valetudinarium 81, 236

washing of the wound 145, 212
wine 52, 66, 67

youth of the warrior 133f., 166, 168, 208

STUDIES IN ANCIENT MEDICINE

1. F. KUDLIEN and RICHARD J. DURLING (eds.). *Galen's Method of Healing.* Proceedings of the 2nd International Galen Symposium. 1991
ISBN 90 04 09272 2
2. HIPPOCRATES. *Pseudepigraphic Writings.* Letters — Embassy — Speech from the Altar — Decree. Edited and translated by WESLEY D. SMITH. 1990.
ISBN 90 04 09290 0
3. ROBERT I. CURTIS. *Garum and Salsamenta.* Production and Commerce in Materia Medica. 1991. ISBN 90 04 09423 7
4. JODY RUBIN PINAULT. *Hippocratic Lives and Legends.* 1992. ISBN 90 04 09574 8
5. RICHARD J. DURLING. *A Dictionary of Medical Terms in Galen.* 1993.
ISBN 90 04 09754 6
6. WILLEM F. DAEMS. *Nomina simplicium medicinarum ex Synonymariis Medii Aevi collecta.* Semantische Untersuchungen zum Fachwortschatz hoch- und spätmittelalterlicher Drogenkunde. 1993. ISBN 90 04 09672 8
7. IRENE and WALTER JACOB (eds.). *The Healing Past.* Pharmaceuticals in the Biblical and Rabbinic World. 1993. ISBN 90 04 09643 4
8. MARIE-HÉLÈNE MARGANNE. *L'ophtalmologie dans l'Égypte gréco-romaine d'après les papyrus littéraires grecs.* 1994. ISBN 90 04 09907 7
9. SAMUEL S. KOTTEK. *Medicine and Hygiene in the Works of Flavius Josephus.* 1994.
ISBN 90 04 09941 7
10. CHARLES BURNETT and DANIELLE JACQUART (eds.). *Constantine the African and ʿAlī ibn al-ʿAbbās al-Maǧūsī.* The *Pantegni* and Related Texts. 1994.
ISBN 90 04 10014 8
11. J.N. ADAMS. *Pelagonius and Latin Veterinary Terminology in the Roman Empire.* 1995.
ISBN 90 04 10281 7
12. IVAN GAROFALO (ed.). *Anonymi medici De morbis acutis et chroniis.* Translated into English by BRIAN FUCHS. 1997. ISBN 90 04 10227 2
13. ARMELLE DEBRU. *Le corps respirant.* La pensée physiologique chez Galien. 1996. ISBN 90 04 10436 4
14. GUIGONIS DE CAULHIACO (GUY DE CHAULIAC). *Inventarium sive Chirurgia Magna.* 2 volumes. Vol. I: Text. Edited by MICHAEL R. MCVAUGH; Vol. II: Commentary. Prepared by MICHAEL R. MCVAUGH & †MARGARET S. OGDEN. 1997.
ISBN 90 04 10706 1 *(I)*; ISBN 90 04 10784 3 *(II)*; ISBN 90 04 10785 1 *(Set)*
15. MARK GRANT. *Dieting for an Emperor.* A Translation of Books 1 and 4 of Oribasius' *Medical Compilations* with an Introduction and Commentary. 1997.
ISBN 90 04 10790 8
16. ARMELLE DEBRU (ed.). *Galen on Pharmacology.* Philosophy, History and Medicine. Proceedings of the Vth International Galen Colloquium, Lille, 16-18 March 1995. 1997. ISBN 90 04 10403 8

17. MARIE-HÉLÈNE MARGANNE. *La chirurgie dans l'Égypte gréco-romaine d'après les papyrus littéraires grecs.* 1998. ISBN 90 04 11134 4
18. KLAUS-DIETRICH FISCHER, DIETHARD NICKEL & PAUL POTTER (eds.). *Text and Tradition.* Studies in Ancient Medicine and its Transmission. Presented to Jutta Kollesch. 1998. ISBN 90 04 11052 6
19. KEITH DICKSON. *Stephanus the Phiolosopher and Physician.* Commentary on Galen's *Therapeutics to Glaucon.* 1998. ISBN 90 04 10935 8
20. PHILIP J. VAN DER EIJK (ed.). *Ancient Histories of Medicine.* Essays in Medical Doxography and Historiography in Classical Antiquity. 1999. ISBN 90 04 10555 7
21. SALAZAR, CHRISTINE F. *The Treatment of War Wounds in Graeco-Roman Antiquity.* 2000. ISBN 90 04 11479 3

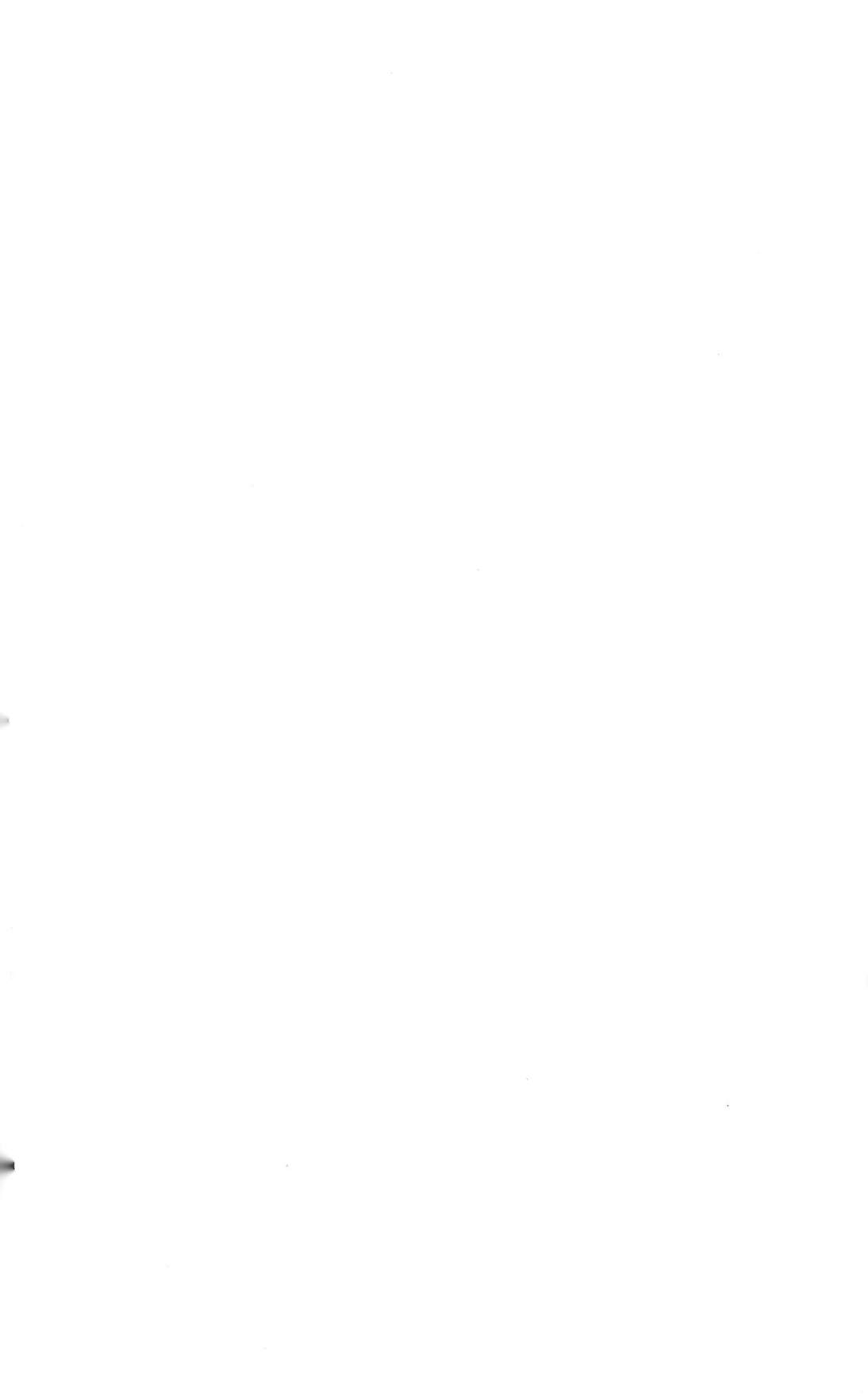